KETO
FOR
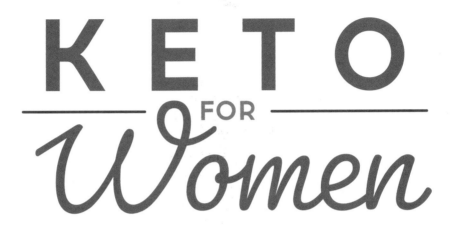
Women

3-Step Guide to Uncovering
BOUNDLESS ENERGY
and Your HAPPY WEIGHT

LEANNE VOGEL

VICTORY BELT PUBLISHING INC.

Las Vegas

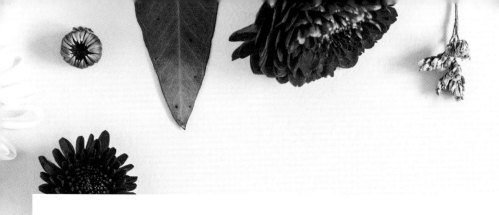

First published in 2019 by Victory Belt Publishing Inc.

ISBN-13: 978-1-628603-70-5

Front and back cover photography and photos of author by Leanne Vogel and Becca Borge
Food photography by Tatiana Briceag
Cover and interior design by Justin-Aaron Velasco
Illustrations by Yordan Terziev, Boryana Yordanova, Charisse Reyes, Elita San Juan, Crizalie Olimpo and Allan Santos

Printed in Canada
TC 0119

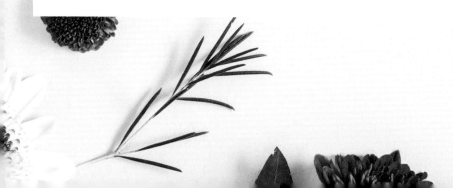

Contents

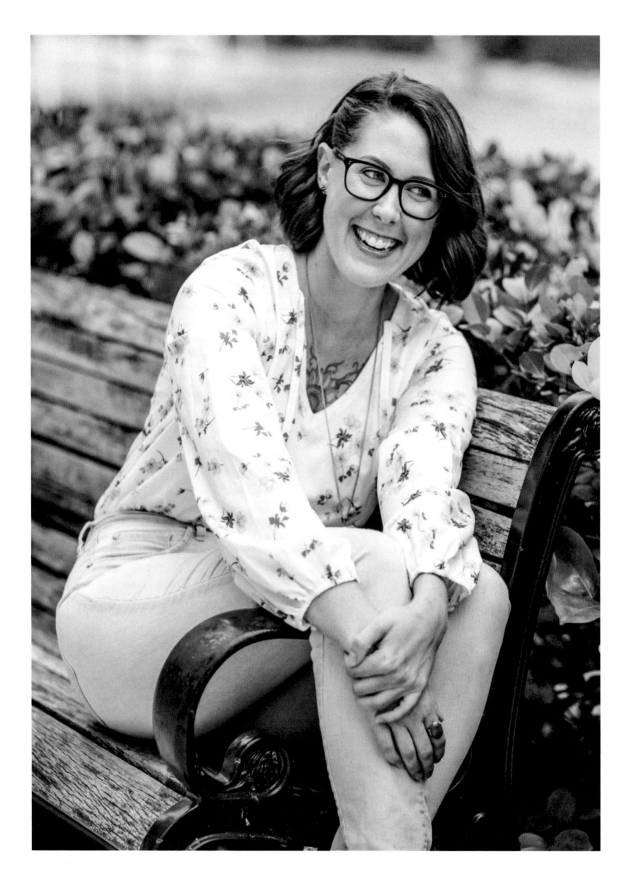

Introduction

I'm in the best health of my life! But before you start thinking that I sport six-pack abs, go to the gym every day because I love it, never deal with sugar cravings, and have a dream marriage, let me tell you, you've got the wrong girl.

I'm a cool size 10 with thighs that touch and arms that jiggle. I'd rather watch Netflix than go to the gym, I don't experience all-out chocolate cake binges anymore, and my husband and I argue over the silliest things, often. But I've learned to take care of myself, know my limits, and respect them.

It took me a long, long time to realize that I don't have to love my body—I just have to accept my body. I don't have to force myself to do things I don't want to do in order to feel like I am taking care of myself. And I don't have to follow a diet perfectly in order to be in the best shape of my life. In fact, by relinquishing the control I held so tightly around how my body looked—the workouts I performed, the food I ate or didn't eat—I am better able to feel my very best.

So yeah, I overeat sometimes, I still get acne, and you'll never see me participate in a belly boot camp again. But where I've said no to a lot of things, I've said yes to a whole host of others.

Yes to dancing in a bikini…in public.

Yes to standing in front of the mirror naked and feeling great.

Yes to doing wild things that scare me, just because I can.

Yes to slumber parties, wine, and non-keto treats.

Yes to feeling free, *finally*.

I think it's important that I tell you this up front because if you're looking for guidance from a person who's got it all together, that's not me. In fact, I don't think that person really exists. Thanks to social media, it's easy to believe that some people always have it all together, but that's not the case. And when we think it is, we can have unrealistic expectations of what life should be like.

No matter how often you go to the gym, no matter how much coconut oil you pound back or how little sugar you eat, life is going to be messy.

I want you to realize that you are already perfect, right now, in this moment. I want to provide you with tools you can use to get closer to yourself, not change yourself. I want you to think for yourself, decide how you want to feel and what action will get you there, and then do that thing because you trust and respect your body.

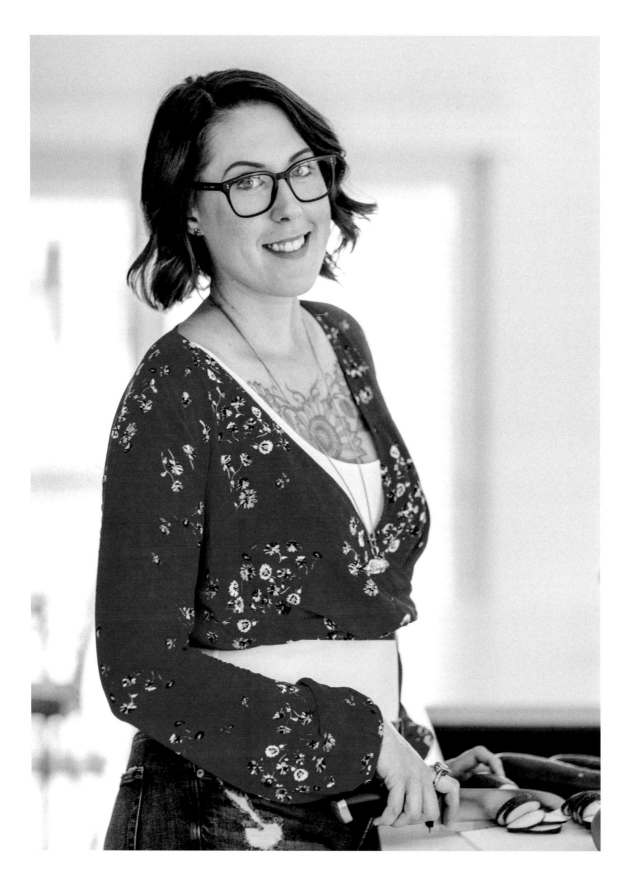

Maybe your goal is being able to run around with your kids. Maybe you want to fit into your old jeans again, walk into a room and radiate confidence, have sex with your partner and feel good about it, or get to a body weight you feel good about. Or maybe you just want to feel better—mentally clearer, physically stronger, more energetic. I want that for you! And my own goal is to give you the tools that you can use to get there.

Hey, I'm **Leanne**

Growing up, I battled with an eating disorder that nearly cost me my life. I've spent years on the path to recovery, slowly stopping the search for perfection and listening to what my body wants on a moment-to-moment basis. I've developed shrewd and nonnegotiable techniques for being honest with myself, true to my body, and brave around food. But it didn't all happen overnight.

Everything came to the forefront when I stopped taking birth control in 2007. My period disappeared and didn't return for eight years. It's not uncommon to have a few months of amenorrhea after stopping hormonal birth control, but in my case, my subtle-but-ingrained disordered-eating tendencies kept me stuck in a pattern of food restriction (which meant not enough calories), too little fat intake, and workout addiction. Those factors prevented my period from returning for a long time.

Now, you may be thinking, *Leanne, why on earth is this a bad thing? No period? Hallelujah! Bathing suits any time you want, white pants without a care in the world...no CRAMPS!* But there's more to your period than you may think. A healthy menstrual cycle means stronger bones, shinier hair, better sleep quality, faster metabolism, tighter skin, stable weight, balanced hunger, less cravings, and, to top it all off, a better sex life.

So yeah, I was willing to give anything just to have a period again. Six years into not having a period, I was sitting in my doctor's office while she ran through the steps I would need to take to *finally* get my health back. The years I'd spent prioritizing body perfection over health would not be so easily reversed.

Of all the options my doctor presented, a low-carb diet was the one I found most appealing, and after much research I eventually decided that a ketogenic eating style—one that's both very low in carbs and high in fat—had the most potential for me. The process of transforming my body from sugar-burning to fat-burning was simultaneously tiresome, confusing, frustrating, and a bit exhilarating. I documented the whole process, from start to finish, in my book *The Keto Beginning* (healthfulpursuit.com/begin).

A month into it, my body had changed in ways I had never expected. Friends, colleagues, and even random strangers started commenting on how "great and skinny" I looked, which only fueled my desire to see how much weight I could lose on this newfound diet. And while you may already be thinking, *Yes, I want that to be me! I want to lose all this weight!* I will ask you to just hold on to that thought for the time being.

I became fearful of carbohydrates, counted calories obsessively, tracked my macros, forced myself to fast even when I was hungry, and developed an insatiable appetite for diet soda. And every couple of weeks, when the cravings got so bad I couldn't handle them anymore, I binged and purged. I was right back in a disordered relationship with food. I perceived my changing body as currency for happiness and healthfulness, when in fact it was anything but.

Despite these negative behaviors, six months into my ketogenic experiment, I was able to stop taking all my ADHD medications, my moods were better, and my hormone levels were much improved. It seemed that things were finally headed in the right direction! But what I wasn't acknowledging (what many of us prefer not to acknowledge) were the inconsistent blood sugar levels, the pins and needles I felt throughout my body, the considerable hair loss, irregular and poor sleep, energy lulls, heart palpitations, and binges, all capped off by the general attitude of self-hate I'd developed about my body.

It was at that point that I decided to combine all I'd learned about the ketogenic diet with the ultra-nourishing practices of holistic nutrition, sprinkled with some intuitive-eating advice and balanced out with a heavy emphasis on self-care. This is how Fat Fueled, my keto rehab program, was born.

There are three pillars to a healthful Fat Fueled lifestyle:

1. Prioritize eating high-quality, nutritious foods over getting the perfect macros (that is, the ratio of fat, protein, and carbs). This means consuming ample plants and few, if any, processed foods.

2. Listen to your body and give it what it needs. This means eating enough, not forcing yourself to fast, and avoiding foods you're sensitive to.

3. Incorporate a cyclical keto practice. This means changing your intake of calories, protein, fat, and carbohydrates as needed to find your sweet spot, which can change according to your activity level and other factors.

By following those three guidelines, in just nine short months, I was richly rewarded with balanced hormones, fewer food sensitivities, strong digestion, healthy moods, and a smile that just wouldn't quit. I wanted to share what I did to get to this place, which is what my next book, *Fat Fueled* (healthfulpursuit.com/fatfueled), was all about.

In 2018, I developed Happy Keto Body (happyketobody.com) as a way to coach women through adjusting the ketogenic diet to work for and support their bodies, a process that's severely lacking in the keto space right now. More than three thousand women have gone through the program to date.

Trying Something **New**

Maybe you're one of the oodles of women out there who are experiencing something similar to my past frustrations and are stuck in the dieting trenches of ketogenic eating. I don't want this for you. Maybe you've never battled with an eating disorder per se, but if you've ever dieted, you've likely developed a relationship with food that centers around shame, guilt, and judgment. And within this experience, on some level, you've probably come to see your body as the enemy.

I have news for you: Food is just food. You can eat whatever you want. The "diet" you are on right now is your choice. You are choosing what to eat, when to eat it, and how much you enjoy it.

When you "slip up," there's no need to judge yourself, hate on your body, feel like you've failed, and then do an egg fast for four days. The guilt you feel after a perceived slipup makes it impossible for you to connect to your body and therefore to maintain self-control, self-esteem, and self-compassion.

Why do we expect to be able to live our healthiest lives when we are constantly consumed with guilt, shame, and failure? We can't. Instead, when we make curiosity—the willingness to experiment and be open-minded, to bend and flex with our goals and be open to new ideas—a priority, we open ourselves up to health at all levels, body and mind.

Instead of thinking of weight loss as the key to health and happiness ("because life will be so much better if I can just lose these last 10 pounds"), try making curiosity and nourishment your top priorities. By doing this, you'll bid goodbye to the shame and judgment you've been directing toward the most important lifelong companion you'll ever have: your body.

Your body wants to be healthy. It wants to be balanced, look good, have energy, and thrive. But many of us are being tricked and misled into doing exactly the things that our bodies don't want. Getting out of your head and into your body is the first major step toward making healthfulness and wholeness your new reality. Sound scary? Don't worry—I've been there, and I'm here to guide you along the way.

There are lots of respected health-and-wellness leaders who are talking about the power of a high-fat eating style. But none of them are talking about making high-fat eating a lifelong practice by breaking free from the diet mentality. And *that's* what I'm here to share with you.

Do we really need an entire book dedicated to doing keto as women? Yes! And I think the size of this book tells you that there's plenty to chat about on this topic. Women experience unique imbalances and frustrations with the keto diet, from weight plateaus that just won't quit to endless sleepless nights to hot flashes that never calm down.

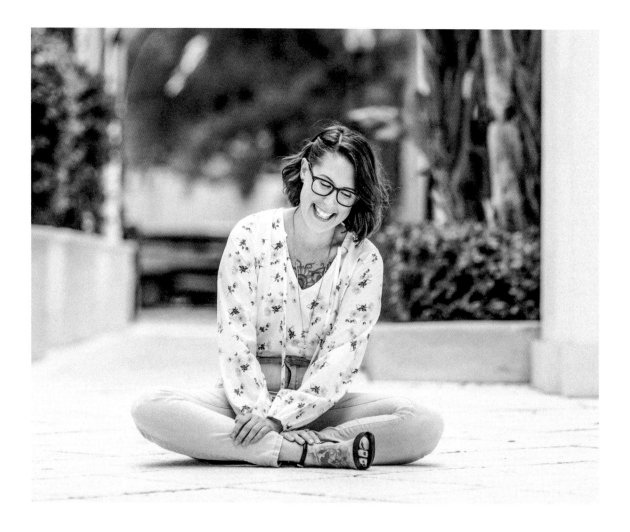

As a keto coach who's worked with thousands of women, I've found that women need different resources than men, which is why I wrote this book!

If you are ready to begin benefiting from a healthy new way of life, built on a solid base of nutritional knowledge with ketosis quietly running in the background, *Keto for Women* will be a thorough resource to support you on your journey.

We can be Fat Fueled, we can listen to and respect our bodies, we can liberate our relationship with food, and we can get into the best shape of our lives—all without counting, measuring, or feeling that we need to think of our bodies as the enemy.

Are you ready? Of course you are.

How to Use This Book for **Awesome Progress**

Are you a 1-2-3-and-done kinda gal? I am. I love processes, steps to success, progress, tracking, and feeling like I'm winning. (Who doesn't want to feel like they're winning?)

When I was setting up the *Keto for Women* program, I wanted you to have goals. I wanted you to feel like you were on your way toward something, not aimlessly drifting in the dark, reading about all sorts of keto health things and picking your way through it all.

Keto for Women has a process, a 1-2-3 process. Each part builds on the last, guiding you through the steps so you feel in control, in the know, and like you're winning. Because after all, if you feel like you're winning, you're more likely to stick it out, trust the process, and start to see actual results.

Here's how the book is organized, so you can make the most of your *Keto for Women* experience:

- Part 1 explains what keto is and why it works, in case the concept of low-carb living is completely new to you. I'll show you why understanding your body is important to your process—when you understand your body, making decisions becomes way easier. I'll explain what keto does to each and every one of your essential hormones and why balancing them is the key to success on keto. And we'll clear up some myths and misconceptions that are likely standing in your way of reaching keto nirvana.

- Part 2 introduces the three sequential steps to becoming a fat-burning female. I'll show you what to eat, how to eat it, and why certain foods will work for you while others will stall your progress. We'll build a meal plan that's easy to follow and get you into ketosis (and keep you there) without stressing out about every—little—thing. We will develop a fasting protocol that helps you hit your goals, keeps you satiated, and doesn't make you go crazy about food. We'll bust through weight plateaus, figure out why you can't lose weight, tackle roadblocks in your way, and develop a protocol that makes eating keto for life so easy.

- Part 3 will help you go the extra mile to improve specific health conditions, including PCOS, autoimmunity, inflammation, horrible experiences with menopause, cardiovascular conditions, gut problems, and more. We'll work together to customize your keto with tiny little tweaks that'll make a world of difference.

So there you have it—everything you need to become that fat-burnin' lady who has it all.

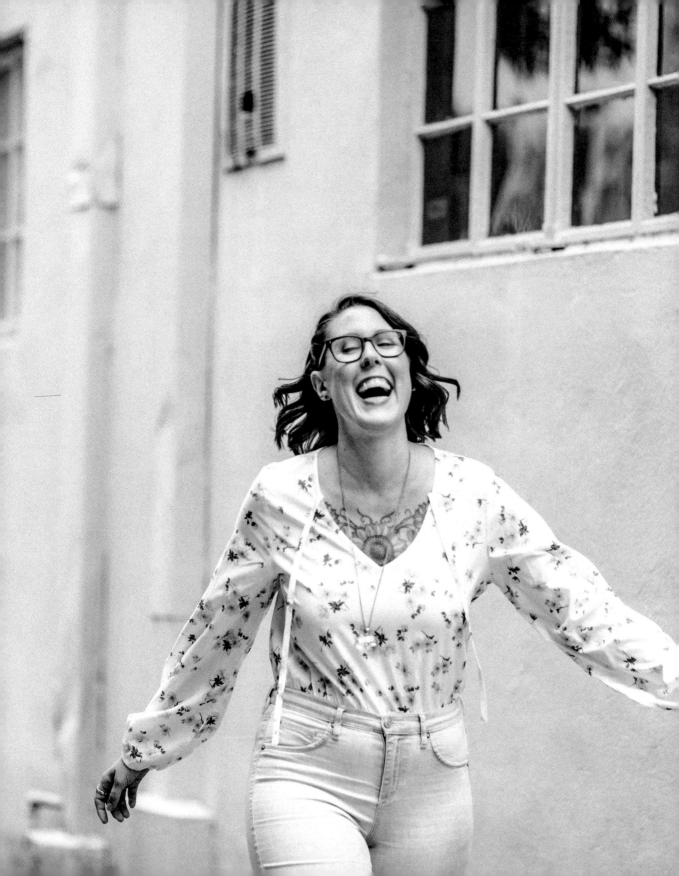

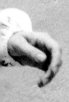

Part 1 — SETTING **THE STAGE**

This part of the book is all about setting you up for success. It'll help you understand how your body responds to keto and what ketones can do for your overall health, and it'll get you excited about what's ahead. Whether you've been eating keto for two hours, twenty-four days, or three years, there's a little something in here for everyone.

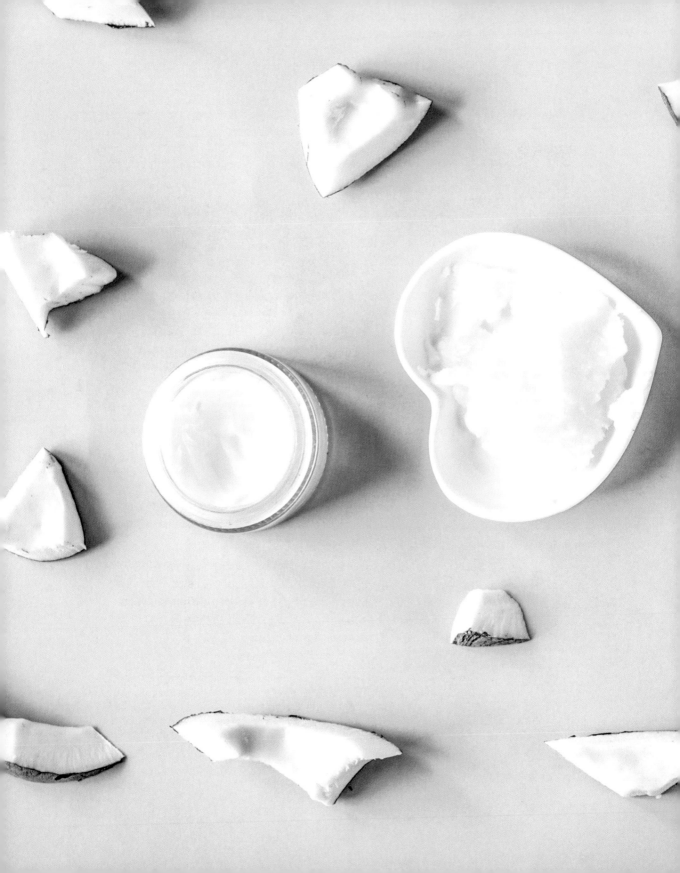

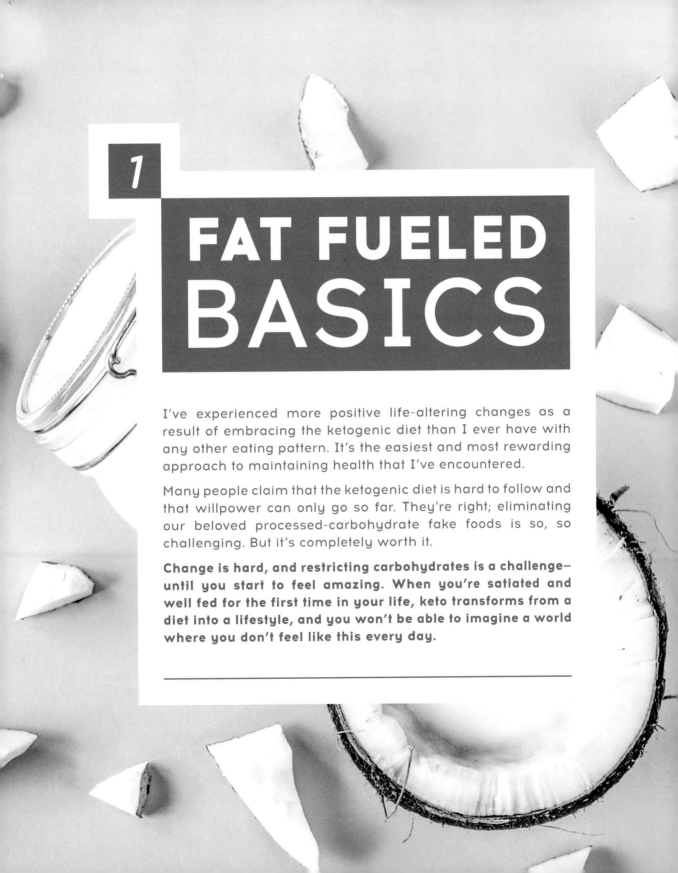

1

FAT FUELED
BASICS

I've experienced more positive life-altering changes as a result of embracing the ketogenic diet than I ever have with any other eating pattern. It's the easiest and most rewarding approach to maintaining health that I've encountered.

Many people claim that the ketogenic diet is hard to follow and that willpower can only go so far. They're right; eliminating our beloved processed-carbohydrate fake foods is so, so challenging. But it's completely worth it.

Change is hard, and restricting carbohydrates is a challenge—until you start to feel amazing. When you're satiated and well fed for the first time in your life, keto transforms from a diet into a lifestyle, and you won't be able to imagine a world where you don't feel like this every day.

Why Your Body
Needs Fat

Conventional wisdom says that eating fat makes you fat. *Au contraire*, I say! Fat is good. Fat makes up the outer layer of every cell in our bodies. Our hormones need it, our muscles need it, and eating too little of it can lead to endless, raging cravings for sugar.

But I didn't always get this. In fact, it took me a long time to get on board with eating fat. Like, at all.

I used to pride myself on my low-fat diet. Heck, I used to make hummus with water instead of olive oil. So why the switch? I realized that a low-fat diet simply wasn't working for me.

When I was looking into switching over to a high-fat keto diet, I was scared. And I'm thinking, if you're considering it, you're probably scared, too. So here are ten reasons why consuming high amounts of fat shouldn't scare you:

1. Eating more fat keeps you satiated and reduces crazy hunger pains, leading to less overeating and bingeing.

2. Eating more healthy fat reduces your blood triglyceride level, a risk factor in heart disease. Low-fat diets, on the other hand, often cause triglycerides to go up.

3. Eating enough healthy fat helps prevent depression, which can be caused by a deficiency of cholesterol and fat in the brain. Too little cholesterol and fat in the brain causes lower levels of the neurotransmitter serotonin, which makes people feel good.

4. Eating more fat helps to raise HDL ("good") cholesterol.

5. Foods high in healthy fats are usually also high in cholesterol, which is used to make hormones. Eating a greater proportion of fat helps balance androgens such as testosterone and estrogen. Losing body fat and maintaining a lean physique are much easier if hormones are balanced.

6. Eating more fat and less carbs reduces insulin levels and leads to stable blood sugar levels. The result? Fewer cravings and steady energy.

7. A diet high in healthy fats increases the size of LDL ("bad") cholesterol. When LDL particles are large and puffy, they cannot easily penetrate the arterial wall, which causes inflammation and can lead to heart disease. The more fluffy LDL particles you have, the lower your risk of heart disease.

8. Fats are loaded with nutrients like vitamins A, E, and K_2.

9. Omega-3 fatty acids help turn on genes that are involved with lipolysis—fat-burning—and turn off the genes involved with fat storage.

10. Fats help you maintain a healthy, balanced metabolism, which in turn helps you maintain your ideal weight.

Important: In a ketogenic eating style, your consumption of carbohydrate decreases to offset the increase in fat consumption. Many of the points listed above are related to the combination of more fat and less carbohydrate.

Still a bit skeptical? Here's a little thing I tried when I was figuring out whether I needed to increase my fat intake: I attacked my cravings first. For a week, anytime I was craving something, no matter what I was craving, I had a high-fat, keto-friendly snack—a glob of coconut oil, an avocado, a couple of spoonfuls of sunflower butter, a handful of macadamia nuts. Within ten minutes, the cravings were gone. This told me very, very clearly that the solution for my cravings was to eat more fat. And that went a very, very long way for me! Try it for yourself and see if you have the same experience.

What Happens When You **Eat Carbs**

Every carbohydrate you eat—whether it's in a handful of candy or an apple—is broken down into sugar in your body. Of course, the apple has lots of healthful nutrients, while the candy has very few (if any at all), but they both still break down into sugar. Once it's broken down into its smallest form, sugar is called glucose.

That glucose enters your bloodstream, and your body produces insulin to move it from the blood to your cells. When you have more glucose than your body needs for immediate energy, the excess is stored as glycogen, first in your liver and then in your muscles. And then, when everything is full, what's left over is converted into triglycerides. The triglycerides are stored in fat cells for later use.

The more we abuse this system by eating foods high in carbohydrates (especially processed carbohydrates), the more damage is done to our cells, our ability to maintain a healthy insulin response (known as insulin sensitivity), and our health overall.

Relying on carbohydrates for fuel:

Is inefficient and unsustainable. We can only store a couple thousand calories of carbohydrates to use at any given time. On the other hand, we have 50,000 calories of fat stored on our bodies to use at any given time.

Increases the risk of heart disease. A high level of triglycerides—an effect of eating more carbs than your body can use—is a major risk factor for heart disease.

Causes blood sugar to constantly fluctuate. This results in endless cravings, the need to eat frequently (sometimes almost constantly), and weight gain.

Reduces nutrient uptake. A diet composed of high-carbohydrate foods can result in a lack of nutrients, including vitamins A, D, and E, and minerals such as calcium, chromium, and magnesium, because it's not varied enough and doesn't provide the necessary amount of fat required to assimilate fat-soluble vitamins.

It saddens me that so many people are just not aware of all this. Many of us think we are doing our bodies a favor by opting for a low-fat muffin, jam, and orange juice—all chock-full of carbs and guaranteed to send blood sugar soaring and then crashing—over a plate of eggs, bacon, and coffee.

What Is **Keto?**

When carbohydrates are your primary fuel source, you're what we call a "sugar-burner."

The opposite is being a "fat-burner," when fat is your primary fuel source. When you become a fat-burner by adjusting your diet, you're in a metabolic state called nutritional ketosis. Why is it called "ketosis"? Because when you burn fat, the liver produces molecules called "ketones," which your body can effortlessly use for energy.

What's a Ketone?

Thousands of years ago, before our ancestors developed the ability to domesticate animals and cultivate crops, they relied on hunting and gathering. Regardless of geographical location, this lifestyle meant a natural balance of protein, fat, and carbohydrates that was very different from what we see today. And they were regularly forced to fast due to the scarcity of food. Combined, these factors meant that glucose often wasn't their primary fuel source. Glucose is the easiest fuel for the body to use, so it's preferred whenever it's present, but when no glucose is available, we can rely on stored body fat for energy. In short, our bodies are hardwired to convert stored fat to energy.

This fat-burning mode produces a metabolic fuel: ketones. While we talk about using fat as fuel, in fact it's ketones—which are produced during the metabolization of fat—that power the body in the absence of glucose.

Fat-burning and ketone production occur anytime your glucose stores are low, especially when you're:

- Fasting

- Engaging in prolonged exercise

- Eating a ketogenic diet

Kinds of Ketones		
Acetoacetate	**Beta-hydroxybutyrate (BHB)**	**Acetone**
Created from the breakdown of long- and medium-chain fatty acids	Moves through blood, allowing it to reach tissues other ketones can't	Created from acetoacetate
Converted to BHB or acetone	When it reaches a cell's mitochondria, it transforms into ATP, what cells use for energy	If not immediately utilized, expelled through breath
If not immediately utilized, expelled through urine		Tested via the breath
Tested via urine		

What You Need to Know About Ketosis

You're in ketosis when you have a certain level of ketones in your blood—above about 0.5 mmol/L. "Nutritional ketosis" is simply ketosis that's induced by diet.

When you're in nutritional ketosis, you use a combination of stored body fat and dietary fat for fuel. The ratio of dietary fat burned to body fat burned is based on a few factors:

- How much fat you eat
- How high your ketone levels are
- What point your body is at in the process of transitioning to preferring fat for fuel

Think of moving into nutritional ketosis as flipping a light switch (your metabolism) from one position (burning sugar) to the other (burning fat). Once the body has made this switch often enough, it becomes easy to alternate between burning primarily fat and burning primarily sugar. This is known as metabolic flexibility.

Tripping this metabolic switch leads to so much more than just weight loss. Once you're in nutritional ketosis, blood sugar stabilizes, insulin levels drop, HDL cholesterol increases (this is a good thing), and the dangerous visceral fat around your vital organs shrinks as it's used for fuel. Many people report a dramatic difference in their metabolic functions, including the ability to:

- Go long periods without food
- Lose weight effortlessly
- Better manage and regulate blood sugar

The easiest way to reach and maintain nutritional ketosis is to follow a ketogenic (literally, "ketone-generating") diet: a low-carb, moderate-protein, high-fat style of eating.

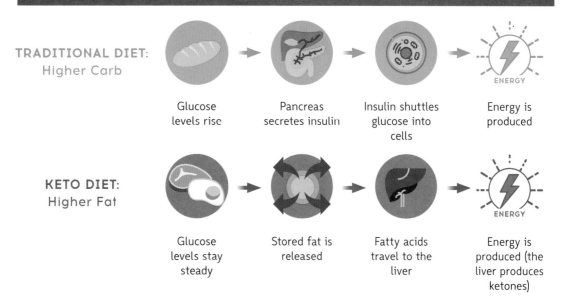

TRADITIONAL DIET: Higher Carb

Glucose levels rise → Pancreas secretes insulin → Insulin shuttles glucose into cells → Energy is produced

KETO DIET: Higher Fat

Glucose levels stay steady → Stored fat is released → Fatty acids travel to the liver → Energy is produced (the liver produces ketones)

Why a Ketogenic Diet Works

A ketogenic diet radically lowers daily carbohydrate intake. With very little glucose coming in through food, the body is forced to use another source of energy: fat. The body does very well in a state of ketosis because most people (yes, even thin people) have plenty of fat stored in their body at all times—roughly 50,000 calories of it, in fact.

So first, you remove the excess carbs from your plate, then your body depletes its glycogen stores. Finally, once your body has used up those stores, it turns to fat as its primary fuel source. Weight loss becomes effortless.

The great news is that weight loss is just one of the benefits of a ketogenic diet. Because when you eat fewer carbs, your body dips into its stores of glycogen. This, in turn, lowers your need to consume carbohydrates for energy, reduces your overall blood sugar because you're not eating all the carbohydrates, and lowers insulin levels. All this to say: keto makes a big change, fairly quickly, to the very core of your metabolism. A ketogenic diet can also be used to help support everything from epilepsy to diabetes to cancer.

Benefits of Going Keto (Beyond Weight Loss)

- You have the freedom to go long periods of time without getting hungry.
- Blood sugar stays stable.
- You understand what you feel like eating and how much you need to eat to feel satiated.
- You have the energy to go on walks with friends and family.
- You actually get full from eating a meal.
- You're ready to move as soon as the alarm sounds.
- You have fewer cravings for sugar.
- You're no longer a slave to your growling stomach.
- Your brain simply functions better.
- You have fewer allergy symptoms.
- You have fewer headaches.
- Your sleep is deep and uninterrupted.
- Skipping meals isn't a big deal.
- You have increased mobility.
- You have clearer skin.
- Your moods are more stable.
- You have balanced blood work and biomarkers, from reduced inflammation to a balanced hormone profile and more.
- You have better mental focus.
- Your memory is sharper.

More Ketones Is Better, Right? Wrong.

Now, if you're like me, at this point you're probably thinking, *If ketones can do all of this, clearly my goal is to get my ketone level as high as possible!* And you'd be sorta right: yes, ketones are beneficial, and yes, if you can get your ketones high enough that you're in ketosis, that's fabulous.

But not at any cost. Later on in the book, we'll chat about the importance of food quality. For now, let me just say something you probably already know: eating real, whole, nutritious food that actual nourishes your body should be a priority. Remember, eating high-quality, nutritious foods is one of the pillars of a healthful Fat Fueled lifestyle (see page 8). If you have to break one of the pillars in order to achieve higher ketones, you're missing the point. Ketones are only a small part to living in a ketogenic body. Your goal should be becoming a balanced fat-burner. And for some, this means having a lower level of ketones. This is okay!

And there are actually some downsides to having tons of ketones. While it may not happen to everyone, higher levels of ketones may actually slow down fat loss. Why? Some bodies perceive ketone levels higher than around 3.0 mmol/L (remember, ketosis starts at around 0.5 mmol/L) as a sign of starvation, which triggers it to break down muscle as the next available source of fuel. When muscle is broken down, glycogen (stored glucose) is released, raising insulin levels. The increase in insulin blocks the release of fatty acids from fat cells—in other words, it's harder to use stored body fat for energy. Both muscle breakdown and insulin spikes are bad things—we don't want either!

TRUTH BOMB

Soon after birth, babies are in ketosis, and they remain so while breastfeeding! Ketones supply the baby with ample energy and help the brain develop.

Ketosis, Keto Adaptation, and Fat Fueled—What They All Mean

Ketosis, keto adaptation, fat fueled... How the heck are you supposed to know what's what? Don't stress; it's not as complicated as it sounds, I promise.

Ketosis: Following a ketogenic eating style puts you into a state of ketosis quite quickly, usually after one to two weeks. When you're in ketosis, you're using fat as energy and producing ketones; officially, it's ketosis when your ketone level is 0.5 mmol/L or higher.

This doesn't necessarily mean that your body is *good* at burning fat, though. When you first enter ketosis, your body isn't very efficient at getting energy from fat. This is because breaking down fat requires different enzymes than the ones needed to break down glucose. Up until now, your body has been focused more on breaking down glucose, so it needs a bit of time to build up a store of fat-converting enzymes. This is one of the main reasons why many people feel tired when they first begin following a ketogenic eating style.

Keto adaptation (aka fat adaptation): Once the fat-focused enzymatic processes have strengthened in your body, your cells change their preferred way of acquiring energy and you become fully keto adapted—fat and ketones aren't just the fuel your body uses in the absence of glucose; they're actually your body's preferred fuel.

Depending on your metabolism, the process of becoming fully keto adapted can take anywhere from a few weeks to a couple of months. This is why it's strongly recommended to stick with keto for sixty days—you need to allow time for your body to become fully keto adapted. Once it is, all kinds of good things begin to happen: your hormone levels balance out, your body carries around less water, your PMS symptoms may subside, you may sleep more soundly and experience a reduction in cravings, and you achieve boundless energy, to name a few.

When you're already keto adapted and you consume more glucose than your body is used to, it will temporarily switch back to using glucose as fuel for as long as it needs to in order to use up the glucose. During this time, your body temporarily suspends ketone production. Stores of glycogen are replenished, leading to water retention, and your insulin level spikes.

The good news is, once the glucose has been depleted, your body is able to return to a state of ketosis much faster than it did in the course of the initial keto-adaptation process because it has already been primed to use fat as energy. This is metabolic flexibility, and it's the end goal—a place we can stay for years and years and that makes it possible to stick with a ketogenic eating style over the long term.

Fat Fueled: Being Fat Fueled (a term I coined to describe a particular way of being keto) is metabolically just like being keto adapted—your body prefers to use fat as a fuel and has adjusted to use fat efficiently. But being Fat Fueled also means that you're focusing on healing the body and adhering to the three pillars of a healthful Fat Fueled lifestyle (prioritizing nutrition, listening to your body, and using cyclical keto—see page 8 for more).

Who Can **Keto**

When what you're doing doesn't seem to be working and you're not feeling 100 percent, then something clearly isn't right, and you owe it to yourself to try something different. There's no sense staying with something that isn't making you happy and getting you the results you want. Keto could be the eating style that works for you.

Until you actually try keto, there is just no way of knowing whether or not it will make you feel great and give you the elusive results you've been searching for. That said, here are some signs that you may be too reliant on carbohydrates and would benefit from keto:

- Your skin isn't looking great. This can be caused by an imbalance of hormones (you'll see acne around the jawline), a lack of skin proteins (you'll see premature wrinkles and aging), and/or inflammation (you'll see breakouts).

- Sweet is not sweet enough—no matter how much sugar is added to food, it could be a little sweeter.

- You have trouble fighting off illness and/or infection. Excess carbs can lead to a weakened immune system that has a harder time protecting the body from harmful germs.

- You struggle with digestive issues, from diarrhea to constipation, bloating, gas, and everything in between. A lack of whole-food nutrition and too much sugar, which can feed less desirable bacteria and yeast, can cause imbalances in the gut.

- Your sex drive is low. High blood sugar levels can shut off the genes responsible for producing sex hormones, causing a drop in your drive to get down and dirty.

- You get a lot of cavities.

- Your cravings are at an all-time high. This is a sign that you're riding the blood sugar roller coaster and need to consume carbohydrates whenever your blood sugar drops.

- Your energy fluctuates during the day. Contrary to popular belief, your energy should be fairly steady from morning to night.

- You're experiencing uncontrollable weight gain. Excess carbohydrates are stored as body fat, primarily in the abdomen, hips, thighs, and love handles.

- Your moods are up and down. Your gut and brain are intertwined. If you're having issues with your brain, look no further than the health of your gut! The gut is where serotonin, the happy hormone, is created, so if it's not healthy, it can cause inconsistencies in our moods.

- You're not sleeping well. With high amounts of sugar comes the inability to sleep.

- You frequently feel bloated. Fructose, a kind of sugar found in fruit and the key ingredient in high-fructose corn syrup, isn't easily absorbed by the body, which can cause bloating.

The above list of symptoms is a good place to start when you're thinking about whether you should give keto a try. But there are also specific groups of women who often benefit from keto. Consider trying keto if you're a woman who:

- Is menopausal

- Struggles with weight

- Is sedentary

- Has epilepsy

- Has a hormonal imbalance (including low estrogen, high progesterone, and cortisol irregularities)

- Has polycystic ovary syndrome (PCOS) or fibroids/endometriosis

- Has type 1 or 2 diabetes

- Has a neurological condition such as Alzheimer's or Parkinson's

- Has cardiovascular disease

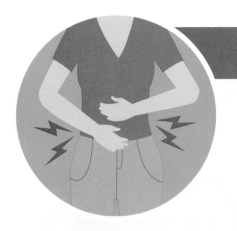

SIGNS THAT IT'S TIME TO LOWER YOUR CARB INTAKE

 MENTAL FOG

 OVERWHELM

 AFTERNOON ENERGY LULLS

 PHYSICAL EXHAUSTION

 DARK UNDEREYE CIRCLES

 POOR DIGESTION

 IRREGULAR MENSTRUATION

 PUFFY, STIFF, AND SORE BODY

 LOUSY IMMUNE RESPONSE

 TROUBLE SLEEPING

 LOW LIBIDO

 WEIGHT GAIN

It would be ludicrous for me to tell you that keto works for everyone and that, if you can just do it *right*, you're bound to experience success. That's not the way the world works. I can't tell you whether or not this will work for you specifically, because you are unique. Only you can truly know you.

What I can tell you is that eating this way has transformed my life and the lives of many other women I've met, some of them in person and many others in Happy Keto Body (happyketobody.com).

2

UNDERSTANDING YOUR BODY

When you understand your body, everything changes. You may think working to understand your body is a waste of time, and I believed that, too, for a long time. After all, why would I need to understand my body when I could rely on someone else to tell me what I needed?

This is what's wrong with women's health today: we outsource. We rely on other people to tell us what our bodies need. We rely on the media to tell us what diet to try and on doctors to tell us what we need to work on, instead of just understanding the very basics so we can make decisions about our bodies on our own.

After all, your body is all you have. And you're the only living thing on this planet that has the capacity to love and care for your body as much as you can. You're with it 24/7 and have a vested interest in success, and you're a pretty smart lady—which means you've got this.

No, you don't need to know all the ins and outs, but if you know the basics, you'll be in a much better place long-term!

How Your
Metabolism Works

Many of us have, at one point or another, jokingly said that we hate our metabolism, that it alone is responsible for our misery. Let's unpack that, because metabolism plays a strong role in weight loss, and the actions you think encourage weight loss could be the exact things affecting your metabolism so that you're unable to lose weight.

Your metabolism determines how your body uses and generates energy, down to the cellular level. Think of it as a finely tuned and highly reactive process that adjusts hormones in response to the various things you do that affect your health. Its goal is to optimize your well-being, but problems can arise when the actions that you take in the name of health send the wrong message to your metabolism.

As an example, let's say that your body burns 2,000 calories every day. You decide that you want to lose weight, so you lower your overall intake to 1,500 calories per day. At first this works and you lose a bit of weight, but then your weight plateaus. In order to push through and lose more weight, you lower your calories even more and start working out more to increase the number of calories you burn. Eventually you're down to just 1,000 calories per day, experiencing erratic hunger cues, working out two hours a day, and cursing the gods for giving you a defective body.

What's happening here? Your metabolism is adapting to the decrease in fuel by adjusting your hormones to decrease your total energy requirements. Instead of needing 2,000 calories per day to maintain your weight, your body now only requires 1,500 calories. And when you get too low in calories, your body will start to completely shut down entire processes, like, for instance, sex hormone synthesis. After all, if there isn't enough fuel to go around, the lowest priorities for your body are libido, glowing skin, and strong bone density.

In this state, women often experience intense hunger and cravings as the body signals that it requires more food, or sometimes the opposite, little to no hunger, as the connection between the body and mind becomes disrupted.

In other words, when necessary, your metabolism's feedback mechanisms allow it to adapt in an opposing direction to the messages it receives, adjusting hormones as it goes. Think of your metabolism as a rebellious teenager—whatever you want it to do, it does the exact opposite.

Understanding your metabolism is the key to determining which weight-loss methods will work best for you and gaining the ability to upregulate your fat-burning potential once and for all. The trick is not to operate at a calorie deficit to the point of damaging your metabolism. The moment you begin experiencing changes in any of the nine metabolic markers listed on page 31, consider it a signal that something may be out of whack, and make an adjustment to address it.

Calorie Restriction

The calorie-for-calorie mentality we've all been so stuck on isn't all that accurate, because there are many other factors that can impact how your body interacts with the foods you eat, including:

- Food quality

- When you eat

- The thoughts and feelings you're experiencing as you eat

- What's going on around you while you're eating

- Your overall mental well-being

- Who you're surrounded by

- Your genes

- Your current and past relationship with food

- How you feel about what you're eating (are you breaking the "rules" or doing something "bad"?)

- What point you are at in your monthly hormonal cycle

- The balanced or unbalanced state and health of your hormones

All of these factors and more affect your individual metabolism. Getting hung up on the number of calories you consume is pointless because it's actually an extremely small piece of the puzzle, and in many cases reducing caloric intake will not lead to any long-lasting, life-altering changes.

The idea of decreasing "calories in" and increasing "calories out" looks at dieting strictly from a "less is best" approach, without taking into consideration what certain hormones—cortisol, adrenaline, insulin, and glucagon—are doing. That approach can result in imbalanced hormones and damaged metabolism, and it leads to cravings, hunger, low energy, weight-loss stalls, weight gain, and more.

And with every calorie that you cut, you are depriving your body of the nourishment that it needs to thrive.

In addition, calorie restriction is relative. Restriction for one person is not restriction for another. And the number of calories your body needs changes depending on what life stage you're in. There's a balance between feeding your body what it needs to thrive (and once you're thriving, weight loss and maintaining a healthy weight are effortless) and underfeeding your body to the point that it cannot thrive (signs of failure to thrive include weight gain), and where that line falls is unique to each person.

Just as we all look different on the outside, we all function differently on the inside, particularly our metabolisms. While the "eat less, exercise more" approach will no doubt work for some people, there are no guarantees it will work for you.

We've been conditioned to believe that if we just eat fewer calories and exercise more, weight loss will magically happen, but that really couldn't be further from the truth.

Instead of looking at calorie restriction as good or bad, I try to view it as an occasional tool used at my discretion with a strategy called intermittent fasting, which we'll cover a bit later on page 138.

An epic decrease in calories—combined with poor food quality, imbalanced hormones, intense training schedules, and copious amounts of stress—isn't good for us. On the other hand, a *slight* decrease in calories—combined with high-quality foods, healthy daily movement, and consistently restful sleep—boosts our quality of life and makes us feel good.

Whether you're happy with the weight you're at, you're looking to lose weight, or you're trying to gain, once you're keto adapted, you will likely notice a dramatic change in your overall food intake as your hunger regulates and your cravings subside. Some days I eat lots; other days I do not. If I add up the week's calories, I find I am usually eating fewer calories than I burn, even as my weight stays steady.

So you see? It doesn't have to be an all-or-nothing thing.

Calorie Deficits for Fat-Burners vs Sugar-Burners

There are plenty of studies that link calorie reduction to improved health and wellness in the context of a ketogenic diet. Compared to a body that's burning glucose as fuel, it is easier for a body in a state of nutritional ketosis to perform at a calorie deficit because it's primed to burn always-ready fat stores as energy. Most sugar-burners can use fat for fuel, but their bodies have a harder time making the switch and using fat efficiently.

Metabolic Markers

Your body has an amazing feedback system in place to alert you to imbalances before they get out of hand. Many of the little signs and symptoms you experience from day to day are the result of your metabolism attempting to communicate with you.

I call the signs that point to whether your metabolism is functioning optimally the nine metabolic markers. If you've been experiencing noticeable fluctuations or changes in three or more of the following markers on a regular basis, it could be your body's way of telling you that your metabolism needs support, whether through a ketogenic diet, a more nutrient-rich diet, an increase in overall caloric intake, or a combination of the three.

The nine metabolic markers are:

1. Hunger

2. Energy

3. Cravings

4. Body weight

5. Water retention

6. Sexual function

7. Mood

8. Digestive function

9. Menstrual function

If you're having an issue with one of the markers, the most common adjustments that lead to success are adjusting macros (see page 126), opting for higher-quality foods (see page 92), eating more, eating less, or exploring food sensitivities (see page 274).

Hunger and Hormones

Hunger is not appetite and appetite is not hunger. We lump them together, but they aren't the same.

Hunger is the physiological need to eat. **Appetite** is the desire to eat and is based not on a physiological need but rather on a psychological need.

For example, say you wake up, skip breakfast, and head to work. Come lunchtime, your stomach's growling. *This* is hunger. You nourish your body with brisket and greens and get back to work, feeling satisfied. But shortly thereafter, a coworker pops into your office with a tray of homemade chocolate-frosted brownies. Even though you're definitely still full from lunch, you're tempted to have a couple. *This* is appetite.

The ketogenic diet helps us get back in the driver's seat of our appetite, so that it's no longer driving us.

There are three main processes that regulate hunger and food intake, all of which are controlled by an area of the brain known as the hypothalamus.

First of all, much as your home has a thermostat, our bodies have an internal "nutrient stat." When the nutrient stat detects that the levels of glucose, fatty acids, and ketones are high, the brain sends out a signal telling the body that hunger is low.

Boosted Initial Hunger on Keto

An increase in perceived hunger is natural during your first couple of weeks on the ketogenic diet, as your body figures out what fuel it's supposed to be using. It is completely normal for you to feel like you want to eat *lots* during this time, but how you respond to your body's hunger signals is your choice. I chose to tough it out and ignore the signals, knowing full well that my body was just confused and that I wasn't actually hungry. Don't worry—the appetite you experience during this transitional period is not an indication that your metabolic hunger marker is off.

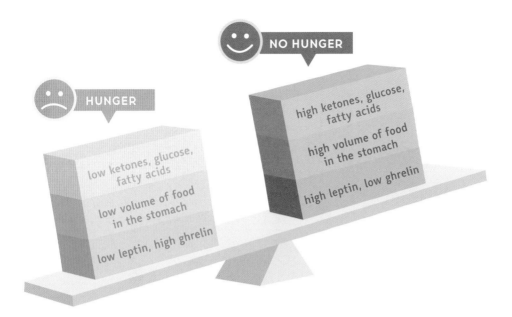

HUNGER

low ketones, glucose, fatty acids

low volume of food in the stomach

low leptin, high ghrelin

NO HUNGER

high ketones, glucose, fatty acids

high volume of food in the stomach

high leptin, low ghrelin

Second, our bodies respond to food mechanically. When we consume a large quantity of food, our stomachs literally expand and our brains receive a signal that we're full. In fact, gastric balloon bariatric surgery, in which a balloon filled with saline is placed in the stomach, reducing the stomach's volume, is based on this biological premise.

Finally, hunger and satiety hormones heavily influence the amount of food we eat. Ghrelin is the hunger hormone and leptin is the satiety hormone—the more ghrelin, the hungrier you are, and the more leptin, the more satiated you are. So it's no surprise that obesity is associated with an impaired regulation of these two powerful hormones.

Dieting significantly affects the expression of leptin and ghrelin. This is likely why the conventional low-fat, low-calorie diet fails—and this is a fact—95 percent of the time. You cut your calories and you initially lose weight, but then your ghrelin goes through the roof. You're hungrier than you've ever been, and you end up eating more and gaining back all the lost weight, plus a few pounds.

What we're aiming for with keto is a way of eating that doesn't negatively alter our hunger hormones, so we can achieve long-term fat loss and a sustainable lean body composition. And if you're worried that eating all the keto things and not actively restricting your calories is going to lead to epic weight gain, studies show that keto individuals who *don't* try to restrict calories actually experience less hunger than those who do!

Support Your Body
by Eating Enough

Your body knows what you need. In fact, it's smarter than you are, and smarter than any health-management program or app in existence. It even knows you better than your momma.

While for some people, there's something to be said for lowering food intake, there are many women out there (perhaps you're one of them) who have been chronically undereating for decades as a means to lose weight, without ever truly succeeding. So perhaps it shouldn't be a surprise that the leading cause of a broken metabolism is eating too little, over and over again, to the point that you're unable to lose weight.

How do you know if you're one of the lucky ladies with a broken metabolism in need of mending? Your body will tell you. Changes in the metabolic markers on page 31 often mean that something needs addressing, but there are also signs that undereating in particular is a problem.

Many of the chronic health symptoms we experience are caused by chronic undereating. The following symptoms could all be signs that you're not eating enough, and some of them may surprise you. If you answer yes to at least a couple of the items below, it might be a good idea to boost your caloric intake over the next ten days and see if things improve.

- **Sleep is miserable.** Not eating enough overall, exercising too hard, and eating too low-carb (we call this a triple whammy) can make it next to impossible to get quality shut-eye.

- **You've been stuck at the same weight** since Britney Spears was doing the *G.I. Jane* look.

- **You're tired.** When you're not eating enough, your body is not getting the nutrients it needs and forces you to slow down to conserve energy.

- **You suffer from chronic constipation.** Lower caloric intake = less volume in your bowel = less movement. Not eating enough can also cause thyroid imbalances, which in turn can cause constipation.

- **You can't get off the blood sugar roller coaster.** Feeling dizzy, sweaty, shaky, or moody (especially if you've been combining undereating with overexercising) could be signs of hypoglycemia, one of the most common side effects of inadequate caloric intake.

- **You liken your mood to the Hulk.** "Moody" doesn't even begin to describe it. If you feel irritable, anxious, or angry whenever you get hungry, it's a likely sign that your body's hangry mode is in control and self-restraint has gone out the window. In this state, coping with stress, resisting impulsivity, paying attention, and regulating emotions become next to impossible.

- **Pregnancy seems unreachable.** Your doctors have told you that you're infertile and have suggested taking birth control pills to regain a normal cycle. Perhaps your menstrual cycle is so irregular that ovulation is impossible to track. Not eating enough lowers your body's metabolic rate to the point that you don't have enough calories (energy) to safely create, grow, and give birth to another human. When this metabolic shift happens, your body will shut down fertility to keep you from getting pregnant, as doing so in this condition could be unsafe for you.

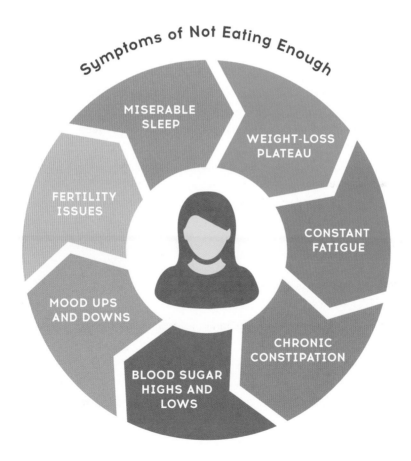

Symptoms of Not Eating Enough

MISERABLE SLEEP

WEIGHT-LOSS PLATEAU

FERTILITY ISSUES

CONSTANT FATIGUE

MOOD UPS AND DOWNS

CHRONIC CONSTIPATION

BLOOD SUGAR HIGHS AND LOWS

So if you haven't been eating enough and you're trying to lose weight without success, before you go any further, you must mend your metabolism.

This took me forever to understand—really, it did. For years and years, I restricted the amount I ate, thinking that restriction would lead to weight loss. You know, calories in, calories out—that whole thing. But what I've come to understand and accept is that my body is not a machine; it is far more changeable and complex. My thoughts, feelings, actions, activities, memories, brain activity—everything!—all have an impact on how much my body needs to eat on a daily basis.

For me, change started with the realization that my body *wants* to be healthy—my body *wants* to have balanced hormones, regulated blood sugar, healthy hair, nourished skin, and happy thoughts. So instead of standing in its way, dictating what I should and shouldn't eat, I decided to just let it flow:

- I gave myself permission to eat whatever I wanted.

- I gave myself permission to eat as much as I wanted.

- I began looking at meals as opportunities to stuff my body with as many nutrients as possible.

- I discovered things outside of food that I loved, like belly dancing, studying German, and hiking.

And to my surprise, I was able to stay true to the Fat Fueled life as I never had before.

Keto is a lifestyle change. It's less about forcing yourself to achieve your dream weight and more about allowing your body to slide naturally into its happy place. The less we force this (or any) eating style on our bodies, the better. My success with this style of eating was ultimately achieved by allowing my body to figure out what it needed and where it wanted to be.

You're probably thinking that living this way will lead to weight gain, right? WRONG! Your body *needs* nutrients to be balanced. If your body's not balanced, it's not focused on weight loss—it's focused on survival.

TRUTH BOMB

Whether you've been restricting calories for a really long time or just a couple of months, it's always the right time to turn your habits upside down and begin giving your body the nutrients that it needs to thrive. A thriving body is a balanced body, and a balanced body is able to maintain a healthy weight range.

How to Boost Metabolism by Eating Enough

If you are currently eating under 1,500 calories per day, you're probably not eating enough. But what's the best way to go about increasing your intake?

Here are the steps you can use to get your intake back to more normal levels and your metabolism functioning as it should:

1. Obey your hunger—eat when you're hungry!

2. During week 1, increase your daily calories by 10 percent. So for example, if your daily intake is 1,000 calories per day, increase to 1,100 calories per day. Remain at this level for 7 days.

3. The second week, increase calories by the same amount—so using the example above, you would increase to 1,200 calories per day. Remain at this level for 7 days.

4. Continue increasing at that pace until you are up to at least at 1,500 calories per day.

5. Stop tracking your food intake. If this thought scares you, start small by not tracking breakfasts, then snacks, then lunch, followed by dinner. So with each step, you're waiting until later in the day to start tracking.

Truths

- Contrary to popular belief, eating a ketogenic diet doesn't automatically mean that you'll lose weight. To put it another way, ketosis doesn't magically lead to successful fat-burning, depending largely on your hormonal balance. (I know this is news that the keto community does not normally share. Consider me the messenger, and please don't shoot!)

- Weight loss is your body's lowest priority when it's trying to heal from a health imbalance of any kind. The only way to easily achieve and maintain your goals is to do so with a balanced body. Once you've achieved a balanced body (using some of the steps I'm sharing in this book), you'll find that your weight should normalize more easily.

- It's very, very likely that your body cannot function on just 1,200 calories. When you're operating at a caloric deficit, you are robbing your body of nutrients it needs to be balanced. And when your body is unbalanced, you are also less likely to lose weight.

All About **Cravings**

As you embark on your keto journey, you're bound to experience cravings here and there, particularly in your first few weeks. Don't worry, these cravings are a natural response to becoming fat adapted. When you're starting out, your body is accustomed to burning glucose as its primary fuel. With keto, you're training it to burn your fat stores instead. As your glycogen reserves are depleted, your body may briefly panic, and the result will be a craving—usually for carbs.

Rest assured, your cravings will subside as you become fat adapted. But they may get worse before they get better.

When a craving hits, there are a number of positive actions you can take.

1 Reach for nutrient-dense foods instead of high-carb bombs.

Great choices are avocados, eggs, salmon, kale, coconut, dark chocolate with no added sugar, bone broth, and fermented foods.

2 Get your hands on a high-fat snack.

You may think you want carbs, but your body really is looking for fat. When a carb craving hits, eat some healthy high-fat foods and watch in amazement as the craving disappears. I like to drizzle coconut oil over macadamia nuts, add a sprinkle of salt, and dig in.

3 Check for hidden sugar.

Cravings, especially carb cravings, are your cue to reassess what you're eating to make sure there aren't any hidden sugars in the foods you're choosing.

4 Up your protein.

Try increasing your protein intake by adding collagen to your coffee, opting for bacon-wrapped chicken breast, or sipping on bone broth between meals.

5 Hold on.

Remove as many temptations from your living space as possible, and be mindful of why you started eating keto in the first place. Maybe you're on this path for weight loss, increased strength, better moods, or reduced anxiety. Keep that goal in mind and let it give you the strength to hang in there.

6 Be open to feeling hunger.

Hunger is a brand-new experience for many of us. Try to embrace it as such. And know that once you become fat adapted, your hunger cues will be subtle, not sharp, as they often are when we're glucose dependent.

Cravings aren't to be feared. Rather, they are your body's way of alerting you to an opportunity to address an issue. They can be understood, embraced, and conquered.

Often what you're craving can tell you a lot about what your body needs. For example, sometimes you experience certain cravings because your body needs a specific nutrient it's not getting.

If you're craving... ♥		Try this 💡
SWEETS	Your diet may be lacking in chromium, phosphorus, sulfur, tryptophan, or carbon.	Eat fresh fruits, chicken, beef, liver, horseradish, kale, raw nuts and seeds, cranberries, cabbage, sweet potato, spinach, and turkey.
BREAD OR SAVORY CARBOHYDRATES	Your diet may be too low in protein.	Eat more protein, such as eggs, fish, chicken, beef, or nuts and seeds.
SALT	Your diet could be deficient in adequate chloride or silicon.	Eat fatty fish, nuts, and seeds. Craving salt can also be a sign of adrenal dysfunction—see page 378.
FATTY AND CARB-HEAVY SNACKS	Your diet may be lacking calcium.	Eat more fat! If the craving for fatty snacks keeps coming, add collards, kale, mustard greens, broccoli, sesame seeds, almonds, and turnip greens.
COFFEE	Your diet may be low in sulfur, salt, iron, or phosphorus.	Eat fish, whole eggs, liver, onions, garlic, bell peppers, greens, seaweed, apple cider vinegar, and spinach.
CARBONATED DRINKS	You could be in need of additional calcium.	Eat leafy greens, sesame seeds, or almonds.
CHOCOLATE	Your diet may be deficient in magnesium.	Eat nuts, seeds, and leafy greens. I'd also suggest adding a magnesium supplement.
CHEESE	You could be lacking in calcium or intimate connection.	Eat more fat, walnuts, and fatty fish. Plus, make sure you get plenty of hugs and intimate snuggles from the people you love. Seriously, these loving actions will actually create the same hormonal response as eating cheese.

Other times, cravings have less to do with food and more to do with situations. As you start to develop an awareness of your cravings, you'll notice that certain circumstances often bring them on. Triggers could be anything from a particular group of friends to the beginning of the fall season to a big family gathering. A little focused attention coupled with a positive action to handle cravings is all you'll need to manage cravings successfully.

For example, if you're finding that you experience more cravings and splurges during weekends when you're running around nonstop, it's an easy fix with a bit more planning. Pack some keto-friendly snacks, like grass-fed beef sticks, packets of nut or seed butters, or your favorite keto-friendly protein bar (my favorite is from a company called Perfect Keto). Or brew some coffee, blend it with your favorite protein powder, coconut oil, and nut or seed butter, and pour it in a thermos to take along with you.

Now, if you're regularly craving and splurging in the evening, this is likely more of an emotional need than a physical one. That being the case, if you've had a rough day at work and just want to park in front of the TV and eat popcorn, ridding your house of popcorn isn't going to be of much use—especially when the grocery store is just down the street.

When we're emotionally exhausted, we'll keep craving and craving until those emotions are processed. Processing emotions instead of covering them up with food may be a totally new concept for you. Trust me, you are definitely not alone.

Gently introduce some self-care into your daily routine before you get home. Go for a walk instead of eating at your desk, take a fifteen-minute break for some quick meditation, or listen to empowering music or relaxing nature sounds on the ride home.

Or perhaps you're simply grieving your favorite foods, like cinnamon rolls, ice cream, chips, or soda. It can be hard to make a drastic switch overnight. So much of this journey is emotional, and that's completely natural. Know that you can always treat yourself to some keto junk food! There are keto-friendly cinnamon rolls, ice cream, brownies, chocolate chip cookies, potato chips, nachos, and more. They shouldn't make up much of your diet, but they can help you satisfy a craving.

With a conversation on cravings comes a need to talk about blood sugar, insulin, and your ketogenic diet, because, as you may have guessed, they are related!

Blood Sugar, Insulin, and **Keto**

You already know from chapter 1 that every carbohydrate breaks down into sugar in the body. After we eat carbs, that sugar enters the bloodstream, causing a rise in blood sugar levels. The rise in blood sugar triggers the production of insulin, a hormone created by the pancreas that helps transport glucose from the bloodstream to cells, which use it for energy.

Insulin is the key that unlocks the doors to your cells, so they can open and allow glucose to enter. Insulin is also a fat-storage hormone: it tells the body, "Hey, there's plenty of glucose available to use, so don't release any from storage. In fact, let's put some of this extra glucose into storage—more body fat!"

Ideally, this process works smoothly, with modest rises in blood sugar and insulin after a meal and steady blood sugar between meals. That's not always the case, though.

Insulin Resistance

When you eat high-carbohydrate foods, your pancreas runs on overdrive to produce enough insulin to take that sugar out of your bloodstream. The problem is that, when insulin is consistently high, cells eventually learn to ignore its signals. It's as if someone were continuously shouting at you; eventually you'd simply tune them out. This is insulin resistance.

When insulin can no longer unlock cell doors for glucose to enter, the result is higher blood sugar levels—along with higher insulin levels, as your pancreas pumps out more and more insulin to try to compensate. If the body continues in this state of insulin resistance for too long, or if it becomes incapable of making enough insulin, insulin resistance turns into type 2 diabetes.

Diabetes

Type 1 diabetes is an autoimmune disease: the immune system attacks the pancreas, destroying its ability to make insulin.

Type 2 diabetes, on the other hand, is generally thought of as a result of diet and lifestyle. When someone consumes too many carbs, sweets, and fruits, or drinks too much alcohol, the pancreas can work so hard to produce enough insulin that it gets burned out. It simply can't keep up with demand.

In both types of diabetes, hyperglycemia, or high blood sugar, is a serious danger—it's a life-threatening condition if not treated quickly. Those with type 1 diabetes require exogenous, or injected, insulin. Those with type 2 diabetes, however, may be able to stabilize their blood sugar and insulin levels and restore the pancreas's ability to produce insulin through diet—more on that in a moment.

Reactive Hypoglycemia

People with reactive hypoglycemia—a drop in blood sugar within four hours of eating—experience blood sugar peaks and valleys because their bodies push glucose into the cells very quickly. This imbalance often causes irritability because their brains are screaming for more sugar. Other symptoms include shaking, sweating, dizziness, and light-headedness. And because people with this condition break down and use carbs so quickly, they are hungry again just one or two hours after eating.

Managing Blood Sugar with Keto

The good news is that a ketogenic diet can help improve all of these issues. Keto keeps blood sugar levels steady, without spikes or drops, because it emphasizes healthful low-glycemic foods, meaning fewer blood sugar spikes, and it encourages your body to use stored fat, an ever-present fuel source—so when you've used up the fuel from your previous meal, your body seamlessly switches to using what it has on hand. This not only helps ward off hunger and cravings and therefore lowers the likelihood that you'll overeat; it also helps improve insulin resistance, type 2 diabetes, and hypoglycemia.

Insulin resistance: Your cells can actually regain their insulin sensitivity if you give them a break from the deluge of insulin. The key here is to eliminate instances where heavy loads of insulin are required to help process your meals—and that means eating less carbohydrate (and replacing it with healthy fats).

Diabetes: By keeping blood sugar controlled and steady throughout the course of a day, keto helps people with diabetes avoid those crashes between meals.

For those with type 2 diabetes, the ketogenic diet may do wonders by reducing the need for insulin and making cells more insulin sensitive.

For those with type 1 diabetes, keto is a very supportive diet as long as blood sugar is monitored *extremely closely, with a doctor's supervision*. Diabetic ketoacidosis (see page 55) is a very real concern for those with type 1 diabetes, and it can be deadly. And if, when you start your ketogenic diet, you continue to inject the same amount of insulin as before, you run the risk of triggering a hypoglycemic coma, which could lead to death! I am not exaggerating; you must be very mindful of blood sugar monitoring and insulin dosage when switching to a ketogenic diet—and you must consult with your doctor.

People with either kind of diabetes need to work closely with their doctors before trying keto. Any medication that affects blood sugar or insulin may need to be adjusted, and that has to happen with your doctor's supervision. I can't emphasize this enough: *If you have diabetes, talk to your doctor before trying a ketogenic diet.*

Reactive hypoglycemia: The best way to avoid a blood sugar crash is to avoid high-carb meals and snacks. Protein and fat are broken down more slowly than carbs, so starting the day with an avocado omelet instead of breakfast cereal will keep you feeling satisfied much longer. On top of that, of course, once you're keto adapted, your body is efficient at using body fat for energy, so when fuel from a meal starts to run out, blood sugar stays steady.

Some doctors recommend eating many small meals a day for reactive hypoglycemia, but I have not found this to be necessary once you've become fat adapted. The only reasons to eat many times during the day are that you are an athlete in training or you have a very physically demanding profession. Otherwise, to kick your hormones into fat-burning mode and stabilize your blood sugar, there should ideally be at least four hours between meals.

It is so amazing just how life-changing the ketogenic diet can be for insulin resistance, diabetes, and hypoglycemia. The stabilizing influence of slow-burning protein and fat definitely improves health and attitude! It's done wonders for my blood sugar—I no longer struggle with hypoglycemia—and I hope it will work for you, too!

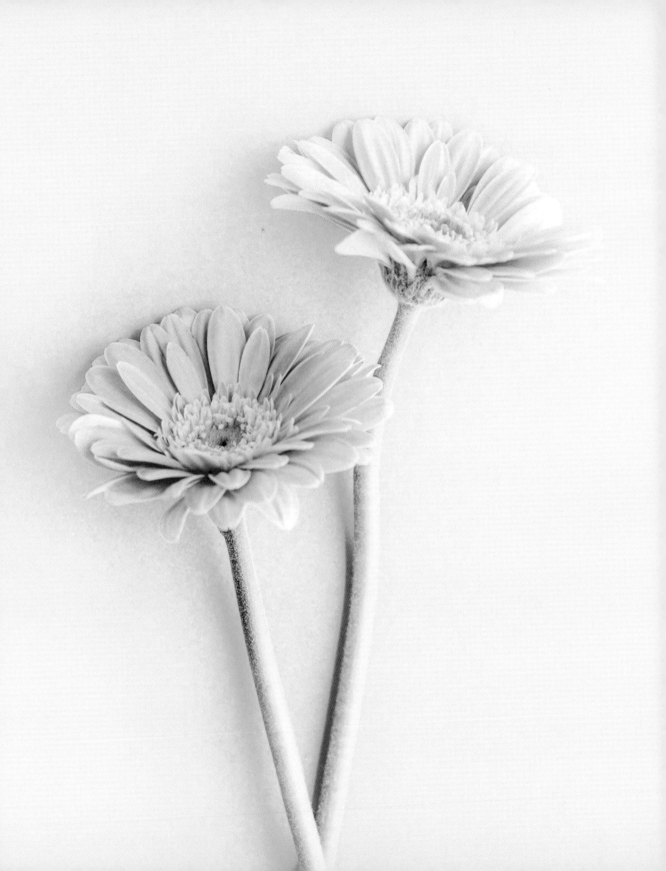

3

AND YOU'RE FEMALE!

I didn't truly appreciate how amazing it was to be female until my period returned after eight years and my hormones started to balance out. Many women I've met feel cursed to be in a body where hormones are able to run rampant and affect quality of life. But when you get right down to it, it's quite a treat to live in a female body. I love that I can be intensely intuitive (especially during menstruation); that my body has systems that cycle with the ebbs and flows of the earth and moon; that I can literally create life; that I have soft and delicate curves, and squishy bits, and stretch marks; that I get to have fun with my hair; that I feel emotions strongly; and that I have a deep urge to nurture those around me.

You may not connect with this list, and that's okay. Make your own list of things you appreciate about your unique body and gender, whatever you align with personally.

This may be the first time you've thought about how lucky you are to be a woman, and that you are! Even though there is struggle over equality and movements like #MeToo are reminding us that harassment and abuse are way too common, our lives as women are full of rich, rich experiences. Let's take a step inward and appreciate this wonderful shell through which we perceive our lives.

And, once we've done that, let's figure out how all of the outside aligns with everything going on inside. By understanding what's going on in your body, you may begin to appreciate all that it does for you while on the ketogenic diet. We'll run through what it means to be a keto woman and how your body responds to keto, we'll bust through some myths that may be standing in the way of your success, and we'll unblock misconceptions that women often struggle with on keto.

What **Keto** Does to a Woman's...

Claims abound that a ketogenic diet will wreck a woman's hormones—specifically, that it affects your thyroid, hypothalamus, pituitary, and adrenal glands. Such claims rest on one of two foundations: alleged scientific or anecdotal evidence.

Let's put these myths to rest for good.

Now, before we dive in, understand that I'm not saying that nutrition can't cause big hormonal problems in women. I'm also not saying that keto is appropriate for every woman. What I *am* saying is that a properly executed ketogenic diet has no observable negative effect on a healthy adult woman's hormones.

Note that I said "healthy *adult* woman." I don't feel that adolescents need to follow a strict keto diet unless it's being used as a therapy for certain conditions, such as epilepsy—and in those cases, keto should be followed under the direction of a health-care professional. Additionally, I absolutely do not recommend that women who are pregnant or breastfeeding start eating keto until they've discussed their options with their health-care team.

...Thyroid

You may have heard the claim that carbs are necessary for thyroid function. This idea is based on the fact that when you reduce carbs and calories, the thyroid marker triiodothyronine, or T3, decreases. Now, this is scientifically accurate—lowered T3 is associated with the ketogenic diet, especially when it's paired with caloric restriction.

However, the problem is that this is often conflated with thyroid dysfunction and hypothyroidism. To be clear, low T3 is not the same thing as hypothyroidism.

Here's a condensed version of how your thyroid gland works: Your pituitary gland secretes thyroid stimulating hormone, or TSH, which causes the thyroid gland to produce thyroxine, or T4. T4 then converts to T3, the active form of thyroid hormone. When you get a thyroid panel on a blood test, it measures TSH, T4, and T3, among other markers.

Hypothyroidism—a nasty dysfunction associated with fatigue, weight gain, hair loss, and depression—is typically diagnosed when there are high levels of TSH and low levels of free T4. What's basically going on in hypothyroidism is that the pituitary gland is asking for more T4 by increasing TSH, but the thyroid gland isn't producing any. Note that T3, the only marker that drops on a ketogenic diet, doesn't have anything to do with this breakdown in communication.

When *only* T3 is low, the thyroid is considered "euthyroid," which simply means "normal." People suffering from hypothyroidism have less energy and lost muscle mass. But low T3 is actually shown to be anticatabolic—it helps preserve muscle—and to improve longevity. And that's in addition to a concurrent increase in energy expenditure. Furthermore, when T3 is low on a ketogenic diet, it will immediately return to baseline after carbs and calories are added.

So, to conclude, a low-carb, ketogenic diet has an isolated effect on T3 and *no effect* on TSH, T4, or the thyroid gland as a whole. You're not developing hypothyroidism if only T3 decreases—a decrease that's easily reversed and actually probably good for you.

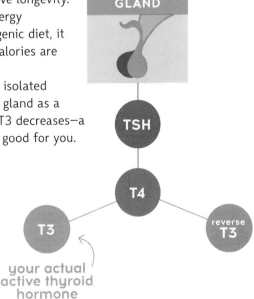

PITUITARY GLAND

TSH

T4

T3

reverse T3

your actual active thyroid hormone

...HPA Axis

The hypothalamus is a gland in your brain that's responsible for secreting hormones. It also communicates with your pituitary and adrenal glands via a pathway that's referred to as the hypothalamic-pituitary-adrenal axis, or HPA axis. Some say that a ketogenic diet interferes with this pathway and leads to utter chaos.

First of all, treat yourself to a direct quote from a study from over a decade ago: "Energy balance in animals on a ketogenic diet appears to be controlled by mechanisms outside of the normal hypothalamic pathways."

Let's unpack that. Molecules called hypothalamic neuropeptides are highly elevated on a ketogenic diet because ketones can cross the blood-brain barrier and signal hypothalamic neuropeptides. These neuropeptides are considered the best, healthiest, and most efficient way to stimulate the hypothalamus.

It's important to note that this increase in hypothalamic neuropeptides *does not* necessarily occur on a high-fat, low-carb diet—which, as we're learning, isn't the same thing as a ketogenic diet. Low-carb doesn't equal ketogenic, high-fat doesn't equal ketogenic—using ketones for energy equals ketogenic.

And what's the verdict on a true ketogenic diet and the HPA axis? There's no evidence that keto affects the HPA axis pathway in any way. The data only show that ketone signaling uses a different—and likely more efficient—pathway.

So it stands to reason that if the function of the HPA axis is not negatively altered but potentially improved on keto, then hormones such as cortisol should be unaffected. Yet some people falsely claim that ketosis itself increases cortisol.

Another false claim is that ketosis decreases leptin, the satiety hormone. There's an article floating around that argues that insulin—which is reduced when you're in ketosis—is needed for leptin production. This is just not true. Moreover, the findings of leptin modulation from ketosis aren't conclusive. Meaning, we don't totally know what keto does to leptin. All we can do now is go off how we feel. If you're satisfied on keto, you're winning! If you're not feeling satisfied, you can adjust some aspects—less fat, more fat, different types of fat—in order to reach the results you want.

What *is* certain, however, is that a ketogenic diet increases overall metabolism, and this happens completely outside of the leptin system. What's *also* certain is that women absolutely, positively suffer massive hormonal consequences as a result of calorie restriction, excessive stress, and high-intensity exercise.

So, to summarize, while a ketogenic diet acts on the hypothalamus in an entirely different way than a nonketogenic diet, there's no conclusive data showing any reduction in hormonal activity in the HPA axis.

...Sex Hormones

A lot of women notice positive changes in their libido when they start a ketogenic diet. This is because a high-carbohydrate diet triggers the adrenal glands to crank out more stress hormones like norepinephrine, adrenaline, and cortisol, and, as you likely know, stress is a total mood killer. Switching to keto reduces those stress hormones.

It also is particularly helpful for menopausal and perimenopausal women because, as menopause approaches, the adrenal glands pick up the slack in producing sex hormones. Keto gives the adrenals a fighting chance to focus on creating sex hormones instead of stress hormones—resulting in a boost in libido, a healthy hormone glow, and balanced, goddess-like moods.

Additionally, researchers have discovered that eating too much fructose and glucose turns off the gene that controls the levels of testosterone and estrogen. Both kinds of sugar are processed and turned into energy in the liver, and if too much sugar is consumed, the liver converts the excess into triglycerides. The researchers learned that when triglycerides are produced in excess, the gene that produces sex hormone binding globulin (SHBG) is turned off.

Here's why that's important: SHBG binds to sex hormones like testosterone and estrogen and carries them into the bloodstream. Only the hormones that are free and unattached to the protein can enter cells. So if the gene is shut down and SHBG isn't being created, then more estrogen and testosterone can enter cells, and this can result in dangerously high hormone levels. On the flip side, when our triglycerides are balanced, SHBG is within a normal range and we have healthy amounts of free hormones and bound hormones.

That balance may not happen right away, though. Once you start burning body fat, you'll simultaneously decrease your body's estrogen production and release the sex hormones stored in fat cells back into your bloodstream. Because of this, all kinds of hormonal weirdness can occur as you become fat adapted, and it might take a little while before you achieve a sustained balance.

...Cycle

Okay, so we know why a ketogenic diet won't harm hormones from a scientific standpoint. But what about the anecdotes? What about all those stories of people suffering negative consequences from keto? Their stories are real, for sure—it's just that the plots are a little misunderstood.

Polycystic ovary syndrome (PCOS), uterine fibroids, and endometriosis can all be improved with a ketogenic diet. This is on top of effortless fat loss, less inflammation, balancing of high cholesterol, *and* improvement of type 2 diabetes, neurological disease, cancer, and insulin resistance, just to name a few.

Here's how it works: The more fat you have on your body, the more estrogen is produced, which, in turn, encourages the body to store more fat, which produces more estrogen—you see where this is going? On top of that, all those fat cells store excess estrogen and other sex hormones. On a keto diet, as you metabolize fat cells for energy, you produce less estrogen and also release the hormones stored in fat cells. There can be some hormonal instability at first as your body adjusts to this new scenario, but eventually it will stabilize and your hormones will level out.

Now, estrogen is not a bad thing. We ladies need it to maintain strong bones, build up our uterine lining before our period, experience fewer hot flashes in menopause, and more. But too much estrogen can lead to increased body fat, impaired thyroid function, lowered insulin sensitivity, and decreased libido, just to name a few concerns.

If you've had an irregular flow for most of your life, a keto diet might normalize it. If you've been on birth control and lost your period, or if you have natural amenorrhea (not uncommon in serious athletes and breastfeeding moms), your period could come back. At first you may have a heavier flow that lasts longer than usual. Once your body adjusts to the changes in estrogen, you can expect your

ESTROGEN POSITIVES AND NEGATIVES

➕ It produces a healthy menstrual flow.

➖ Too much can cause weight gain.

➖ Too little can cause weight loss and inability to maintain healthy weight.

➕ When balanced, it creates a healthy libido.

➖ Too much increases the risk of cancer.

➖ Too little causes bone density issues.

period to return to normal, or even end up being better. Many PMS symptoms, such as backache, acne, and cramps, often improve, though ketosis doesn't cure bloating, which is the result of a surge of estrogen that happens during that part of your cycle.

It's true that hormone changes during your period affect insulin sensitivity. A surge or drop in blood glucose during this time is normal for all women, regardless of diet. After your period, it should get back to regular levels.

Some women have reported to me that when they started eating keto, their cycles initially lengthened to thirty-four to forty (or more) days. This isn't unusual; as you change from a sugar-burner to a fat-burner, there are changes throughout the body, and that can include delays and changes in cycle length. These changes may persist for a few months but usually regulate themselves once the body adapts to nutritional ketosis. Some women also experience some initial moodiness along with elevated or decreased libido when they go keto. These swings are completely normal—once your body adjusts, things will return to normal.

A well-formulated ketogenic diet will help balance out the hormones involved in your menstrual cycle, so that pretty soon your hormones will be just as nature intended.

...Menopause Experience

Some women have an almost fatalistic outlook on menopause; others are enthusiastic optimists. The reality is, menopause is going to change things, and how they change is different for every woman. Let's talk about some common changes.

Many women believe that they can eat the same way they always have during perimenopause (the several-year period before menopause, during which the ovaries make less estrogen) and menopause while maintaining their weight. Unfortunately, this is not true. For most women, when estrogen drops, metabolism drops with it—and it doesn't help that muscle mass declines as we age. The more muscle we lose, the less energy our bodies need for general metabolism. So during perimenopause and menopause, many women experience weight gain, particularly around the abdomen, and also find it is much harder to shed those unwanted pounds. After menopause, a woman's risk of elevated cholesterol, high blood pressure, cardiovascular disease, and type 2 diabetes all increase. These effects are likely related to the lack of estrogen, which can make blood vessel walls less flexible. How can we combat these problems?

A ketogenic diet is always my go-to suggestion as a starting point for menopausal dietary changes. During menopause the body seems to become much less tolerant of carbohydrates and sugars, and it may not even tolerate as much protein as it once did. Exercise is especially important for postmenopausal women, particularly weight-bearing exercise, which improves muscle mass and bone strength.

But we also need to accept our changing bodies. We need to understand that the body is wise and may be hanging on to a few extra pounds to protect us, not just to stress us out. Many studies show that older individuals who carry a bit more weight on their frame tend to live longer. Slowing down the metabolism might be nature's strategy for keeping you around longer in your new healthy body.

I encourage you to find a place of acceptance and calm in this transitional stage. It is still of course recommended to avoid obesity, smoking, and a sedentary lifestyle in order to reduce your risk of cardiovascular disease, but if none of those things apply to you and you're only carrying five to ten additional pounds after menopause, try not to look at it as a negative.

Menopause will bring changes and challenges, but the ketogenic diet can help you switch gears smoothly to continue enjoying a healthy and happy life. For more on menopause, see page 359.

...Pregnancy & Breastfeeding Experience

Having been keto since 2014, if I were to get pregnant tomorrow, I would continue eating the way I have been. I really wouldn't change anything, except maybe I'd consume a larger quantity of food. Same goes for breastfeeding—I'd just keep eating keto, perhaps eating even more fat than I do now to keep up with the demands of having a rich milk supply.

However, if you're currently pregnant or breastfeeding and you're thinking about starting keto, it may not be the best time. There's a lot going on in your body right now, and introducing something brand-new while you're going through a major life transition probably isn't the best choice. However, if you're gung ho about it, chat with your primary health-care practitioner. In the case of breastfeeding, if you're given the go-ahead, just be cautious not to forcefully lose weight at the get-go. But if you've been keto awhile and are now pregnant, or about to be, and you're wondering whether you can eat keto throughout the process, you absolutely can—I've worked with many women who have. Just make sure you chat with your health-care provider to ensure that the foods you're eating will help you reach your personal health goals.

There's reason to believe that pregnant women who follow the ketogenic diet may be giving their children a mental health advantage. A study found that mice who were exposed to the ketogenic diet in utero were less likely to exhibit anxiety and depression symptoms after birth. They also showed elevated levels of physical activity, which is no doubt a boon to mental and physical health.

Don't Lose Weight When Breastfeeding

You don't want to lose copious amounts of body weight all at once when you're breastfeeding; it can disrupt the quality of your breast milk and affect your baby. Instead, load up on healthy fats to get your body primed for fat-burning, ensuring you're eating as much as you need to breastfeed. Then, when you're ready, you can lower your intake, adjust your macros, and begin losing weight.

When you're breastfeeding, you need fat—a lot of fat. So you've come to the right place! Here are some strategies you can follow, keeping in mind that slow and steady wins the race, especially if you're starting keto for the very first time.

- Now is *not* the time to be restricting calories. In fact, you need an additional 500 calories per day when breastfeeding!

- The more fat you eat, the creamier your milk will be and the easier it will be to fill up your baby!

- For encouraging milk production, chasteberry, flaxseed, brewer's yeast, and nutritional yeast all work well. Brewer's yeast can be added to baked goods or mixed with spices as a coating for chicken. Nutritional yeast can be used as a topper on salads or a coating for chicken livers.

- Snacking is a great thing. When you're hungry, eat. Snacks like full-fat coconut milk, fat bombs, whipped avocado mousse, and fatty green shakes go a long way.

Misconceptions and **Fears** Standing in Your Way

So many women aren't finding success on the keto diet because they're still terrified to eat fat, they don't have the right information for their bodies, they're not eating enough, they're training too much, or they're eating the wrong kinds of fat. The reasons are endless, but the solution is simple: education. Yes, you read that right! All you need to do is learn. Soak up every bit of information and decide whether a course of action fits your life. Simple as that!

In this chapter, I'll explore every concern or misconception I've heard women mention about the ketogenic diet since I started Happy Keto Body (happyketobody.com) in 2018.

Let's clear the air a bit, shall we?

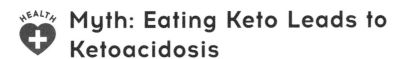 Myth: As Long As You're Eating Lots of Fat, You're Good!

While keto is gaining in popularity, there are still a lot of people who don't understand what it is. There are a couple of common misconceptions about what keto is—that you eat fat all day, or that it must include french fries and/or gorging on butter and cheese.

Sadly, when you search for "keto diet" on the internet, many of the articles against keto use this imagery. So it can be difficult for people to get an accurate understanding of what keto is.

So if someone approaches you with a negative comment about the way you've chosen to eat, instead of getting your back up and feeling offended, remember that they may not know what you're actually doing (even though they may pretend they do!). While you can technically reach ketosis by scarfing down Crisco and drinking diet soda, I wouldn't recommend it. The results we see and how good we feel on keto are directly related to the quality of foods we choose and whether they interact well with our bodies.

Myth: Eating Keto Leads to Ketoacidosis

Some people like to bring up diabetic ketoacidosis as a risk of a ketogenic diet.

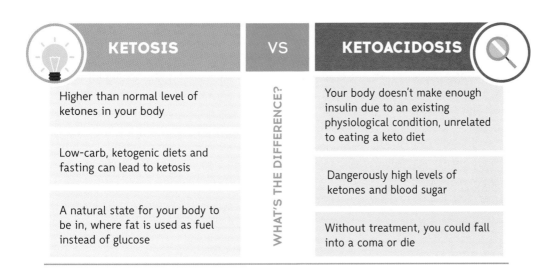

KETOSIS	WHAT'S THE DIFFERENCE?	KETOACIDOSIS
Higher than normal level of ketones in your body		Your body doesn't make enough insulin due to an existing physiological condition, unrelated to eating a keto diet
Low-carb, ketogenic diets and fasting can lead to ketosis		Dangerously high levels of ketones and blood sugar
A natural state for your body to be in, where fat is used as fuel instead of glucose		Without treatment, you could fall into a coma or die

Ketoacidosis is a dangerous condition in which both ketone levels and blood sugar are extremely high at the same time. In nutritional ketosis, on the other hand, ketone levels are elevated (though not nearly as high as they are in ketoacidosis—about 3 mmol/L compared to 30 mmol/L) and blood sugar is *low*.

Ketoacidosis affects people with diabetes or impaired liver function, and as long as your pancreas functions normally, it's almost impossible to achieve.

However, it's always best to chat with your health-care professional before adjusting your diet. And if you do have diabetes or impaired liver function, *definitely* see your doctor before trying keto. Any medication that affects your blood sugar can become very dangerous when you change your diet, so talk to your doctor about this, and always keep an eye on your blood sugar level.

✚ Myth: Too Much Fat Is Terrible for You

If all keto fat sources were trans fats, those man-made fats found in margarine and shortening, it would absolutely be dangerous. However, a healthy keto diet avoids trans fats and emphasizes healthy, high-quality fats, such as avocado oil, coconut oil, olive oil, and grass-fed meats. Omega-3 fatty acids, abundant in foods like salmon, sardines, walnuts, and flax seeds, even help turn on genes that are involved with burning fat and turn off the genes that store fat.

High-quality fats are safe and help keep you satiated longer, which reduces hunger pangs and cravings, and therefore the likelihood that you'll binge on carbs and take your body out of ketosis. And if you're concerned about how the high percentage of fat on keto affects cholesterol and heart disease, don't be. I'll explain why it's not a concern on page 58.

On the flip side, a deficiency of dietary fat can lead to low cholesterol, which is not necessarily the good thing it's been touted as—it's been shown to play a role in depression, anxiety, and inflammation.

Moreover, tons of studies have been done in the last thirty years that prove that a keto diet is healthier and more effective at improving overall health than a low-fat diet.

The key is that the fats you consume have to be high-quality fats from whole foods, which lower inflammation and regulate sex hormones and fat-burning hormones.

♥ Myth: Eating All Those Fats Must Cause Liver Damage!

There are two non-alcohol-related liver problems in which fatty deposits accumulate in the liver: nonalcoholic fatty liver disease and nonalcoholic steatohepatitis. Some people are concerned that a high-fat diet could contribute to those fatty deposits in the liver, so let's explore that.

For fat deposits to form on the liver, all of these conditions must exist at the same time:

1. The body is experiencing insulin resistance (see page 41).

2. Fat-burning is in full swing.

3. There's a high amount of inflammation in the body, caused by decades of consuming inflammatory grains, sugars, dairy, and alcohol.

4. The body is under oxidative stress, caused by decades of consuming vegetable oils and avoiding antioxidant-rich foods. The following also play a role: cigarette smoke, physiological stress, environmental toxins, shift work, and chronic infections.

On the keto diet, numbers 1, 3, and 4 are all improved, though of course it takes time to heal damage. But after a few months on keto, the only one of these that should be in play is number 2, fat-burning. In the absence of the others, fat deposits don't form on the liver.

It's true that some studies indicate that saturated fat is associated with liver imbalances. But some studies show the opposite: in one study, participants ate a diet consisting of over 40 percent saturated fat and saw a significant *improvement* in liver fat deposits compared to participants on a low-fat diet.

So what gives? My guess is that when a study connects saturated fat consumption and liver imbalances, participants are consuming saturated fat from unhealthy sources. As sad as it makes me to admit it, not many people are proud of eating beef tallow! In the standard American diet, most saturated fats come from processed foods.

Myth: Keto Harms the Kidneys

One of the common "keto diet dangers" touted on the internet is the misconception that the keto diet will affect your kidney health, and if you already have a kidney imbalance, it should be avoided at all costs. There are two myths that surround this belief: the development of stones due to high protein intake and low electrolyte intake, and an increased acidity of your urine causing kidney stress. Let's unpack each so you can make an educated decision on whether to avoid keto because of your kidneys.

Kidney stones are a painful experience, so when someone tells you that the diet you're on can cause them, you probably wouldn't be apt to keep eating that way. Here's why people say that keto causes kidney stones: keto is high in protein, they believe, which requires your kidneys to work harder, forcing your body to excrete excess amounts of calcium, sodium, and potassium, which leads to lower blood pressure and stresses your kidneys out even more. However, keto is not a high-protein diet, electrolyte supplementation is advised, and even if you ate ample protein and didn't supplement with electrolytes, studies show that a high-protein diet is not harmful for renal function in individuals with renal dysfunction.

Next up, increased urine acidity, which changes the pH of your urine to be acidic, overworking the kidneys. The problem with this misconception is that increased urine acidity only happens in ketoacidosis (see page 55), not in nutritional ketosis.

In the end, carbohydrates will damage the kidneys more in the long term than meat will. Focusing on your potassium intake on keto will naturally support the kidneys. As long as you are eating enough greens, you should be getting the proper amount of potassium to keep your body happy.

If you have concerns, chat with your primary health-care practitioner so that you can develop a keto approach that suits your needs.

 # Myth: Keto Increases Your Risk of Heart Disease

The fear that eating keto raises your risk of heart disease probably comes from a truth: keto can raise your cholesterol. But that's far from the whole story, and in the end, a keto diet will actually make you *less* likely to get heart disease.

But before we get into the truth about cholesterol, keto, and heart disease, here's a factoid to remember: the vast majority of the cholesterol in the body—about 80 percent—is actually made by the liver. What we ingest with our food is a paltry 20 percent of what's circulating. So adjusting your diet is generally going to have a fairly minimal effect on your cholesterol level.

All About Cholesterol

Cholesterol has a bad reputation, and that's so unfortunate because it's actually a pretty cool thing. Cholesterol is necessary for all body functions, including the production of bile, which in turn is essential for breaking down fat. Without cholesterol, white matter, which insulates nerves and brain cells, cannot be produced. Cholesterol is also needed for the production, development, and healthy functioning of virtually every hormone in your body, including estrogen, progesterone, testosterone, and cortisol. As women, ensuring we have enough cholesterol is crucial for overall health. So you can see why trying to lower your cholesterol could be dangerous.

Lowering cholesterol robs your body of the ability to perform many important processes, such as the processing of vitamin D, fat digestion and absorption, inflammation reduction, and nerve insulation.

While we tend to refer to a singular "cholesterol level," there are more things at play when it comes to how our cholesterol is transported and its potential risk to our health. You may have heard of HDL, the "good" cholesterol, and LDL, known as the "bad" cholesterol. HDL and LDL are actually not cholesterol themselves; they're molecules called lipoproteins that shuttle cholesterol all over the body.

HDL is known as the better of these two lipoproteins because it carries cholesterol back to the liver, which flushes it from the body. LDL, on the other hand, has the potential to cause damage. But before you start freaking out about your LDL level, know that there are actually two kinds of LDL cholesterol, and the type you have makes a big difference. Pattern A is large and fluffy, and pattern B is small and dense. Pattern B is the one that's dangerous: it's the only kind that embeds itself into the walls of your arteries and, in the presence of oxidative damage and inflammation, causes plaque to form.

Eating plant-based processed oils—like corn oil, soy oil, and cottonseed oil—does reduce LDL cholesterol. But this is because free radicals in the oils damage and break down the large, fluffy LDL A, the kind that's *not* dangerous. The amount of small, dense LDL B actually *increases*. And so does the risk of heart disease.

When you have your cholesterol measured in a blood test, the "total cholesterol" number represents LDL cholesterol, HDL cholesterol, and other lipoproteins that carry cholesterol throughout the body. It is the commonly accepted benchmark for heart disease risk—the lower the number, the conventional thinking goes, the lower your risk. But it's better to get an NMR LipoProfile test, which provides a full panel of cholesterol-related measurements, including total cholesterol, LDL, HDL, and triglycerides, as well as lipoprotein sizes.

Today, we have a far better indicator of cardiovascular risk than total cholesterol: the ratio of triglycerides to HDL. If your triglyceride/HDL number is less than 1.0, you are in a great place.

There is a direct correlation between carbohydrate intake and triglyceride level: the more carbs you consume, the higher your triglycerides—and the higher your triglycerides, the greater your risk of heart disease. If your triglycerides are over 100 mg/dL (1.1 mmol/L), you may be eating too many carbohydrates.

The Truth About Heart Disease

Studies show that only half of patients who have heart attacks have high cholesterol. Given that, it's not surprising that cardiovascular disease is likely more a problem of inflammation and oxidative stress than one of elevated cholesterol.

Molecules called free radicals are behind oxidative stress: they can damage cells, DNA, enzymes, pretty much anything in your body. When LDL cholesterol becomes embedded in arterial walls, it joins with free radicals, causing inflammation—which narrows the arteries. If no free radicals are present or they've been neutralized by antioxidants, this won't happen. So to keep your heart and arteries healthy, keep oxidative stress at bay by consuming as many antioxidants as possible. On the flip side, if you're already experiencing issues with your cardiovascular system, working toward reducing inflammation and oxidative stress side by side is the one-two punch that your body needs to heal.

A lot of us don't truly appreciate how powerful inflammation is. I'll go fully into the topic starting on page 251, but now's a perfect time to chat about how cholesterol helps to control inflammation and how a high total cholesterol number could be a sign of increased inflammation in the body.

All cholesterol but LDL pattern B actually works to reduce overall inflammation. Think of inflammation as the fire and cholesterol as the firefighter: the firefighter doesn't cause the fire, but where there's a fire, you'll also find lots of firefighters. Whenever you have high amounts of cholesterol, it could be a sign that your body is fighting inflammation. If you only take steps to lower your cholesterol, without finding and treating the source of the inflammation, you are putting your body at an even higher risk.

How to Reduce Oxidative Stress

- Supplement with glutathione, one of the most powerful antioxidants.

- Avoid sugar.

- Balance your blood sugar.

- Meditate to reduce stress.

- Avoid excess toxins (see page 312).

- Eat glutathione-rich foods like walnuts, spinach, tomatoes, and asparagus.

- Eat sulfur-rich foods so you can produce your own glutathione. Sulfur-rich foods include garlic, onions, avocados, and cruciferous vegetables.

- Consume antioxidant-rich foods such as beets, kale, berries, tomatoes, nuts and seeds, green tea, cinnamon, ginger, and turmeric.

The best way to reduce inflammation is to take the following steps:

- Avoid sugar.

- Keep stress low.

- Get enough quality sleep.

- Limit your exposure to toxins and chemicals.

- Incorporate lots of colorful veggies and healthy fats into your diet.

- Follow the strategies and adjustments starting on page 251.

Heart disease is almost always preventable and treatable with diet and lifestyle alterations.

For heart attack or stroke patients who are unwilling to change their diet and lifestyle, statin drugs reduce absolute risk of a secondary event by about 5 to 10 percent. So, technically, statin drugs can help prevent another heart attack or stroke if you've already had one—but the data is unclear on whether that will actually extend your life. What the data is very clear about is that when it comes to efficacy as well as safety, reducing your risk for cardiovascular disease using diet and lifestyle absolutely trumps using statins.

What Happens to Cholesterol on Keto

What happens to your cholesterol when you are consuming a high-fat diet? Good things, because the quality of fat you're eating, the volume in which you're eating it, the reduction in carbohydrate, the elimination of processed foods, and the ample intake of nutrient-rich vegetables all have positive effects:

- The number of smaller, denser LDL B particles decreases.

- HDL increases.

- Triglycerides decrease.

This can all happen alongside an increase in total cholesterol. Don't panic! It doesn't mean your risk of heart disease has increased. Remember that the ratio of triglycerides to HDL, not total cholesterol, is the best gauge of heart disease risk—you want that ratio to be less than 1.0. Since you're likely to see an increase in HDL and decrease in triglycerides on keto, that number should be looking pretty good.

How Sugar Causes Inflammation

Nothing raises blood sugar faster than sugary foods and drinks, and a rise in blood sugar causes several changes that increase inflammation:

- More pro-inflammatory molecules called cytokines

- More uric acid, a trigger for inflammation and insulin resistance

- More LDL B, which increases C-reactive protein, a marker for inflammation

- More advanced glycation end products, which trigger inflammation

- Increased gut permeability, which allows more particles through the gut lining, leading to increased inflammation

So what do you do if, despite following the ketogenic diet, your cholesterol remains high and your doctor advises you to start taking a statin? Do a bit more testing with your doctor. Running panels for homocysteine, apolipoprotein A and B, lipoprotein A, and CRP may help paint a picture of your true risk for cardiovascular disease.

Also, imaging tests like coronary calcium scans and angiograms can be incredibly valuable tools in assessing your true risk. If all these things indicate high risk, then you probably do need to consider a statin—maybe you're that one it is going to help.

Myth: Keto Doesn't Work Long-Term

You may have come across the theory that a ketogenic diet is a good short-term fix for weight loss but shouldn't be practiced for extended periods of time. One reason cited is rooted in the purported health risks of eating keto: the false notion that eating even good-quality dietary fat leads to heart disease. This is ironic because a lot of diseases are a result of inflammation, and a well-formulated ketogenic diet significantly lowers inflammation.

Many people also say that keto is simply impossible to practice long-term, as if it's too challenging to follow day in and day out forever. As a woman who's been eating keto since 2014, I can tell you that eating keto long-term is absolutely doable—but only if you make it work for *you*. Whether you're able to practice keto long-term comes down to personalization. You have to adjust your macros for your individual needs and develop a positive relationship with the idea of "failure." Life happens; you'll eat cake sometimes and jump out of keto for a hot minute, and that's part of the journey. Understanding that and not letting it derail you is what makes keto doable long-term. The slipups don't need to slow you down.

The keto lifestyle is just that, a lifestyle. It leads to both short-term benefits—like reversing metabolic syndrome, healing autoimmune issues, and losing weight—*and* long-term health by protecting against Alzheimer's, cancer, diabetes, coronary artery disease... The list goes on.

Myth: Getting into Ketosis Is Easy for Everyone

Some people have a relatively easy time getting into ketosis and becoming fat adapted. Others, not so much. Moreover, there's no set time frame for how long the process will take. You may be fully fat adapted in as little as two weeks. However, if you're overweight and/or insulin resistant, it could take as long as eight weeks.

Unfortunately, some people may cite the side effects you may experience while adapting as evidence of a problem with keto as a whole. What's more, a lot of the studies on ketogenic diets are conducted for only a few weeks, which is certainly not enough time to measure all of keto's amazing benefits post-adaptation. Yes, our bodies can run on ketones, but they can't make the switch from glucose-burning to ketone-burning instantly.

Most of the negative effects you hear about are part of the process of becoming fully fat adapted. While you're adapting, you may experience fatigue, headaches, low energy, muscle cramps, gas, diarrhea, bloating, mood swings, or impaired cognition. You may also notice an increase in cholesterol, triglycerides, and other blood markers. Additionally, when your body switches its fuel source to fat, the liver releases much of the salt and associated water it was holding onto when you were eating high-carb.

If you follow the suggestions outlined in this book, these issues will not only dissipate after fat adaptation, but they should improve as you stay on keto. Other diets can't promise that. And thankfully, most symptoms can be alleviated with some extra salt and potassium, lots of water, and oodles of alkaline foods, like kale, avocado, and spinach.

If you're experiencing problems on keto after a few months, here's what's probably going on:

- You're not actually in ketosis yet.

- You're not eating enough.

- You're training too hard.

- You're forcing yourself to fast.

- You're eating processed foods like nitrate-rich bacon, hot dogs, diet soda, cream cheese, and other nutrient-devoid "food" items.

- You're eating too many foods you're sensitive to.

- You're releasing toxins stored in fat cells as the fat is metabolized.

When you see people ranting in forums on the interwebs about negative effects of keto, they likely aren't in ketosis, are chronically calorie restricting, are overtraining, or are overstressed—or all of the above.

Here's how it often plays out: Someone's doing super-intense HIIT workouts. They begin to eat what they think is a ketogenic diet, but they're restricting calories in an effort to lose fat, and they're eating a low-quality diet because they're following an unhealthy plan they found online. They're stressed because they're not losing fat, so they work out even harder and get even more stressed because of their lackluster performance in the gym. Then they start having energy and fatigue problems, and voilà—the ranting ensues.

These anecdotes aren't pointing to a problem with the ketogenic diet. They're pointing to a systemic mismanagement of overall health.

The most unfortunate effect of all the uninformed "keto is bad for women" claims is that they prevent women from reaping all the amazing hormonal rewards a ketogenic diet can offer. A ketogenic diet is one of the best ways to reduce triglycerides and blood sugar and increase HDL cholesterol. You'll see improved energy, better moods, and stronger focus, as well as reduced cramps and chronic pain. Just get over the hump of adapting and you'll be well on your way!

Myth: All That Meat *Must* Be Causing Inflammation

Whenever people seem concerned that the meat I'm eating must surely be causing inflammation, in their eyes it's almost always about red meat.

In most people, red meat is no more inflammatory than other meats, and it's potentially less inflammatory than carbohydrates and refined oils. A 2007 study concluded that increasing red meat consumption by replacing carbohydrates with red meat actually reduces markers of inflammation. I know—I'm blowing your mind left, right, and sideways.

Charred Meats and Inflammation

Advanced glycation end products (AGEs) are molecules that can cause inflammation, and they're often created by overcooking meat. Eliminate the risk of char by marinating cuts of meat in an acidic marinade and adding a little apple cider vinegar or lemon juice before cooking.

Then there is the concern surrounding the omega-6 content of animal protein, specifically arachidonic acid (AA), an essential omega-6 fatty acid and a vital component of the membranes of most cells in your body. Although we need AA, our bodies cannot create it, so we have to get it from our diet. When injury or irritation occurs, this fatty acid gets converted into important inflammatory molecules that help restore damaged tissues. AA plays a role in the inflammation-signaling process, the body's defense against foreign invaders, the activation of immune cells, muscle contractions, and so much more.

The concern about AA is that it's an omega-6 fatty acid, and omega-6s are often seen as bad because they do increase inflammation. That's important to encourage healing, but some people worry that high AA intake also increases overall systemic inflammation. There is no consensus on that, though one study found that AA does not increase the concentration of inflammatory markers and may even reduce inflammation. We do know, however, that a deficiency in omega-6 fatty acids like AA can damage the central nervous system, compromise immune response, and trigger learning disorders such as ADHD and dyslexia.

So you see, there's a lot more to it than just eating red meat or not. It all comes down to quality. And if quality meat is at the forefront, I feel that there's certainly no reason to worry about eating red meat.

Myth: A Ketogenic Diet Is High in Protein

The ketogenic diet is not a high-protein diet but rather a moderate-protein diet. So we're not chowing down on meat day in and day out. However, the ketogenic diet does advocate animal protein consumption, which is a concern for some. Keep in mind that a key feature of keto is *high-quality* protein. Opting for grass-fed and grass-finished beef, pasture-raised pork, and free-range chicken; staying away from processed meats that have nitrates; and avoiding charred meats goes a long way toward making your meat consumption healthful rather than harmful.

Myth: Protein Spikes Blood Glucose, So Limit Your Protein

This fear stems from a misunderstanding of gluconeogenesis, the process by which the body can make its own glucose from amino acids (the building blocks of protein) or fats. The term literally means "the generation of new sugar," and word on the street is that even small amounts of protein above your immediate needs will be turned into glucose through spontaneous gluconeogenesis and kick you out of ketosis. This belief makes protein intake a hot topic in keto, or at least a confusing one. There's a lot of fearmongering surrounding ketogenic diets and protein intake, to the point that some people aren't eating enough protein to support their keto bodies.

Here are the facts: Gluconeogenesis is demand driven, meaning that when the body needs more glucose, it'll produce more glucose—no matter how much protein you're eating. Studies have shown that increases in protein intake have little to no effect on the rate of gluconeogenesis. Many people can eat 150 grams of protein in one sitting with an insignificant effect on blood sugar.

So gluconeogenesis is not the enemy of a ketogenic diet. In fact, it's what makes the keto diet possible. Without it, on a keto diet, your body wouldn't have enough glucose to fuel the parts of your brain that require it.

Additionally, most of the gluconeogenesis that occurs when you're fat adapted doesn't use protein. When fats are broken down, glycerol is stripped from the triglyceride molecule, freeing three fatty acid molecules to be used as fuel. The glycerol molecule is sent to the liver, which uses it to form glucose.

There's a related misunderstanding about why people with type 1 diabetes need to take insulin when they eat protein. It's not because the protein will spike their blood sugar.

You see, when you eat protein, two hormones are released: insulin and glucagon. Insulin helps the uptake of amino acids in muscle cells—a process that makes fewer amino acids available for gluconeogenesis. Glucagon counters that by stimulating the uptake of amino acids into the liver to make gluconeogenesis possible.

The release of these two competing hormones is a smart move by the body. Aside from their effects on amino acids, insulin lowers blood sugar levels while glucagon raises blood sugar levels. So in someone without diabetes, releasing both hormones ensures that blood sugar doesn't drop to dangerously low levels.

But in people with type 1 diabetes, whose bodies don't produce insulin, the release of glucagon after eating protein would cause a blood sugar spike—there's no simultaneous release of insulin to lower blood sugar. Additionally, the amount of protein used for gluconeogenesis would increase because there's no insulin to counter the glucagon. This is why people with type 1 diabetes need to take insulin when eating protein, not because protein spikes blood sugar.

⊕ Myth: The Brain Needs Sugar to Function Properly

If you're on a well-formulated ketogenic diet and in a fat-adapted state, your brain will run primarily on ketone bodies. Nevertheless, every human brain does need some glucose to function properly. If you're no longer consuming a lot of glucose, where's the brain getting its supply?

Gluconeogenesis, of course. It's really as simple as that.

So that debunks the "your brain needs sugar" myth. But your brain doesn't only get by on ketones—it *thrives*.

Many people follow the ketogenic diet specifically to help improve their mental performance. The following four factors are just some of the benefits that help the brain.

- Balanced blood sugar. On a very-low-carb diet, you avoid blood sugar spikes, which would leave you feeling exhausted and drained throughout the day.

- Better function with ketones. Ketones are a great source of fuel for the brain, even better than glucose—it simply functions better on ketones.

- Nutrient-rich energy from fats. An increased intake of healthful fatty acids can benefit the brain's function overall.

- Boosted mitochondrial function. Ketones improve the efficiency of mitochondria, the energy factories in cells. That has a particularly strong effect on the hippocampus, the part of the brain associated with memory and emotional regulation.

So not only will your brain survive on a ketogenic diet, it'll flourish, with improvements in cognition, mental acuity, focus, moods, and so much more.

There is also an ever-growing body of evidence that many mental illnesses can be managed with diet, lifestyle, minerals, and vitamins. Conventional drugs certainly have a place in treating severe mental illness, but we can do so much to optimize our moods and emotions without drugs.

Research has shown that a ketogenic diet is beneficial for Alzheimer's, which is now being referred to as "type 3 diabetes" or "insulin resistance of the brain," and bipolar disorder. These two diseases share a similar characteristic: in both, parts of the brain atrophy.

In addition, balancing blood sugar, replenishing minerals and vitamins, and healing the gut—key aspects of keto—are all proven to help us feel better and happier. And let's not forget the power of mantras and daily affirmations to keep us thinking positively, hopefully holding negative thoughts at bay.

Myth: I'm Going to Lose 5 Pounds a Week

First of all, just because you're in ketosis doesn't mean you're going to lose weight. Having a good number of ketones is only one piece of the puzzle. Other super important pieces are (1) being fat adapted, which takes time, (2) having stable insulin and blood sugar levels, which also takes time, and (3) having balanced hormones.

Furthermore, how much weight you can expect to lose on the ketogenic diet varies from person to person, depending on how your particular body works, your starting weight, your health status, your happy weight (the weight your body feels and operates best at), your caloric intake, and the quality of the food you eat.

In particular, losing weight may take longer for those who are insulin resistant than for those who are insulin sensitive. Studies show that in people who are overweight and insulin resistant, there are fewer mitochondria—the parts of the cell that generate energy—and the mitochondria they do have don't function optimally. Mitochondria help break down fat for fuel and play a huge role in the formation and utilization of ketones. So if you're overweight and/or insulin resistant, the bad news is that you're at a disadvantage for becoming fat adapted. The good news, however, is that a ketogenic diet improves both the number of mitochondria and their function. Any disadvantage can be overcome—it's just going to take some time.

On the other hand, insulin-sensitive people—aka your friends who can eat whatever they want and stay lean—will likely do well on any diet as long as they have the ability to properly digest, absorb, and metabolize any ratio of macronutrients.

It's not fair, I know. But all is not lost. If you're overweight and insulin resistant, you absolutely *can* lose fat, and you can get healthier than you ever thought possible. It's just going to take time. The true metabolic advantages of a ketogenic diet may take several weeks to manifest.

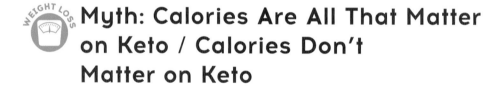

Myth: Calories Are All That Matter on Keto / Calories Don't Matter on Keto

The classic "eat less, move more" approach to weight loss is based on the "calories in, calories out" mentality—the idea that losing weight is simply a matter of consuming fewer calories than you burn. But your body is far more complicated than that. The ketogenic diet is better described as an endocrine model of weight loss: the idea that your hormonal responses to food affect hunger, weight gain, and weight loss. For this reason, keto does not need to be about restricting calories. Instead, you can eat foods that will get your hormones to do the weight-loss work for you.

See, your body has different hormonal responses to different foods. For example, protein stimulates the release of glucagon, a hormone that signals the body to burn stored fat. Fructose, meanwhile, doesn't lower the hunger hormone ghrelin as other foods do—you're just about as hungry when you finish your fruit salad as you were before you took the first bite. So the foods we eat can help or hurt our weight-loss efforts by affecting our hormones, regardless of calories.

The ratio of macronutrients—carbs, proteins, and fats—you consume also has an impact on your appetite and weight. Fat is more satiating than carbs or protein, so when fat makes up a greater percentage of your diet—as on keto—you'll eat less and feel more satiated.

What we're aiming for with the ketogenic diet and its high percentage of fat is natural hunger suppression, so that we eat less *effortlessly*. We then find ourselves in a calorie deficit without even trying, losing weight while feeling completely satiated. But this ideal state gets a bit muddled when you're having difficulty becoming fat adapted, having issues with your metabolism, or experiencing hormonal fluctuations—particularly if you're a woman.

Women are especially subject to hormonal fluctuations that influence hunger, so if you're forcing yourself to eat the same number of calories every day, it can be very difficult to get in touch with your own feelings of hunger and satiation, so that you're eating the amount of food your body really needs. You'll naturally be hungrier at certain times in your cycle than at others, so if you're eating according to your hunger—as you should—your calories will vary from day to day. And many people, regardless of gender, have wrecked their metabolisms through repeated starvation dieting and bingeing. This yo-yoing can create leptin resistance, and if you're resistant to leptin, the satiety hormone, it can be even more challenging to know when you are satisfied.

Of course, if you eat more than your body can handle, on any diet, you will gain weight. So if you aren't seeing the results you want on keto or you're having trouble getting into ketosis, yes, you might be eating too many calories. That being said, if you're only focusing on calories, you're missing the big picture.

The point I really want to drive home is that our bodies are not machines. Our thoughts, emotions, activities, hormonal profiles, circadian rhythms, food choices—they all have an impact on our energy requirements and therefore on how many calories our bodies need from day to day. The reason keto is beneficial *regardless* of calories is that it balances blood sugar and, as long as you're focusing on high-quality foods, provides your body with the building blocks it needs to regulate hormones, stabilize your appetite, and make reaching your happy weight so, so easy.

There's much more to weight loss than calories in, calories out. Supporting hormones, balancing macros, and boosting metabolism are also crucial pieces to the weight-loss puzzle. A ketogenic diet offers a positive weight-loss experience and lifelong maintenance because it meets our bodies on *their* terms.

Myth: You Have to Be in Ketosis to Burn Fat

You don't have to be in ketosis to burn fat. By and large, fat-burning comes down to insulin sensitivity, balanced hormones, and the consumption of high-quality foods that minimize inflammation. Even if your ketones don't rise to the levels that other people's do, you are still able to burn fat. Think about it for a second: if having high ketone levels were the only way to lose fat, no other diet out there would work. And we all know people who have lost weight on other diets.

Remind yourself of this when/if you get down on yourself because your ketones fell below the threshold for ketosis. There's so much more to the ketogenic diet than your ketone levels, and everything you're doing is priming your body for a fat-adapted state. Eating keto is going to balance your insulin level, and when insulin is balanced your body isn't in fat-storage mode anymore. Once this happens, your body will release fat stores regardless of your ketone level.

TRUTH BOMB

Regardless of your ketone levels, you can see the benefits of eating a ketogenic diet. If you're feeling better than you did before you started, that's a huge victory.

Think of ketones as an added benefit to the whole deal—like a therapeutic dose of healing ninjas running through your body and repairing it. Those ninjas are awesome, but they're not necessary for losing weight.

It may be a good idea to step away from the numbers from time to time and remember why you're really here. For me, it's optimal brain function—and I have that. No matter what my body may look like on a daily basis, I have a highly active brain and balanced moods. And for me, that's more than enough.

Myth: BMI Is Important

Most of us are all too familiar with the body mass index, or BMI. News stories about the average American's BMI abound; charts online will tell you your BMI; there are even BMI calculators specifically geared toward women.

The only problem is that BMI is a completely useless measurement. It doesn't differentiate between fat and muscle. Twenty-five pounds of fat acts a lot different than twenty-five pounds of muscle around strong, dense bones—and has an entirely different set of health implications.

However, going by the body mass index scale, if you're six feet tall and two hundred twenty-one pounds of solid muscle, you're obese. Pretty absurd, right? On the other hand, you could have a BMI that falls within the normal range and yet be very unhealthy by any other objective measurement.

BMI also fails to factor in where your body holds onto fat. Excess visceral fat—the kind stored around your waist—is much more dangerous than excess fat elsewhere.

This erroneous formula often misinforms people, particularly women, of their true body composition and can encourage body dysmorphia and body image issues. You may be quite healthy, but if your BMI says you're overweight, it can feel like it's just one more standard you're not measuring up to.

So why do we use the BMI at all? Well, because it's easy. Instead of taking a close and careful look at your overall health and body composition, you just plug your height and weight into a formula. To really know yourself and your state of health requires a bit more introspection than that.

I'm sure the BMI was created with the best of intentions—it's important to keep regular tabs on your health. But for practical applications, it's very misleading.

Myth: Exogenous Ketones Will Sabotage Your Keto Efforts

We've talked about ketones as molecules that are produced when you burn fat. Surprise! You can ingest ketones, too. These are known as "exogenous ketones"—ketones that originate outside the body—and they can make getting into and staying in a fat-adapted state much easier.

Unfortunately, some people seem to think that exogenous ketones will stop you from burning fat and making ketones. Here's the flawed logic: "Exogenous ketones contain energy. Body fat is stored energy. If you consume energy, you can't burn stored energy. Ergo, if you consume exogenous ketones, you can't burn body fat."

This simply isn't how the body works. The natural extension of that logic would dictate that anyone who eats anything would never be able to burn any stored fat. Unless every person who has ever lost weight has done so by water fasting, I don't think that logic holds up.

So, before we go any further, *no*, exogenous ketones do not stop you from burning fat. Your body can use both your body fat and exogenous ketones for fuel at the same time, and believe it or not, it can use some carbohydrates at the same time, too! As long as one scoop of exogenous ketones doesn't contain an infinite amount of energy, you'll be able to supplement with it and still lose weight. In fact, exogenous ketones can indirectly encourage fat-burning by increasing your energy, encouraging you to be more active, clearing your mind, improving your mood, and so much more.

What's more, exogenous ketones curb food cravings and promote appetite control. This means you eat less overall and tap into your fat stores. And they provide the body with easily accessible energy, encouraging more movement. The more you move, the more your blood flows, the higher your metabolism, and the more fat you burn.

Of course, exogenous ketones aren't some sort of magic fat-burning pill. They're just one tool in your ketogenic toolbox. You need to be eating real food in rational amounts, moving often, sleeping well, and decreasing stress before you're going to lose any appreciable amount of fat.

If you're supplementing with exogenous ketones and you suspect that they're making you gain weight, it's likely due to some hidden ingredient—certain brands contain a ton of artificial sweeteners. My favorite brand of exogenous ketones is from Perfect Keto (see healthfulpursuit.com/ketones) because of their commitment to quality ingredients and the fact that they don't use any artificial gunk.

Myth: You Have to Limit Dietary Fat to Burn Body Fat

Are Exogenous Ketones Right for You?

How can you know if exogenous ketones are something that you'd benefit from? Here are a couple of signs:

- You want to try fasting but can't seem to go too long without eating.

- You have a health condition that would improve with high ketone levels, and you can't quite get there with diet alone.

- You've been struggling with keto flu for days and days and just can't seem to shake it.

- You're thinking about trying keto but want to know what it feels like before you dive in. (Knowing what ketosis feels like can also inspire you to keep going once you do dive in.)

You can potentially, possibly, *maybe* play around with your fat intake to find a sweet spot that'll lead to faster weight loss.

Hopefully, you're picking up on the fact that you should use this strategy with caution. Some people have success with it, but most don't. That being said, let's get into it.

In order to get into a ketogenic state, you've got to eat fat. And, in the first one to four weeks, you have to eat enough fat that your body is encouraged to enter fat-burning mode quickly. Weeks after achieving fat-burning status, you may find that you require less fat to stay in ketosis.

Essentially, the strategy of reducing dietary fat is based on the idea that if you eat too much fat, your body won't have a chance to tap into its fat stores. While slightly flawed in logic—eating less fat may increase your appetite, causing you to eat more overall—this approach has worked for those who were eating far too much fat.

So how do you determine just how much fat to eat on a ketogenic diet? Check out page 157 for a table that provides fat-intake ranges that might allow your body to burn a touch more body fat.

But before you give that a go, keep in mind that an overwhelming percentage of people aren't eating *enough* fat on keto, not too much. It's more likely a lack of fat that's preventing you from optimizing your fat-burning and losing more weight. Be mindful when adjusting your fat intake—if your numbers are already on the chart and things are going well, please don't use this resource.

 # Myth: Calorie Counting Is More Important Than Healing Your Body

Let's say that your body needs to heal itself—from a low sex-hormone profile, high sex-hormone profile, leaky gut, adrenal dysfunction, candida, mitochondria decline, you name it—and you're limiting your food intake to 1,200 calories per day. First of all, as chapter 1 explained, any weight loss is going to be short-lived because your resting metabolism will adjust to the new caloric norm.

And if your body is dealing with a crisis, such as an inflammatory condition or any of the issues I just mentioned, weight loss is not its number one priority. In fact, by reducing your calories you're making it that much harder for your body to heal. Without plentiful nutrients, positive lifestyle factors, and a healing environment, the condition will just exacerbate and you'll be even more imbalanced...and you'll probably weigh the same, or more.

As long as your body is dealing with imbalances or any kind of threat, it will hold on to your weight as a protective mechanism against the strife and starvation that it thinks might be coming.

This isn't to scare you; it's just a thing I see *all* the time—women feel as if they need to weigh less in order to be happy when *actually* they're unhappy because their DHEA (a hormone that is responsible for sex drive, muscle building, and a graceful aging process) is low because their adrenals aren't functioning optimally, because their thyroid is off, because they don't eat enough or don't eat enough nutrient-dense food.

The only way to mend all these imbalances is to eat more nutrient-dense food.

Many people don't believe that the health problems they encounter when they go keto could be caused by a lack of calories and nutrients. But then they eat more food, increase their carbs, and stop tracking—and their symptoms magically improve. And, once their bodies heal—which can take a couple of weeks or longer—their weight effortlessly readjusts.

When you ditch the rules about how many calories you should eat, you give yourself permission to understand what makes your body happy. And while you may think "no rules" equates to a free-for-all with ice cream, candies, chips, and soda, you and I both know that that doesn't make our bodies happy—we get constipated, headaches, moody, bloated... This is not a happy body.

While you're healing your body with nourishing fats, make a point of reminding yourself of these three truths:

1. Time spent obsessing over your body is time not spent doing things you love. Ask yourself, "What am I willing to give up to achieve the body that I'm after?" and "What am I missing out on by obsessing over weight loss and changing my body?" It could be spending time with your kids, enjoying an early-morning run, or being intimate with your partner. Are you willing to continue sacrificing these life experiences to attain the "perfect" body?

2. Weight loss is your body's lowest priority when it's trying to heal an imbalance. Trust that your body wants to be healthy and support its healing process. Once you're in a better-balanced space, you'll find that your weight will normalize quite easily. Think: NO MORE FIGHTING!

3. It's very, very likely that your body can't function on just 1,200 calories. When you're operating at a caloric deficit, you're robbing your body of the nutrients it needs to be balanced. When your body is unbalanced, you are less likely to lose weight.

Myth: I Have to Train Hard to Lose Weight

The phenomenon of overtraining is a result of all the "eat less, move more" nonsense. Don't get me wrong, physical activity is wonderful and essential, but overtraining will damage your hormones—this includes decreasing female reproductive ability, increasing cortisol, and affecting the function of the thyroid gland. And as a result of these internal changes, you may experience weakness, fatigue, low energy, amenorrhea, and low moods.

Have you ever heard the adage "Six-packs are made in the kitchen"? It's true! Ask any physical coach, athlete, or weekend warrior and they'll agree: what you eat has far more power over how you look (and what weight loss you experience or don't experience) than any physical activity. So, as with any project, you need to find the right tool for the job.

By pairing keto with a balanced workout or movement plan, you can be sure to reach your goals without pushing yourself beyond your physical limits and dealing with health imbalances as a result. *How* you pair your workouts with keto depends on what workouts you're performing. If your movement of choice is high-intensity interval training or heavy lifting, a classic approach to the ketogenic diet may not be for you. For ways to adjust your keto diet to better meet your goals and complement your movement, head to page 207. On the other hand, if a runner's high is where it's at for you or you thrive on aerobic activities, staying the course with your ketogenic diet is the way to go.

 # Myth: Keto Is an Acidic Diet

If you recall your high school chemistry, alkaline and acidic are on opposite ends of the pH scale—a balanced pH is 7, a pH of 0 is completely acidic, and a pH of 14 is completely alkaline.

The body is naturally alkaline, but diets high in processed foods tend to make us more acidic, which causes a whole host of issues, like bone loss, muscle loss, and a depressed immune system. You can test your pH with a urine-testing kit. The goal is to have a urine pH level between 7.0 and 7.5.

A traditional ketogenic diet that's *not* based on whole foods—one with a limited focus on food quality, an abundance of processed snacks, cured meats, and multiple fatty coffees a day—is acid-forming. An acidic diet can increase aging, affect hormones, increase inflammation, slow down detoxification, lead to infertility and PMS, affect nutrient absorption, cause horrible menopause symptoms, and more.

On the flip side, when an alkaline diet is combined with a low-carb diet, many women experience a reduction in any health symptoms because it's nutrient dense and has fewer toxic substances. An alkaline ketogenic diet—like the diet you'll see in the Fat Fueled Food Pyramid on page 85, with a focus on nutrient-rich (and alkaline-forming) non-starchy vegetables, fresh herbs, grass-fed and pasture-raised proteins, and low-fructose fruits—can have some amazing effects on your body, including slowed aging, balanced hormones, reduced inflammation, and better detoxification. It supports your overall health by increasing nutrient absorption, which can reduce symptoms associated with PMS, menopause, and infertility.

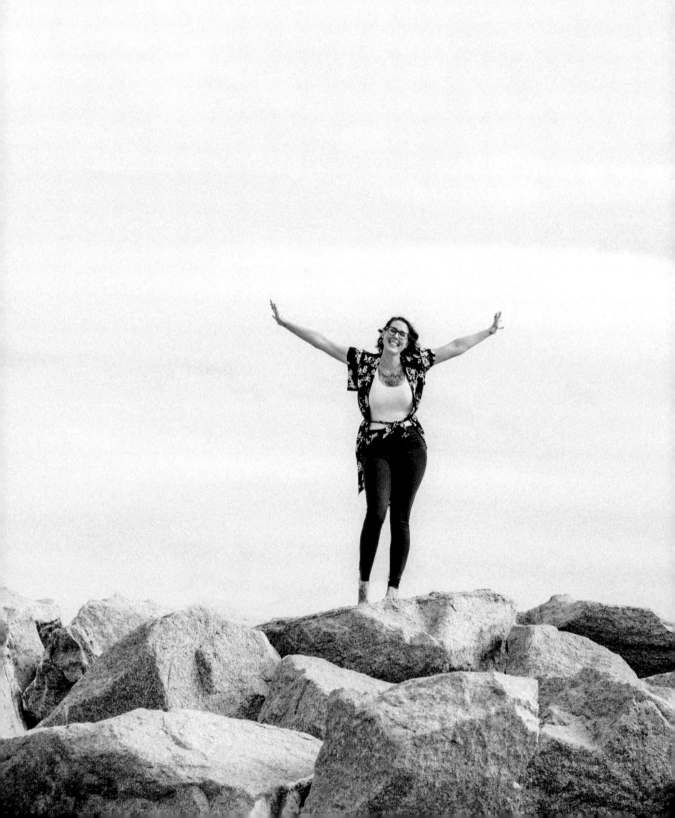

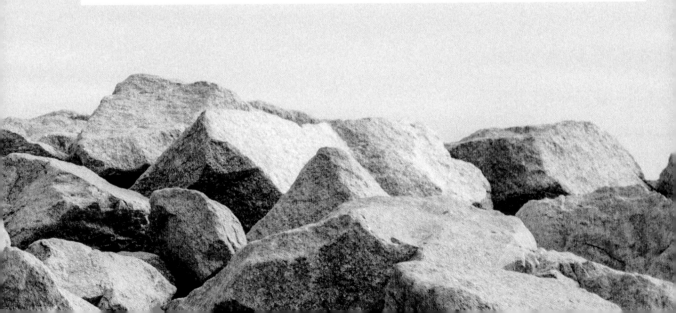

— *Part 2* —
THREE STEPS TO
FAT FUELED FREEDOM

I am not the type to tell you that if at first you "fail," you just need to push harder. I really don't think that improving our lives should be about pushing. Instead, I believe it should be about grace and ease, and we know that we're headed in the right direction when changes come almost effortlessly.

Approaching your ketogenic diet with grace and ease will help you stay with it over the long term and lead to positive results.

Ten years ago, I ate McDonald's cheeseburger meals every day, loved my East Side Mario's endless breadsticks and unlimited pasta, and never said no to a Slurpee. To go from a McDonald's-every-day mentality to preferring a low-carb, high-fat eating style that emphasizes whole, nutrient-dense foods took me about ten years. Of course it doesn't have to take you *that* long (I didn't know how to nourish my body properly, or what to do or where to go to learn how), but it would still be unreasonable to assume that such a major change could possibly happen overnight and then beat yourself up when it doesn't.

If the thought of "changing everything" and becoming strictly keto makes you feel stressed and anxious, it doesn't mean you're a bad person. The fact that you even have an inkling of where you want to go—and you've picked up a guide like this to get you there—is most of the battle! Now you just need to apply a little patience as you go through the process, and you'll be able to reach your body's happy place with self-care, kindness, and a little self-forgiveness.

If your previous experience with keto lasted just two days because on day two you succumbed to your craving for insert-favorite-treat-here, or life got in the way, or you felt like it was too much effort to cook for your entire family *and* make a separate meal for yourself, keep reading.

Many women feel like they fail on keto because they bite off more than they can chew. We ladies, you see, we're so, so good at multitasking and taking on the world that we often forget that there's a process to things. Your ability to take on the world is a great gift in many cases, but the last time you tried to overhaul your lifestyle in seven days, how'd that work out for you? I'm guessing it lead to "failure"...yeah?

Regardless of what brought you here, you can follow three steps to enjoy the health and happiness that a keto lifestyle brings.

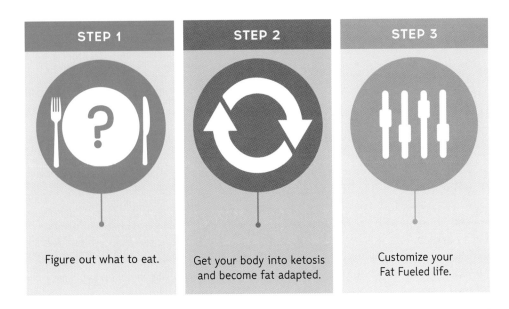

STEP 1	STEP 2	STEP 3
Figure out what to eat.	Get your body into ketosis and become fat adapted.	Customize your Fat Fueled life.

The next three chapters will walk you through these steps in order, but you can always kick off where you're at. If you're quite familiar with low-carb eating, you may be ready for step 2. If you've been eating keto for a while, you may be ready for step 3. Most times, women combine steps 2 and 3 as they're becoming fat adapted and learning how to listen to their body.

Don't rush to move from one step to the next—you can spend as long as you need to at each step, until you feel comfortable. Keep your eyes on the prize: healing!

8 Keys to Bliss for the Keto Woman

- Eat nutrient-rich food.
- Keep your carbs low.
- Keep your healthy fats high.
- Remember that you are unique.
- Respect your body.
- Eat when you're hungry.
- Eat until you're satisfied.
- Choose love.

4

STEP 1: FIGURE OUT WHAT TO EAT AND HOW TO MAKE IT

Average time: 1 to 4 weeks

If you're already eating keto, you may be thinking you've graduated this step and are planning to skip on over to step 2 without batting an eye. But wait! The Fat Fueled woman does things a little differently, and you might actually learn a thing or two by starting with the basics. For starters, step 1 is all about focusing on nourishing whole foods, something you may not be practicing fully. So hold on to your avocado, and let's get this party started.

You may also think that focusing only on what to eat four weeks or longer is a waste of time. Please, don't think that! Remember, this is a lifestyle change, not a race to the finish line. (Psst—there is no finish line.)

Focus on Changing What You're Eating, Not How Much

Step 1 is all about food quality and learning how to prepare high-quality foods easily. If adding macro counting into the mix is too much right now, don't worry about that! In step 2, we'll run through how to start counting and tracking your intake of fat, carbs, and protein. For now, the most important thing for your success is understanding what to eat and how to prepare it, so that you can stick with keto long-term.

You're here because you're fed up with living the way you have been, rushing through life, never feeling like you're actually winning at something. This ends now. You *can* change, you *can* be happy, you *can* have energy, but it's not going to be an overnight thing. Embracing this concept, and reminding yourself of it often, will take the anxiety, stress and overwhelm out of the shift you're making for yourself.

Soak up the information in this chapter. Even if you already focus on eating whole foods, I bet you could benefit from adjusting some of the foods in your life. Perhaps you don't eat as many sulfur-containing vegetables as you could, or you're overeating mercury-rich foods. All of these little microadjustments make getting into ketosis, staying there, and using it to heal your body that much easier.

The rest of this chapter will walk you through what foods are keto-friendly and health promoting and how to prepare them. Overall, here's the process you'll go through as you're focused on step 1:

1. Sort the items in your fridge and pantry, getting honest about what doesn't belong: processed foods, sugary drinks and treats, and so on. Keep them around for the family, donate them to a friend, or use them up—whatever makes the most sense for your budget.

2. Start understanding how to swap out nonsupportive foods with supportive foods (see page 104).

3. Learn how to prep supportive foods (see page 105).

4. Get comfortable with the changes through time and practice.

5. Stay focused on food—don't worry about your ketones, weight, goals, and so on. Just eat well.

6. Once you feel super confident that you have the food part down, move on to step 2.

What to **Eat**

It's important to understand that when someone says a certain food isn't "keto," what they really mean is that the food is avoided on *their* version of the keto diet.

Remember, ketosis is a metabolic state, just like being a sugar-burner. Burning glucose requires that you eat carbohydrates. Being in a state of ketosis, at its most basic, requires that you eat fat (there is more at play here, like fasting and limited carbohydrate intake, but you get the point).

There are approximately a zillion ways to feed a glucose-burning body. The only thing they have in common is that glucose is the primary fuel source, not fat. And you probably know people who have been on a glucose-fueled diet and reached their goals, found success, and are really happy and healthy.

Similarly, there are many, many versions of a ketogenic diet, and just because some keto expert tells you that certain foods aren't keto doesn't mean you can't achieve your goals while eating those foods. It simply means that this person has decided that their particular version of keto is best. And that's fine, but that doesn't make their rules right for everyone.

So, as you forge ahead with this chapter and learn what foods I recommend, remind yourself that this is only one way of doing things and that you have the right to adjust things as you see fit. My approach is based on the success I've seen with my health, but it may need to be adjusted for your needs.

"Is It Keto?" Is the Wrong Thing to Ask

It's easy to fall into the trap of thinking of the keto diet as having "good" foods that keep you in ketosis and "bad" foods that kick you out of it.

But there really are no foods that automatically kick you out of ketosis. Said another way, there are no foods that are guaranteed to bring your level of measurable ketones to zero after you eat them. Heck, even honey, white sugar, and candy won't necessarily knock you out of ketosis. It's all about balance.

Instead of asking if something is a "good" food or a "bad" food, ask yourself:

- Is the food nutritious?
- Is the food best for my physical state? Does it bring me closer to my goals for healing my body?
- Does this food make me feel good?
- How much of this food am I able to eat without it affecting my ketone level?

The Fat Fueled Food Pyramid

Keto for Women is not about "junk food today, whole-food keto tomorrow." It's not a sudden, overnight switch—it's a gradual transition from one eating style to another. Depending on where you're at, it could be a drastic change, and the idea that you could magically unlock the secrets to having the best and healthiest life ever in the span of roughly forty-eight hours simply isn't realistic.

I find the easiest way to move toward change is to follow a template that can grow with you, which is why I developed the Fat Fueled Food Pyramid. It can be challenging at first to figure out what to eat and how much. Having the pyramid to guide you makes it that much easier to embrace this lifestyle without needing to incessantly count and track what you eat. Don't worry, if tracking and counting works for you, we'll get there in step 2, but for right now, the most important thing to focus on is what to eat—and this pyramid will make it a breeze.

The pyramid outlines how to prioritize your foods following my dairy-free, whole foods–loving approach, making it possible to achieve all of the factors crucial to lifelong health: a natural, effortless reduction in calories, boosted healthful-fat intake, reduced carbohydrate intake, and increased greens. As a whole, this approach leads to stable blood sugar, optimal cell health, ample action in the mitochondria (the energy centers of cells), and more. But your particular diet may require some tweaking, as we'll cover in step 3.

Avoiding Sneaky Sugar

The place I see people making the most mistakes during their first few weeks on keto is grabbing foods that they think are safe but that are loaded with sugar. Many foods sneak in the carbs, so take a careful look at these following products:

- **Products labeled "low-carb."** There is no standard definition of "low-carb," so don't just assume it's safe. Read the label!

- **Spices.** Onion and garlic powder, ginger, allspice, and cinnamon have carbs in them, but if you're just using a sprinkle, they're usually fine.

- **Condiments.** The stuff in bottles at the store often contain added sugars or are made with harmful oils.

- **Chocolate.** Chocolate is actually fine on keto so long as it's very low in sugar or completely sugar- and sweetener-free.

- **Medicine.** Some cold medicines, cough syrups, and similar over-the-counter medications contain sugar to make them more palatable. Keep an eye on this when you're sick.

The Fat Fueled Food Pyramid

 THE EXTRAS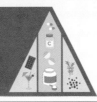

 LOW-FRUCTOSE FRUITS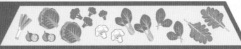

 PROTEIN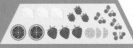

 NON-STARCHY VEGETABLES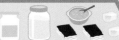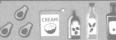

 HEALTHY FATS

 WATER

THE EXTRAS

- **Indulgences:** alcohol, dark chocolate, sweeteners, whole-food keto treats
- **Supportive supplements:** multivitamins, omega-3s, probiotics, superfood powders
- Dried herbs and spices
- Fresh herbs
- Condiments

LOW-FRUCTOSE FRUITS

Berries, grapefruit, lemons, limes

PROTEIN

- **Plant-based:** natto, nuts, seeds, tempeh
- **Animal-based:** bone broth, collagen, eggs, fatty fish, free-range chicken, grass-fed beef, organ meats, pasture-raised pork

NON-STARCHY VEGETABLES

Broccoli, Brussels sprouts, cabbage, cauliflower, leafy greens, onions

HEALTHY FATS

- **Plant-based:** avocado oil, avocados, coconut cream, coconut oil, olive oil
- **Animal-based:** duck fat, ghee (if you're not sensitive to dairy), lard, tallow

WATER

Because meats and fats tend to be expensive while carbs are notoriously cheap, you may be thinking your grocery bill is going to skyrocket. Remember that when you're on keto, you eat *far less* than you do when you're eating carbs every two to three hours. Honestly? It all evens out!

But if you're freaking out, here are a few ways to stay cost-conscious when grocery shopping:

- **Keep your eyes open for deals.** Coupons, sales, and manager cuts (look for meat-manager specials) can help you stay within your budget.

- **Buy in bulk, cook, and freeze.** Buying lots of an item at once can save you some serious cash. Put aside a few hours on the weekend to cook up big batches of dishes to last you through the week.

- **Make dishes from scratch.** Individual ingredients are often cheaper than processed, prepared products, and you can control exactly what goes into the final dish.

Keep these things in mind, and you'll be on your way to planning a great and healthy keto diet!

The Extras

When you're looking at extras like herbs and spices, supplements, wine, and condiments, the most important things to remember are that sugar hides in everything and fake/nasty ingredients are everywhere. Always read the label!

Sauces and Condiments
Many store-bought sauces and condiments have added sugars, so when you can, make your own so you know exactly what's in them. Always double-check nutrition labels if you do need to buy them in the store.

Sweeteners
While sweeteners aren't optimal for whole-body healing—they take up vital space in your diet that could be used for more nutrient-rich items—suggesting that you go 100 percent sweetener-free for life is a bit too much for most of us to handle, especially if you have sweet tooth like me!

Some sweeteners are better than others when it comes to blood sugar, insulin, and ketosis. Especially if you're just getting started with keto, you'll want to choose one of the following sweeteners and keep it on hand to satisfy a sweet craving when it hits.

Erythritol: A sweetener produced by fermenting corn or wheat starch. Most brands on the market today are made from corn and include a touch of monk fruit. I enjoy using granulated and powdered erythritol in baking; it's a 1:1 replacement for sugar.

Monk fruit: Sourced from the luo han guo fruit, monk fruit has a better flavor profile than erythritol or stevia. It doesn't have an odd aftertaste and mixes well into any recipe or drink. Like erythritol, it's a 1:1 replacement for sugar.

Stevia: Made from the stevia plant and available as a powder or a liquid. I personally find stevia to be overpoweringly sweet, so I don't enjoy baking with it, but a drop or so can work well to sweeten drinks.

There are many other sweetener options out there that I don't recommend for various reasons. Allulose is difficult to find. Xylitol can cause digestive upset and is sourced from birch, which many people are allergic to. Other types of sweeteners, including aspartame, sucralose, acesulfame K, and sorbitol, may spike glucose, cause diarrhea, and/or cross the blood-brain barrier (which terrifies me—this barrier exists to protect the brain from toxins and pathogens while allowing nutrients to reach the brain).

Alcohol

Alcohol is good for you in moderation. Studies focused on the health benefits of having a drink every now and then have found that it may reduce the risk of these health concerns:

- Bone atrophy
- Cognitive impairment
- Coronary heart disease
- Erectile dysfunction
- Type 2 diabetes

But notice that I said "a drink every now and then" and "may." I wouldn't plan a bender with your pals in the name of strengthening your bones. And if you're someone who doesn't respond well to alcohol or doesn't know when to stop, I'd avoid it. In fact, I personally have avoided alcohol for a very long time. (Not counting the glass of wine I had to celebrate signing the deal for this very book.)

Wine: It's Not Just About Carbs!

Wine has no nutrition label and no ingredients label. How do you know what you're really drinking? In short, you don't. And there are a ton of potential wine ingredients that you'd probably be best avoiding. How do you find a good wine? Look for wine that is:

1. Organic or biodynamically farmed: This means it's free of most spray chemicals, including pesticides, herbicides, fungicides, insecticides, and chemical fertilizers.

2. Dry farmed: Dry-farmed vines get their water from natural rainfall, which requires the roots to dig deeper to search for water. The deeper the roots go, the more nutrients they have access to, which makes for a healthier wine.

3. Additive-free: Additives are sometimes used to change flavors, add coloring, increase sweetness, and a whole lot more, but you don't want to put them in your body. Additives include (but are not limited to) sulfites, grape juice concentrate, tartaric acid, oak "essence," colorings, commercial yeast, acetaldehyde, albumen (egg white), ammonium phosphate, ascorbic acid, defoaming agents, gelatin, granular cork, milk products (pasteurized whole, skim, or half-and-half), and soy flour.

4. Low in alcohol content: Alcohol is toxic. So are water and oxygen in the wrong dosage. Dosage matters. Low-alcohol wines allow you to enjoy the benefits and taste of wine without feeling like you just got hit over the head.

5. Sugar-free: When wines are allowed to fully ferment, all the naturally occurring sugars are converted to alcohol. With no residual sugar remaining in the wine and no additives thrown in to sweeten it, a wine is sugar-free. Most American wines are not sugar-free.

TRUTH BOMB

If you've been on a low-carb, ketogenic diet for some time, remember: you're now a lightweight! Be careful the first time you drink after becoming fat adapted, because your body may not be able to handle as much as it used to.

All of alcohol's potential health benefits—and then some—can also be achieved by following a high-fat, ketogenic eating style. And if you're trying to lose weight or become fat adapted, drinking may limit your progress. And when I say "may," I mean, "will."

Here's why: Alcohol is the first fuel the body burns, before carbohydrates or fat, and while your body is burning alcohol for energy, it will not burn fat or glucose. If you're already fat adapted, this does not completely stop fat burning but rather pauses it until the alcohol is used up.

But! There is good news, sort of. Once the alcohol is burned through, you will immediately go back into ketosis, as long as you were in ketosis before the drink. And for some people, drinking alcohol can jump-start weight loss that continues for weeks—though for others, it can stall weight loss for days.

TRUTH BOMB

Alcohol is dehydrating, so be sure to drink extra water either before you drink, while you're drinking, or immediately after.

 ## Low-Fructose Fruits

Low-fructose fruits like berries and grapefruit can add flavor to infused water, work well as a topping on low-carb cereal or porridge (I like to make my cereals and porridges with nuts, seeds, and coconut), or make a fabulous dessert with coconut cream.

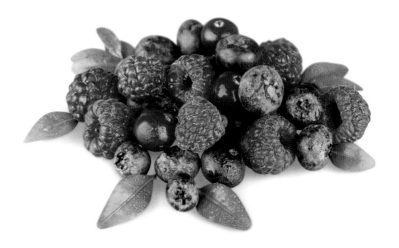

Choosing Alcohol Mindfully

Enjoy having a drink with friends now and again? Here are the most popular items to choose from and the impact they'll have on your low-carb, ketogenic life.

Note: Because there are so many brands and types of drinks, some of the categories here give a range of calories, carb counts, and sugar amounts. Also, many companies do not provide nutritional information for their products. The ranges given here were prepared with the information available, but some products will likely fall outside these ranges.

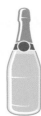

CHAMPAGNE
serving: 4 fl. oz. (120 ml)
calories: 90
carbs: 1.6 g
sugar: 0.8 g

Best choices: brut natural or brut

Do you find dry champagne too dry? Try adding a drop of NOW Foods alcohol-free stevia. It sweetens it up, sugar-free style.

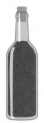

RED WINE
serving: 5 fl. oz. (150 ml)
calories: 125
carbs: 3.8 g
sugar: 0.9 g

Best choices: pinot noir, merlot, or cabernet

Organic red wine boasts more antioxidants and fewer toxins, making it a better-for-you beverage.

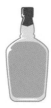

WHISKEY, BRANDY, SCOTCH, COGNAC
Based on 80 proof, 40% alcohol
serving: 1 fl. oz. (30 ml)
calories: 64
carbs: 0 g
sugar: 0 g

Research has found antioxidants in bourbon, Armagnac brandy, and cognac.

Best choices: whiskey with Zevia cola; brandy with apple cider vinegar, water, and stevia; scotch with Zevia ginger ale and lime juice; cognac with water, lemon juice, and stevia

Best Low-Sugar Mixers

- Citrus essential oils
- Coconut milk
- Cucumber juice
- Kombucha
- Lemon juice
- Lime juice
- Mineral water
- Seltzer water
- Soda water
- Unsweetened cranberry juice
- Water kefir
- Zevia (stevia-sweetened soda)

You can also garnish drinks with watermelon slices, infuse them with fresh herbs, or add stevia drops.

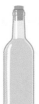

WHITE WINE
serving: 5 fl. oz. (150 ml)
calories: 120
carbs: 3.8 g
sugar: 1.4 g

White wine is lower in phenols and antioxidants than red wine.

Best choices: sauvignon blanc, chardonnay, or pinot grigio

LIGHT BEER

serving: 12 fl. oz. (350 ml)
calories: 104
carbs: 6 g
sugar: 0.3 g

What makes a light beer? It's in the alcohol content. Anything under 5% alcohol is considered light.

Light beer has the same lowered phenol and antioxidant activity as white wine.

Beer has gluten! If you're avoiding gluten, hard cider is a better choice.

Best choices: Bud Select, MGD, Michelob Ultra, Coors Light, Beck's Premier Light

VODKA, GIN, CLEAR RUM
Based on 80 proof, 40% alcohol

serving: 1 fl. oz. (30 ml)
calories: 64
carbs: 0 g
sugar: 0 g

These options are lacking in antioxidant activity.

Best choices: herb-infused vodka and water, gin with mineral water and lemon slices, rum and Zevia cola

HARD CIDER

serving: 12 fl. oz. (350 ml)
calories: 99–200
carbs: 1–30 g
sugar: 1–24 g

Offers an impressive antioxidant boost, but watch out for dry ciders that have a considerable amount of sugar!

Best choices: Strongbow Low Carb, Mercury Dry, Bulmer's Original

BEER
Not including craft beers and IPAs, which pack a lot of carbohydrates

serving: 12 fl. oz. (350 ml)
calories: 150
carbs: 9–13 g
sugar: 0–10 g

The color of the beer doesn't always indicate the carb count.

Beer has gluten! If you're avoiding gluten, hard cider is a better choice.

Best choices: Rhinebecker Extra or San Miguel

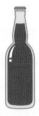

STOUT

serving: 12 fl. oz. (350 ml)
calories: 200
carbs: 20–25 g
sugar: 10–15 g

Stout has gluten! If you're avoiding gluten, hard cider is a better choice.

Best choices: Guinness Draught or Brooklyn Dry Irish Stout

UMBRELLA DRINKS

serving: 12 fl. oz. (350 ml)
calories: 300–780
carbs: 30–90 g
sugar: 13–85 g

Included so that you can see the amount of sugar. So much sugar. SUGAR!

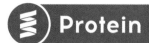

Protein

Protein is an essential part of a keto diet. If you eat too little protein, there's a risk that your body will use proteins from muscle tissue to make glucose (through gluconeogenesis; see page 65).

Animal Protein

It is *very* important to pay attention to the source and quality of your meat. There is a growing body of evidence that over the long term, eating poor-quality meat may be detrimental to your health.

When it comes to beef and bison, always choose grass-fed and grass-finished. Grass-fed animals ate (no surprise) primarily grass, and grass-finished animals weren't fed grains before slaughter. (An animal could be grass-fed but not grass-finished—grass-fed cattle are often fed grains for the last few months of their lives to fatten them up.) Also look for free-range, pasture-raised animal protein. These animals eat a natural diet and consume fewer chemicals, hormones, and steroids, so they're not passed on to you. Choose darker meats, as they tend to be fattier, and eat plenty of fatty fish.

Red meat is fine to consume, but if you're eating meats that have been processed (such as sausage and cured meat), watch out for added carbs, sugar, and nitrates. Choose fattier cuts of steak or ground beef with a higher amount of fat. Lamb is also a great option.

Here's how to choose your animal protein:

- Beef: Look for the fattiest cuts of grass-fed *and* grass-finished options.

- Eggs: Get them free-range if possible.

- Fish: The fattier, the better. Always go for wild-caught instead of farmed when possible. Avoid fish that are high in mercury, a neurotoxin that's associated with neurological and kidney disease (see the box on the facing page).

- Organ meats: Look for grass-fed *and* grass-finished. The liver, heart, kidneys, and tongue are loaded with healthy minerals.

- Pork: Look for the fattiest cuts of pasture-raised pork.

- Poultry: Look for the fattiest sections of free-range chicken, duck, and wild birds—dark meat with the skin on is best.

- Shellfish: Crabs, lobster, clams, and oysters are all good options.

- Bone broth (made from beef, pork, or poultry bones), uncured bacon, and filler-free sausage are all great options as well.

Avoid High-Mercury Fish!

The following fish are higher in mercury than others and should be avoided if possible:

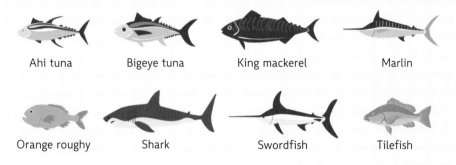

Ahi tuna   Bigeye tuna   King mackerel   Marlin

Orange roughy   Shark   Swordfish   Tilefish

Processed Meats

Deli meats, hot dogs, and cured bacon are a staple in many keto households, and I enjoy my fair share now and again. However, I always opt for nitrate-free options and am mindful of my overall intake. Nitrates themselves are not bad, but they turn into nitrites in the body, and that can be a problem.

Nitrites are formed when nitrates interact with the iron present in the meat to create free radicals. In the body, nitrites can cause damage to cells and increase your risk of hypothyroidism. They also may be linked to diabetes, Alzheimer's disease, and cancer.

Now, before you go to the internet machine and type in "nitrate-rich food" and swear off anything with a nitrate, it's worth mentioning that while plants such as beets, celery, lettuce, spinach, and radishes do in fact have nitrates, because of the vegetables' antioxidants, the nitrates transform into nitric oxide, a molecule that's responsible for many healthful body functions, including increasing circulation throughout the body.

So what does all this mean? Eat conventionally raised processed meats very sparingly. But before you start thinking bacon is off the table, uncured bacon is good, and pork belly is a must on the ketogenic diet.

If no nitrates are used in the makin' of your bacon, you're safe!

If you treat bacon like a condiment, you can probably splurge and get the expensive pasture-raised stuff. Just don't go all-out on bacon, day in and day out. Bacon all day, every day doesn't leave space for other nutrient-dense options in your meals.

Conventional Beef vs. Grass-Fed and Grass-Finished Beef

There's a big difference in quality between conventional and grass-fed, grass-finished beef.

CONVENTIONAL BEEF	GRASS-FED, GRASS-FINISHED BEEF
High levels of omega-6 fatty acids, which cause inflammation	Healthy ratio of omega-6 to omega-3 fatty acids
Less conjugated linoleic acid (CLA), a potential cancer fighter	Good amounts of CLA
Less antioxidants and vitamins	Rich in vitamins B_1 (thiamine), B_2 (riboflavin), and E, calcium, magnesium, potassium, iron, zinc, sodium, and phosphorus
Treated with exogenous growth hormones and antibiotics	No hormones or antibiotics used (in the case of organic certified)
High levels of bacteria	Few bacteria
May contain traces of antibiotic-resistant bacteria	Not applicable
Lectins in the grains that the cattle eat cause gut irritation in humans	Not applicable

Non-starchy Vegetables

Vegetables undoubtedly have carbs in them, but non-starchy veggies have less, and some come with a powerful nutrient punch that can mean the difference between struggling to meet your goals on keto and getting there with flying colors. Yes, they really do make a difference.

If you only eat two types of vegetables on your keto diet, these are the ones you want to focus on: sulfur-rich veggies and leafy greens.

Sulfur-Rich Vegetables

Sulfur is a mineral whose benefits are a bit...hidden. Unlike magnesium, which will soften your stool, or zinc, which is amazing (and quick!) for stabilizing moods, sulfur often goes unnoticed, but it offers great benefits for those who consume it regularly.

Sulfur plays a crucial role in the synthesis of glutathione, an antioxidant, and taurine, an amino acid that supports the cardiovascular and central nervous systems. It strengthens hair, is necessary for the production of insulin, and does so much more.

TRUTH BOMB

Sulfur is essential! It's one of the most abundant minerals in the human body, contributing about 1/3 pound (140 grams) of your overall weight.

Sulfur-rich vegetables include:

| Bok choy | Broccoli | Brussels sprouts | Cabbage | Cauliflower |

| Garlic | Leeks | Onions | Shallots |

Make the Most of Your Sulfur-Rich Veg!

The way you prepare sulfur-rich vegetables makes all the difference. Not preparing them properly can reduce the sulfur, or make it so that the sulfur isn't absorbable. Preparing food using the following methods ensures that your body is able to assimilate as much of it as possible!

VEGETABLES	HOW TO PREP	BENEFITS
Broccoli	Steam until bright green and al dente.	Boosts the immune system
Brussels sprouts	Steam until al dente.	Improves memory and focus
Cabbage	Slice and let sit for 10 minutes before lightly steaming until al dente.	Protects mitochondria for better energy
Cauliflower	Cut into small pieces or pulse florets in a food processor. Let sit for 10 minutes before lightly steaming until heated through but not mushy.	Reduces inflammation
Bok choy, leeks, garlic, onions, shallots	Mix raw into salads and dressings. When cooking, slice and let sit for 10 minutes before applying heat.	Good for the nerves, kidneys, liver, and brain

Leafy Greens

There are so, so many types of leafy greens that it's hard to give a succinct list, but here are some you may be familiar with:

- Arugula
- Baby greens
- Beet greens
- Chard
- Collards
- Endive

- Kale
- Lettuce
- Mustard
- Parsley
- Spinach
- Sweet potato leaves

Greens offer an essentially noncaloric, nutrient-dense way to pack your keto diet full of minerals, like magnesium, calcium, potassium, and manganese. Think of them as whole-food supplements gifted to us by Mother Nature herself.

In addition, pairing greens with meals helps to encourage spontaneous caloric restriction because of their volume—you feel like you've eaten lots, a great strategy if weight loss is your goal. There's nothing you need to do to realize this. Just eat greens, and they'll do the rest.

Ideally, you should aim for 2 to 3 cups of leafy greens a day.

Healthy Fats

Saturated and monounsaturated fats are chemically stable and less inflammatory than other fats, so they are the best kind you can eat.

Fat Increasing Your Cholesterol?

Not everyone handles saturated fat well! Most people thrive on it, but if you have a certain genetic marker, you'll realize very quickly that a typical keto diet is not working for you—your body just can't process saturated fat. If your cholesterol is skyrocketing on keto, or your weight is going up and up and up, you may have the APOE4 gene; head over to page 176 for more info and try doing keto Mediterranean style, with loads of fatty fish, avocado, olives, and olive oil.

FATS AND OILS

SATURATED FATS

CONSUME OFTEN
- Solid at room temperature
- Great for higher temperature cooking
- Have gotten a bad rap over the years, but they're actually awesome for our health
- Great for the heart, liver, brain, nervous system, and more
- Help increase HDL cholesterol

EXAMPLES OF SATURATED FATS:

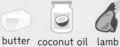

bacon beef butter coconut oil lamb tallow/suet

MONOUNSATURATED FATS (MUFAS)

CONSUME OFTEN
- Typically liquid at room temperature and solid when chilled
- Moderately stable and good for light cooking between 320°F (160°C) and 350°F (177°C)
- Look for keywords like "cold-pressed," "centrifuge-extracted," and "expeller-pressed"—there's little chance of consuming oxidized fats, which can cause cell damage

EXAMPLES OF MONOUNSATURATED FATS:

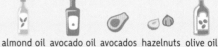

almond oil avocado oil avocados hazelnuts olive oil macadamia nuts

POLYUNSATURATED FATS (PUFAS)

USE SPARINGLY
- Always in a liquid state
- More likely to become oxidized during heating, so they're not good for cooking
- Foods containing these oils, such as salmon, trout, hemp seeds, chia seeds, and flax seeds, should be minimally heated, just until cooked.

Omega-3 and Omega-6
- The body cannot produce them, yet they're required for normal body functions.
- A 1:1 ratio of omega-3 to omega-6 will ward off inflammation
- A ketogenic diet that's high in saturated fat and low in processed oils is naturally balanced in omega-3 and omega-6.

EXAMPLES OF POLYUNSATURATED FATS:

salmon flax

Polyunsaturated Fats: Omega-3 & Omega-6

Polyunsaturated fatty acids (PUFAs) are essential in your diet—the body cannot produce them on its own, and they're necessary to support the heart, brain, and eyes from degeneration.

However, two of the most important PUFAs, omega-6 and omega-3, are often out of balance on the standard American diet. We get way too much pro-inflammatory omega-6 and not nearly enough anti-inflammatory omega-3, leading to a higher risk of cardiovascular disease, cancer, and inflammatory and autoimmune diseases. On the flip side, getting more omega-3 suppresses these effects. Also, if that's not enough to convince you of their importance, omega-3 fats help turn on the genes that are involved with fat-burning. So eating food high in omega-3s, like wild salmon and shellfish, is going to work in your favor!

If you don't like fish, you can get omega-3 in a supplement. Although you hear about some nuts and oils (like walnuts, almonds, pine nuts, sunflower oil, and corn oil) being high in omega-3s, many—especially processed oils—are also high in inflammatory omega-6s. Eat fatty fish, avoid snacking on too many nuts, and don't overindulge in desserts that include a lot of almond flour, and your omega fatty acids should be balanced.

If you like to fry your food, always go for non-hydrogenated lard, tallow, ghee, or coconut oil. These fats have higher smoke points than others, which means they oxidize less and won't cause inflammation.

Refined Oils

Some oils are naturally good, and some oils are naturally bad, and some oils are just not awesome when they're heated beyond a certain temperature. One of the main characteristics of a detrimental oil is that it's unstable when heated—polyunsaturated fats are particularly sensitive to heat and become unstable when heated. In order to extract oil from a seed, heat is often used, and if this seed contains a high amount of polyunsaturated fat, the extraction process will make the oil rancid and highly inflammatory. Often these unstable oils are used for high-heat cooking, frying, and baking, which only creates more inflammatory factors.

Oils to avoid include soybean, rice bran, wheat germ, peanut, sesame, corn, grapeseed, cottonseed, and safflower, as well as vegetable shortening, margarine, and vegan spreads. These oils have high ratios of omega-6 to omega-3 and lots of processed ingredients (in the case of the spreads and margarines), and many are genetically modified and use chemicals to extract the oil from the seed, which is even worse than using heat.

Oils you do not want to cook with include unrefined avocado oil, olive oil, almond oil, and MCT oil. These oils are perfectly safe when chilled or at room temperature, but they should never be heated because their smoke points are lower than others. The lower the smoke point, the less safe the oil is to cook with because heat causes it to become rancid, so it will cause free-radical damage in your body when ingested.

When you're shopping, look for these keywords on labels—they're all signs of a good oil: cold-pressed, centrifuge extracted, extra-virgin, unrefined.

Dairy

I hate to be the bearer of bad news for milk enthusiasts, but there is evidence that drinking milk can lead to a whole host of health issues, including respiratory conditions, digestive upset, increased risk of cancer, and increased inflammation.

We're told to consume dairy because it's high in calcium, and calcium is good for the bones, right? Well, it turns out that consuming more dairy doesn't necessarily lead to better bone health. Dozens of studies have concluded that eating a lot of dairy has very minimal impact on bone strength and thus will not reduce your risk of breaking a bone.

In fact, in cultures where people consume less than 300 milligrams of calcium daily from food, there's actually a lower rate of bone fractures than in cultures where calcium consumption is higher. Now, granted, these cultures are in warm environments where vitamin D from the sun is plentiful—vitamin D also helps bones, so it may have compensated for the lower calcium intake. But it is very easy to receive 300 milligrams of calcium through the diet without dairy. In fact, dairy pushes us over the limit of how much calcium our body needs.

And taking calcium supplements may actually be harmful. Several studies have shown that not only do they have a minimal impact on bones, leading to no change in fracture risk, but they also may lead to more plaque buildup in the arteries, increasing your risk for heart attack and stroke.

Researchers also suggest that a high intake of milk might have undesirable effects because it contains D-galactose. From what we know right now, chronic exposure to D-galactose is damaging to health. Even a low dose of D-galactose induces changes that resemble natural aging in animals, including a shortened life span, oxidative stress, chronic inflammation, degeneration of the nervous system, and impairment of the immune system. Dairy has also been labeled as a key trigger of irritable bowel syndrome symptoms and other digestive conditions, so if you're dealing with a gut issue, avoiding dairy may give you some relief.

Of course, the best-known reason to avoid dairy is lactose intolerance, which can cause cramps, stomach pain, bloating, gas, diarrhea, and nausea. Did you know that an estimated 75 percent of the world's population has some degree of lactose intolerance? Figuring out if you're one of them usually requires removing dairy from your diet for a couple of weeks, having a touch of dairy, and then seeing how your body responds.

A1 vs. A2 Dairy

If you're in love with dairy and can't give it up but feel it may be contributing to imbalances in your body, look for dairy made from A2 milk. There are two kinds of casein, the main protein in milk: A1 and A2. There's some evidence that milk that has only A2 casein may not cause the discomfort some people experience after consuming dairy.

Let's say you still want to treat yourself to dairy once in a while. That's fine! But dairy products made with conventional milk are usually pasteurized, which lowers overall nutrient density, and they may contain hormones, chemicals, and antibiotics. So if you're going to do dairy, purchase products prepared with raw milk sourced from grass-fed and grass-finished cattle or, alternatively, locally produced products, so you can chat with the makers about the quality. It's the best way to ensure you're eating a superior product that'll do more good than harm.

Humans are the only mammals on the planet to drink milk after infancy, so if we follow Mother Nature's guide, adults should probably stop drinking it. On top of that, consuming dairy is consuming milk from another mammal, milk that's meant to grow a baby sheep, cow, or goat. Think about it for a second: Would you drink pig's milk? What about pigeon? How about cockroach? For serious. These animals do in fact make milk for their young.

Finally, some research suggests that consuming milk products may increase your risk of developing cancer. Milk products may contain contaminants, such as pesticides, that have carcinogenic potential, and growth factors, such as insulin-like growth factor 1, which has been shown to promote the growth of breast cancer cells.

What we were taught to believe about the need to consume dairy is not accurate. Our bodies need calcium, there is no doubt about that, but it's better to get it from fish and greens than from dairy.

Bottom line is, if you are taking a calcium supplement, stop. If you are drinking milk, stop. And if you want healthy bones, exercise—weight-bearing exercises are excellent for improving bone health—and change your diet a bit.

CALCIUM CONTENT IN LOW-CARB FOODS
PER 100 GRAMS

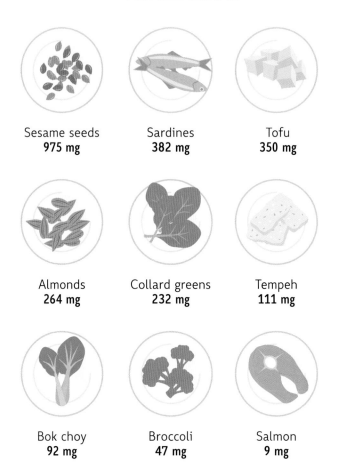

Sesame seeds
975 mg

Sardines
382 mg

Tofu
350 mg

Almonds
264 mg

Collard greens
232 mg

Tempeh
111 mg

Bok choy
92 mg

Broccoli
47 mg

Salmon
9 mg

💧 Water

When women come to me with health imbalances, my first question is, "How much water are you drinking?" For real, so many of our health imbalances and little issues are because we don't drink enough water.

Your body stores glycogen (the storage form of glucose) in water, so it only makes sense that as you start eating keto, your body doesn't hold on to as much water as it did when it was in a glucose-burning state. As your body burns through glycogen without replenishing it, your water stores get depleted as well. This is why many people see epic weight loss during the first couple of weeks on keto—it's water weight! Losing that water weight is also a contributing factor to the keto flu, which can be caused by mild dehydration and can be shortened tremendously by drinking more water.

Ensuring you're well hydrated also assists with balancing your appetite—what you think is hunger often turns out to be thirst—and helps you metabolize fat more efficiently, since burning fat requires that more water be present.

The easiest way to check your hydration level is to note the color of your urine next time you head to the washroom. If it's light in color, like chamomile tea, you're hydrated! The darker the color—the closer it gets to the color of apple juice—the less hydrated you are and the more water you have to drink.

Five liters (5.2 quarts) is my lucky number. I know—that's a lot of water! To make drinking water a habit and get into a rhythm, I set up a water schedule in my calendar that alerted me to drink at certain times. It took about two weeks until drinking before I was thirsty started coming naturally. You see, if you wait until you're thirsty to drink, it's often way past when you should have had a sip or seven. Don't wait until you're dehydrated to hydrate!

My water schedule:

- Wake up: 1 quart (1 liter)

- After working out: 1 quart (1 liter)

- After coffee: 1 pint (475 ml)

- 1 hour after first meal: 1 quart (1 liter)

- 1 hour after second meal: 1 pint (475 ml)

- 2 hours before bed: 1 quart (1 liter)

Best Exercises for Strong Bones
Balancing
Climbing stairs
Dancing
Rebounding (mini trampoline exercises)
Step aerobics
Tennis

The Fat Fueled Food Pyramid in Detail

THE EXTRAS

INDULGENCES

Cacao powder

Cacao nibs

Erythritol

Monk fruit

Stevia

CONDIMENTS

Apple cider vinegar

Balsamic vinegar

Coconut aminos

Horseradish

Hot sauce

Ketchup (no sugar added, or make your own)

Mustard

Pickles

Relish (no sugar added)

Salad dressing (made with 100% avocado oil or olive oil)

Worcestershire sauce

DRIED HERBS AND SPICES

Allspice powder	Dried basil	Ground cinnamon
Bay leaves	Dried ground oregano	Ground cloves
Cajun seasoning	Dried ground rosemary	Ground nutmeg
Cardamom	Dried ground thyme	Onion powder
Cayenne pepper	Dried oregano leaves	Red pepper flakes
Chili powder	Dried rosemary leaves	Sea salt
Chinese five-spice powder	Dried thyme leaves	Seasoning salt
Coriander powder	Garlic powder	Smoked paprika
Cumin	Ginger powder	Turmeric
Curry powder	Ground black pepper	Vanilla powder

FRESH HERBS

Basil	Rosemary
Chives	Sage
Cilantro	Tarragon
Dill	Thyme
Mint	
Oregano	
Parsley	

SUPPORTIVE SUPPLEMENTS

Superfood powders like spirulina, bee pollen, mushroom elixirs

Daily supplements like a multivitamin, omega-3 oil, probiotics

LOW-FRUCTOSE FRUITS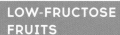

Blackberries

Blueberries

Cranberries

Grapefruit

Lemons

Limes

Raspberries

Strawberries

PROTEIN

PLANT-BASED

Almonds (whole, butter, milk)	Natto
Brazil nuts (whole, butter, milk)	Pecans (whole, butter, milk)
Chia seeds (whole, milk)	Sunflower seeds (whole, butter, milk)
Flax seeds (whole, milk)	Tahini (whole, butter, milk)
Hazelnuts (whole, butter, milk)	Tempeh
Hemp seeds (whole, butter, milk)	Walnuts (whole, butter, milk)

ANIMAL-BASED

Bone broth

Collagen

Eggs

Fatty fish

Free-range chicken

Gelatin

Grass-fed beef

Organ meats

Pasture-raised lamb

Pasture-raised pork

Wild game

NON-STARCHY VEGETABLES

HIGHER PRIORITY

Arugula

Baby greens

Beet greens

Bok choy

Broccoli

Brussels sprouts

Cabbage

Cauliflower

Chard

Collards

Endive

Garlic

Kale

Kimchi

Leeks

Lettuce

Mustard greens

Onions

Parsley

Sauerkraut

Shallots

Spinach

LOWER PRIORITY

Artichoke hearts

Asparagus

Bell peppers, green

Capers

Celery

Cucumbers

Daikon

Eggplants

Fennel

Kohlrabi

Lettuce

Mushrooms

Okra

Radishes

Rhubarb

Turnips

Zucchini

HEALTHY FATS

PLANT-BASED

Avocado oil

Avocados

Cacao butter

Coconut butter

Coconut cream

Coconut meat (shredded, fresh, pulverized)

Coconut milk

Coconut oil

Macadamia nuts (whole, oil, butter, milk)

MCT oil

Nondairy yogurt

Olive oil

Olives

ANIMAL-BASED

Duck fat

Ghee (if you're not sensitive to dairy)

Lard

Mayonnaise (made with 100% avocado oil or olive oil)

Tallow

FOOD SWAPS

SWAP OUT THIS	→	FOR THIS AWESOME THING!
Burger buns		Portobello mushroom caps, iceberg lettuce, bacon woven together and cooked, eggplant slices
Fat-free mayo		Mayonnaise made with 100% avocado oil, or homemade
Fat-free yogurt		You can sweeten any of these options with stevia: **If doing dairy:** full-fat plain Greek yogurt* **Dairy-free:** chia pudding, dairy-free yogurt (my favorite brands are Coyo and Yoso)
Grains (including oatmeal and granola)		Flax seeds, hemp hearts, chia seeds, nuts
High-sugar drinks (including fruit juice, soda, and energy drinks)		You can sweeten any of these with stevia or monk fruit: Mineral water, lemon juice, lime juice, cold-brewed teas
Legumes		Nuts and seeds
Mashed potatoes		Steamed and mashed cauliflower
Nonfat milk		**If doing dairy:** High-fat dairy, such as heavy whipping cream* **Dairy-free:** Lite coconut milk, almond milk, hemp milk
Pasta		Low-carb noodles (such as kelp noodles or konjac noodles); spiral-sliced zucchini, turnip, and jicama
Potatoes and other starches		Cauliflower, radishes, turnip, jicama, rutabaga
Protein powder (whey or otherwise)		Collagen
Rice		Grated and steamed cauliflower, rutabaga, and turnips
Sandwich wraps		Butter lettuce, collard greens
Sugar (including maple syrup, honey, coconut nectar)		Stevia, monk fruit, erythritol
Sweets (including fruit snacks, sugar-free candies, and granola bars)		Dark chocolate (no added sugar); a handful of berries, nuts, or seeds
Vegetable oils (for cooking)		**If doing dairy:** Ghee* or butter* **Dairy-free:** Avocado oil, coconut oil, butter-flavored coconut oil, red palm oil, bacon grease, beef fat/tallow
Vegetable oils (for salads)		Olive oil, MCT oil, avocado oil
Vegetables: Beets, carrots, corn, parsnips, peas		Asparagus, broccoli, cabbage, cauliflower, cucumber, kale, onions, romaine lettuce, spinach, tomatoes, and more

best if grass-fed and grass-finished

How to **Make It**

Let's keep things really simple here. I could load you up with recipes and resources, meal plans, food lists, and everything in between, but that wouldn't actually teach you anything. Instead, here's a strategy I've used since 2008, after I graduated from nutrition school. It's wildly effective and will actually teach you how to feed yourself with what you have on hand.

Instead of stressing over recipes, shopping lists, and meal plans, *focus on surrounding yourself with nourishing food*, then learn how to throw it all together easily.

Think of your ketogenic diet as being made up of the following five meals:

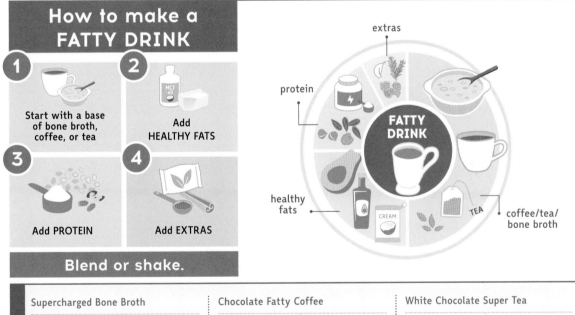

How to make a FATTY DRINK

1. Start with a base of bone broth, coffee, or tea
2. Add HEALTHY FATS
3. Add PROTEIN
4. Add EXTRAS

Blend or shake.

Examples	Supercharged Bone Broth	
	Base	Bone broth
	Healthy Fat	Lard
	Protein	None (bone broth itself is a protein)
	Extras	Mushroom elixir, turmeric, ground black pepper, salt

Chocolate Fatty Coffee	
Base	Coffee
Healthy Fat	MCT oil
Protein	Collagen, hemp seeds
Extras	Cacao powder, stevia

White Chocolate Super Tea	
Base	Tea
Healthy Fat	Cacao butter
Protein	Gelatin
Extras	None

How to make a SHAKE

1 Start with a base of tea, water, coffee, or nondairy milk

2 Add HEALTHY FATS

3 Add NON-STARCHY VEGETABLES

 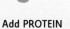
4 Add PROTEIN

5 Add LOW-FRUCTOSE FRUITS

6 Add EXTRAS

Blend or shake.

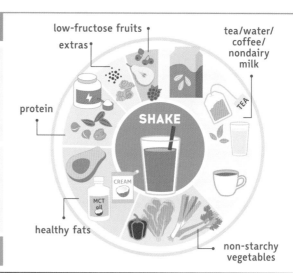

low-fructose fruits
extras
tea/water/coffee/nondairy milk
protein
SHAKE
healthy fats
non-starchy vegetables

Examples

Raspberry Lime Green Smoothie	
Base	Water
Healthy Fat	MCT oil powder
Non-starchy Veg.	Kale
Protein	Sunflower seed butter
Low-Fructose Fruits	Raspberries
Extras	Lime juice, mint leaves, salt

Ultra-Fatty Smoothie	
Base	Coconut milk
Healthy Fat	Avocado
Non-starchy Veg.	Spinach
Protein	Almond butter
Low-Fructose Fruits	None
Extras	Stevia

No-Fruit Buzzed Smoothie	
Base	Chilled coffee
Healthy Fat	Coconut cream
Non-starchy Veg.	None
Protein	Collagen
Low-Fructose Fruits	None
Extras	Bee pollen, cinnamon

How to make a SAUCE/DRESSING

1 Start with HEALTHY FATS

2 Add ACID

3 Add CONDIMENTS

4 Add other EXTRAS

5 Add NON-STARCHY VEGETABLES

Stir or blend.

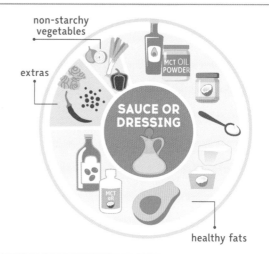

non-starchy vegetables
extras
SAUCE OR DRESSING
healthy fats

Examples

Zinger Creamy Dressing	
Healthy Fats	Mayonnaise
Acid	Apple cider vinegar
Condiments	Mustard, horseradish
Extras	Salt
Non-starchy Veg.	Chives

Balsamic Dressing	
Healthy Fats	Avocado oil
Acid	Balsamic vinegar
Condiments	Coconut aminos
Extras	None
Non-starchy Veg.	None

Spicy Veggie Dip	
Healthy Fats	Avocado, MCT
Acid	Lime juice
Condiments	Hot sauce
Extras	Erythritol, cayenne, garlic powder, chili powder, salt
Non-starchy Veg.	Spinach

How to make a HOT MEAL

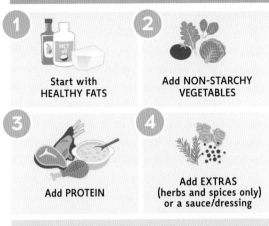

1 Start with HEALTHY FATS

2 Add NON-STARCHY VEGETABLES

3 Add PROTEIN

4 Add EXTRAS (herbs and spices only) or a sauce/dressing

Heat the healthy fat, add the protein, and sauté or boil. Add the vegetables and extras and sauté or boil until heated/cooked through. You can also approach these options as soups or stews, or cook items separately for better presentation.

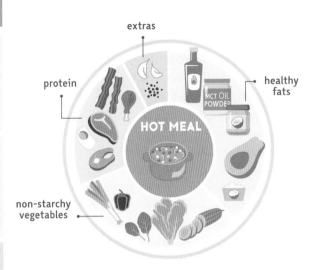

Examples	Sautéed Kale and Spiced Chicken Thighs		Cabbage Soup		Wilted Spinach and Ground Beef	
	Healthy Fat	Coconut oil	**Healthy Fat**	Lard	**Healthy Fat**	Avocado oil, avocados
	Non-starchy Veg.	Kale	**Non-starchy Veg.**	Cabbage	**Non-starchy Veg.**	Spinach, tomatoes
	Protein	Chicken thighs	**Protein**	Bone broth	**Protein**	Ground beef
	Extras	Turmeric, cumin, salt	**Extras**	Oregano, salt, ground black pepper	**Extras**	None

How to make a COLD MEAL

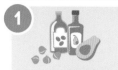

1 Start with HEALTHY FATS

2 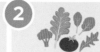 Add NON-STARCHY VEGETABLES

3 Add PROTEIN

4 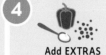 Add EXTRAS (herbs and spices only) or a sauce/dressing

Combine the liquid ingredients in a large salad bowl. Stir to combine, then add the remaining ingredients and toss to coat.

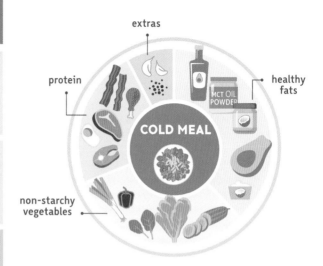

Examples	Creamy Tahini Vegan Salad	
	Healthy Fat	Olives, olive oil
	Non-starchy Veg.	Lettuce
	Protein	Cooked tempeh, sesame seed paste
	Extras	Red pepper flakes, apple cider vinegar

Crunchy Greens for Days Bowl	
Healthy Fat	Macadamia nuts
Non-starchy Veg.	Broccoli, asparagus, arugula
Protein	Hard-boiled eggs
Extras	Mayonnaise, ground black pepper

Boosted Coleslaw	
Healthy Fat	Avocado oil, avocados
Non-starchy Veg.	Spinach, tomatoes
Protein	Cooked ground beef
Extras	None

Step 1 **Problems** and **Solutions**

As you make the transition to a whole foods–based ketogenic diet, there are some common side effects and imbalances you may experience. In this section I'll give you my best tips for managing and minimizing them. Be sure to also review the problems common in step 2, starting on page 163, as some people experience certain issues before others. Of course, you may not experience anything other than pure bliss, endless energy, and crazy libido!

Keto Flu

As you begin to lower your carbohydrate intake, you'll likely experience at least some symptoms, especially if the carbohydrates you were regularly eating before embarking on your journey were refined, high in sugar, or loaded with grains.

So if you're feeling a little groggy, tired, or dizzy, and you've been thinking and dreaming of all things pizza, pasta, ice cream, and tacos, don't worry—there's nothing wrong with you! You're just experiencing a touch of the keto flu.

Symptoms of the keto flu include:

- Brain fog
- Carb cravings
- Dizziness
- Fatigue
- Flu-like symptoms
- Inability to focus

- Insomnia
- Irritability
- Nausea
- Shakiness
- Stomach upset
- Weakness

If you're avid about exercise and hit the gym regularly, you may also notice some lost strength and endurance.

The keto flu is pretty common and tends to go away after a few days to a few weeks. There are two main reasons why people experience the keto flu:

The ketogenic diet is a diuretic. This means that you'll urinate more, which can lead to a loss of electrolytes and water. Dehydration and depleted electrolytes can leave you feeling really poor—nauseous, headachy, tired.

Your body is transitioning from being a sugar-burner to being a fat-burner. When you first start eating keto, your body is still equipped to process a higher intake of carbs and a lower intake of fat. It takes time for your body to create the enzymes needed to utilize fat fully. While your body adjusts, your brain may run low on energy, which means you may feel groggy, tired, or fatigued, or even have a headache.

While the keto flu tends to last less than a week or two, you can do a few things to minimize its duration and feel better faster.

1. **Increase your intake of electrolytes.** With the reduction of insulin that naturally occurs on a low-carb diet, your body is no longer able to store as much sodium as it could before. Plus, as you shed water weight, sodium and other electrolytes are being flushed out of your cells. To replace your electrolytes, focus on electrolyte-rich foods such as greens, dark chocolate, nuts, seeds, and salt! Add Himalayan salt to water, add fresh lemon juice to water, or boost your water with an electrolyte supplement (make sure it's sugar-free with no fillers!). This will replenish your depleted electrolyte levels and make you feel a great deal better.

2. **Drink copious amounts of water.** While it's true that being dehydrated *can* boost ketones, unfortunately it can also make you feel like…hot garbage. Drink and drink and drink some more.

3. **Eat more fat.** As your body adjusts to the change in fuel source, eating more fat will help it adapt faster.

4. **Eat enough.** When you first start eating high-fat, low-carb, it's easy to fall into a pattern of not eating enough as your body sorts out your new appetite on keto. Aim for at least two solid meals per day, with a focus on whole foods, and things will level out in a matter of weeks.

5. **HIIT your way through.** Engage in periodic high-intensity interval training, which works to lower glycogen stores quickly, encouraging your body to become fat adapted faster!

6. **Supplement with carnitine.** Carnitine facilitates the adaptation process by helping the body to shuttle fatty acids into the mitochondria, which produce energy.

7. **Supplement with exogenous ketones.** Ketone supplementation can be quite a fabulous thing (as long as you are selective in the supplements you use). It can help you to begin to experience all of the benefits of nutritional ketosis before you have even become completely fat adapted, and it may boost your body's ketone levels enough to help you overcome any keto flu symptoms. My favorite brand is Perfect Keto exogenous ketones (healthfulpursuit.com/ketones). Medium-chain triglyceride (MCT) oil can also help boost ketone levels temporarily.

8. **Boost your intake of non-starchy vegetables.** The keto flu can be the result of cutting carbs too low, too fast. By increasing your non-starchy vegetable intake, you'll boost your carbs slightly—and also get more micronutrients.

There are four reasons that might explain why you aren't experiencing the keto flu.

1. You preemptively followed the advice on page 110, especially for increasing your electrolytes and water intake.

2. You're not in ketosis yet. This is okay. Remember, you don't *have* to be in ketosis to become fat adapted or lose weight.

3. Your body's hormonal and enzyme processes are naturally handling the switch with ease.

4. You were already eating a relatively low-carbohydrate diet. Perhaps you were eating a Paleo diet for some time before making the switch to keto.

Fruity Breath

When I started experimenting with ketosis, I experienced fruity breath for the first five days. (I like to call it dragon breath because it sounds a little more hard-core.) It wasn't pleasant for me, and even less so for anyone in close proximity to me (my poor husband—bless his heart).

Fruity breath is the result of acetone, a ketone body, being released in the only way it *can* be released, through your breath. Don't worry, it should vanish in a couple of days.

If you're still dealing with fruity breath two, three, or even four weeks into your keto journey, here are some strategies you can try:

- Chew on fresh mint leaves.

- Carry peppermint essential oil around with you and add a drop to your tongue when needed. (It's also great for your digestion!)

- Check your protein intake. Excess protein can make fruity breath worse. Reduce your protein intake a little to see if that helps.

- Drink plenty of water.

- Consume fermented foods such as kimchi, sauerkraut, and kombucha.

- Start taking a probiotic.

- Scrape your tongue with a tongue scraper (you can find them at any drugstore).

Brain Fog

When you've been powering your body and brain with glucose, you are familiar with the way your systems react when you're beyond hungry. You know—that fuzzy-headed, "I need something right now or else" feeling? Or when you've had a long day and your brain just seems to be giving out? This is the brain's way of shouting, "I need more glucose!" Because up until now, that's the only fuel it has ever known.

The best solution here is to simply keep eating fat! Your brain will adapt to its new fuel and your head will be clearer than ever before.

Sluggishness

I'm not one to sugarcoat things, so I'll just come out and say it: I felt like crap for the first week on the keto diet. I was very sluggish, and I had a hard time concentrating—or even moving. Once my body was drained of glucose and made the switch to using fatty acids as fuel, the sluggishness went away.

Stay mindful of your electrolyte intake (preferably in the form of whole foods, such as leafy greens, nuts and seeds, olives, seaweed, celery, and avocados) and know that this, too, shall pass.

Constipation

There are a few reasons you might get a little backed up on a ketogenic diet:

1. You're eating more whole foods than you're used to. A boost in whole foods generally equals a boost in fiber, something your body may not be used to. And an increase in fiber, at least in the beginning, can cause constipation.

2. You're eating less plant-based food than you're used to. This is actually the opposite of the scenario in #1: if your increase in whole foods has all been on the meat side, you may be getting less plant-based food, which may mean a reduction in fiber.

3. You're not drinking enough water.

If you've been fat adapted for a while and are constipated, or you have a long history of constipation, here are some tricks and tools that you can try to help you stay regular.

Supplements

- Mix 1 teaspoon of ground psyllium husk in ½ cup (120 ml) water every morning and let it sit for 1 minute before drinking. (If you're practicing intermittent fasting, this will not break your fast.)

- Take magnesium oxide daily.

- Add 3 cups (720 g) of Epsom salts to a hot bath before bed. The magnesium in the salts is absorbed through the skin, making them an excellent magnesium supplement. Allow the salts to completely dissolve, and stay in the tub for at least 30 minutes. Add hydrogen peroxide to help your body soak up the magnesium better.

- Take 1 to 5 grams of vitamin C powder per day, any time *other than* after a workout.

- Take 1 tablespoon of apple cider vinegar before each meal to aid in digestion.

- Try 1 to 2 capsules of a probiotic, taken in the evening.

- Take the recommended dosage of a good-quality digestive enzyme before or after every meal.

Lifestyle

- Begin each day with a session in front of a full-spectrum light or 20 minutes walking in the sun.

- Spend 20 to 25 minutes in a near-infrared sauna, one to three times per week.

- Break up your day with five-to-ten-minute meditation sessions on a Yantra mat. (Yantra mats can help facilitate a meditative state for those who find it difficult to get into the groove.)

- Chew your food thoroughly—at least twenty chews per (not-too-large) mouthful.

- Eat in a calm, quiet environment whenever possible.

Nausea

You might be surprised to hear that eating too much fat makes me nauseous. It's not a fine line—I have to eat a *lot* in order to trigger this. I've learned over time that maintaining a 90 percent fat macro does not sit well wih my body, and anything over 220 grams per day is definitely overkill. Now I know! So be aware that you, too, will have your limits, and be prepared to adjust your intake according to the messages your body sends.

Disaster Pants

When you first start eating more fat, your body might thank you by giving you diarrhea. Although I've never experienced this, my husband Kevin has, so I know how frustrating and unpleasant it can be. Your body reacts this way to an increase in fat intake because it isn't yet able to produce and store enough bile to break down all the fat you're eating.

To counteract this effect:

- Reduce the amount of fat you're eating by at least 10 percent.

- At the same time, boost the amount of fermented foods in your diet in the form of kombucha, water kefir, sauerkraut, kimchi, or your favorite fermented vegetable.

- Drink unpasteurized sauerkraut juice (the water from the bottom of the jar).

- Add apple cider vinegar to your drinks and salad dressings.

- Consider trying an ox bile supplement.

Stay on the lower amount of fat for seven days—or until you are feeling the effects of these changes—before gradually increasing your fat intake back up to where it was.

Feeling Like You're Undereating or Overeating

Believe it or not, once your body is fat adapted, the amount of calories you actually consume from day to day becomes largely irrelevant. I'm not sure exactly how it works, but basically, I experience a different kind of energy burn in ketosis than I did in my glucose-burning state. I have days when I eat significantly less than what I think my body might require, and days where I eat 1,000 calories more than I estimate I have burned. It makes no difference—since becoming familiar with what nutritional ketosis feel like in my body, I've been able to replicate it every day. Whether I am over or under my expected number of calories doesn't seem to matter—my weight, energy levels, and body functions stay consistent.

Being able to step away from the "I have to eat now" mentality and the many other restrictions and rules that used to inform my daily food choices has been the most freeing aspect of keto for me. As I've gone further in my keto journey, it's become easier for me to respect when I'm hungry, when I'm not, and the amount I need to eat to feel satisfied.

Eat when you feel hungry, just to the point of feeling satisfied, and get on with life. No weighing, tabulating, or calorie counting needed. If old habits are hard to break and you just can't resist counting calories, don't freak out if they're super high or super low. It's just the normal ups and downs of nutritional ketosis!

Hunger

When you first get started on keto, feelings of hunger—sometimes extreme—are to be expected, at least for the first couple of days. You can either try to ignore them or indulge them by consuming more fat. On the flip side, some people experience a drastic decrease in their hunger levels as they become fat adapted. In both cases, give your body a chance to catch up and trust that what you're eating is fueling and nourishing you. If you're not hungry when everyone else is eating, that's okay. If you're hungry in the middle of the afternoon, that's okay, too. Be open to these changes in your hunger levels, and to gradually redefining your relationship with food. Listen to your body—it knows! If you're hungry, eat. If you're not, don't.

Heartburn

Prior to going keto, I'd never experienced heartburn, ever. Three days in, when it happened to me for the first time, I thought I was dying. I was so concerned that I went straight to my doctor, who quickly diagnosed what I was experiencing and prescribed antacids—which I didn't take. Instead, I supplemented with apple cider vinegar, licorice tea, and fresh ginger steeped in hot water.

Fortunately, this unpleasantness only lasted a couple of days and never came back. If you've been experiencing heartburn during your transition and you're concerned, seek medical attention as needed to relieve your symptoms and calm your fears.

Keto Rash

Prurigo pigmentosa, aka "keto rash," is a bumpy red rash that can develop anywhere on the body. Although very rare, it sometimes occurs in response to following a strict ketogenic diet, one that's 80 percent fat or higher.

The fact that it doesn't affect everyone who's in ketosis tells me that it's not necessarily *caused* by ketosis but may be a potential by-product of ketosis when certain conditions are met.

There are a lot of theories about which conditions, when coupled with ketosis, might cause keto rash. Below, I've listed only those potential triggers that I've encountered firsthand:

- Abundance of *H. pylori* (the bacteria that cause ulcers)
- Candida die-off or aggravation
- Imbalanced gut bacteria
- Autoimmune disease
- Stress
- Toxins from fat cells
- Intermittent fasting
- An allergenic response to a new food you've been eating on keto

Some of the resources out there recommend going on a round of antibiotics to address keto rash. I feel like this advice is a bit over the top, but if it's a treatment you want to consider, chat with your doctor about it. In my experience, keto rash is most often a symptom of an underlying imbalance that antibiotics won't address. However, in the case of candida-influenced keto rash, a round of fluconazole (a prescription antifungal medication) will often do the trick.

How to Overcome Keto Rash

- Acupuncture
- Address any candida imbalances (see page 267).
- Drink bone broth daily.
- Heal any gut imbalances (see page 256).
- Relieve stress (see page 164).
- Rotate the types of fats you're eating.
- Stop intermittent fasting.
- Supplement with activated charcoal, glutathione, and/or grapefruit seed extract.

Try one solution at a time, and sit tight for one to two weeks to see if things improve before reassessing. It's best not to try more than one possible remedy at once so that you can see what's helping and what isn't. Generally, the rash will go away after a couple of weeks.

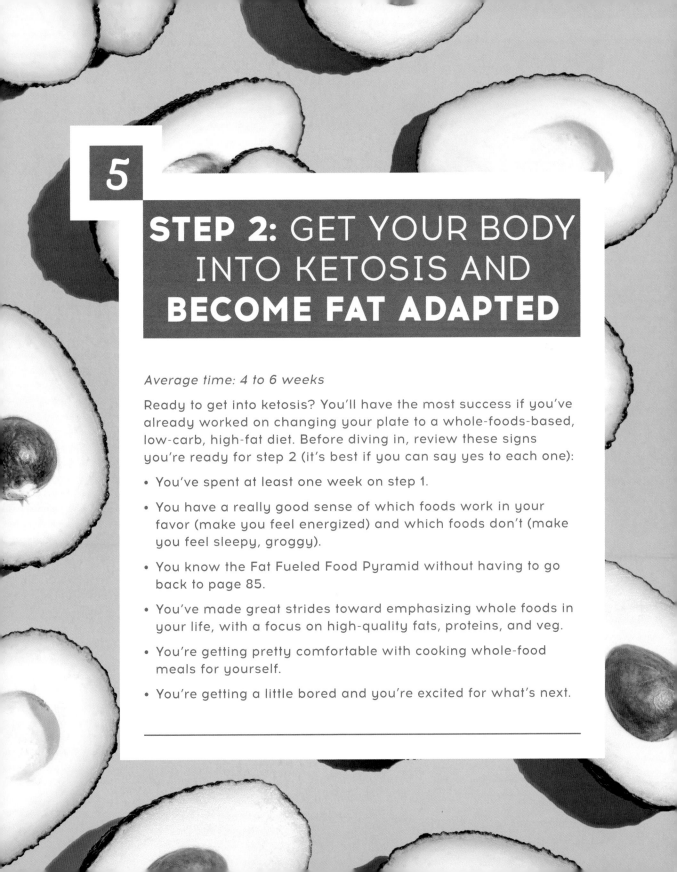

5

STEP 2: GET YOUR BODY INTO KETOSIS AND BECOME FAT ADAPTED

Average time: 4 to 6 weeks

Ready to get into ketosis? You'll have the most success if you've already worked on changing your plate to a whole-foods-based, low-carb, high-fat diet. Before diving in, review these signs you're ready for step 2 (it's best if you can say yes to each one):

- You've spent at least one week on step 1.

- You have a really good sense of which foods work in your favor (make you feel energized) and which foods don't (make you feel sleepy, groggy).

- You know the Fat Fueled Food Pyramid without having to go back to page 85.

- You've made great strides toward emphasizing whole foods in your life, with a focus on high-quality fats, proteins, and veg.

- You're getting pretty comfortable with cooking whole-food meals for yourself.

- You're getting a little bored and you're excited for what's next.

Now that you know how to feed yourself with whole foods, it's time to understand how to use those foods in different quantities to nudge your metabolism into a state of nutritional ketosis. Without knowing the food aspect (step 1), the nutritional ketosis aspect (step 2) can be pretty daunting. But you're a pro now!

You can expect to spend one to two weeks tweaking your ratio of carbs, fat, and protein until you reach ketosis. Then you can expect to spend another two to four weeks waiting for fat adaptation to take hold. It may take more time; it may take less. It depends on many factors, but this shouldn't discourage you.

No matter what meters, checklists, and your keto friends say, the simple act of eating low-carb and high-fat has amazing benefits.

Try not to get stuck on the numbers. You spent *years* burning glucose as your main fuel. It'll take you a while to switch to fat. But each healthy behavior is a step in a loving and positive direction.

Once you learn how to make small tweaks to what you're eating to get into ketosis (it's easy!), it's important to understand what other factors can speed up or slow down your progress toward fat-fueled freedom.

Let's dig in!

How to Tell Whether You're in **Ketosis**

If you followed step 1, you may very well already be in a state of ketosis. It's okay if you are, and it's okay if you're not.

Whether you're working to attain a state of ketosis or have already achieved it, there are three factors that will help you gauge how well your body is responding to your efforts:

- Ketone level: You want a moderate amount of ketones, though not at the cost of food quality, mental health, or social health.

- Blood glucose level: You want your blood glucose to be moderately low so that your insulin is low, which allows for an increase in fat-burning. While low blood glucose isn't a sure sign of being in ketosis, it'll help you understand how your body is responding to the new way of eating. For more on insulin and blood glucose levels, head back to page 41.

- Feedback from your body: The way you feel can tell you where you are in the process of becoming keto adapted.

At the outset of my keto journey, I used a blood ketone meter, blood glucose meter, and urine ketone strips to help me understand quantitatively how my body reacted to different scenarios. With the help of these tools, I discovered very quickly how my body reacted to different amounts of protein, fat, and carbs; stress; exertion; keto sweeteners; alcohol; and more. Without them, it would have been difficult for me to learn as much about my body as I did in such a short time.

You can choose to have this kind of relationship with testing, or you can avoid testing completely and just go by how you feel. What you choose is entirely up to you!

These days, just as I refrain from jumping on the scale two hundred times a day, I refrain from testing. I remind myself that, for me, frequent testing for ketones and blood sugar is not conducive to a healthy relationship with food or eating, or to my commitment to a balanced life and a peaceful mind. You may do well on testing, but once you know what nutritional ketosis feels like in your body, I really encourage you to rely on *that* as your guide. Remember, more than a new diet, this is a lifestyle change. It's supposed to free up time and make you feel good.

Ketone Level

You're officially in ketosis when your blood ketone level is over 0.5 mmol/L. So it makes a certain amount of sense—especially when you're new to keto—to test your ketones to find out exactly what your level is.

I recommend testing ketones three times per day:

- No more than two hours after you wake up, on an empty stomach and before physical exercise

- Two hours after physical exercise, to see how your body settles after physical exertion

- Two hours after your final meal, to see how it compares to your start-of-day level, which shows you what influence food had on your ketones throughout the day

There are several ways to test your ketones, including a few that don't require blood.

Blood Ketone Meter

A blood ketone meter tests for the ketone beta-hydroxybutyrate in your blood and is the most reliable and accurate approach to ketone testing. Unfortunately, it's also the most expensive. The reusable meter is about $35, and the nonreusable test strips range from $1 to $4 each. If you test twice a day, that will add about $240 a month to your monthly budget. Yikes!

When I first started eating keto, I purchased a meter and tested once a day at various times. I recorded my results and why I thought my ketone level had increased or decreased. I did this for thirty days, long enough to give me a good idea of the foods and activities that likely affected my ketone level. I'd advise you to do the same, as this information can be invaluable to your progress!

TRUTH BOMB

Just because you're not generating a lot of ketones doesn't mean you're not cashing in on the benefits of ketosis. A lot of us get caught up in the numbers when it's not necessary. If you're feeling good and getting the results you want, who cares?

These days, I test once a week or even less. Frequent testing in the beginning gave me a solid understanding of what helped raise my ketones and what did the opposite. Now that I know how my body feels and performs in ketosis, it's pointless for me to keep testing—I just know what nutritional ketosis feels like. When I'm on the mark, I can tell. When I don't feel it, I know where I fumbled and what I need to do to get back on track. Testing my blood and tracking my results when I first started out helped me immensely in developing this awareness.

WHAT LEVEL OF KETOSIS IS OPTIMAL?

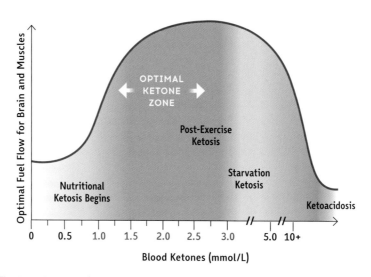

Source: *The Art and Science of Low Carbohydrate Performance* by Jeff S. Volek and Stephen D. Phinney

Breath Ketone Meter

A breath ketone meter is a fabulous tool for testing your ketones. There are various forms of breath monitors—some plug into your computer to display the results, others have apps, and some just display your ketone reading with a pattern of flashes and colors of light. But the premise is the same for all of them: blow into the device, and it tells you the concentration of ketones in your breath.

The key to making this a more accurate test is ensuring that you blow into the unit the same way every time. A change in the strength, length, or intensity of the blow can throw off the results. When done properly, its accuracy is comparable to blood ketone meters.

If you're deciding between a breath ketone meter and urine ketone strips, breath testing will give you far more accurate results!

Urine Ketone Strips

These strips are often inaccurate and may not work for the vast majority of people. Their major downfall is that they only test for *excess* ketone bodies, which are excreted through the urine. They tell you nothing about the big picture of your ketone generation.

Once you're keto adapted, your body will be using most of the ketones produced, not excreting them in the urine. In this situation, the urine ketone strip test could display high ketones one day and no ketones the next. You might be wondering what you did wrong when, in actuality, this drastic change could be telling you that you're becoming *more* fat adapted as your body learns how to use the ketones instead of dumping them. (If I were to test my urine for ketones right now, after eating this way for three years, the test would come back with small traces of ketones, but my blood would show a ketone level around 2.3 to 2.8 mmol/L.)

However, if you're just starting the ketogenic diet and spending upwards of $300 on blood ketone testing for the first month is out of the question (I wouldn't blame you!), urine ketone testing is a reasonable alternative that can at least give you some idea of where you're at for the first few weeks. But don't freak out when you wake up one day and your test says you're no longer in ketosis! This will happen eventually, and when it does, you'll have to decide whether you want to begin to fly by your instincts (you should have a good idea of what ketosis feels like by that point) or switch to another testing method to keep yourself motivated and on track.

Blood Glucose Level

A reduction in blood glucose is the body's natural reaction to a low-carbohydrate eating style and is the key to encouraging fat-burning. As you begin eating keto, you may notice that your blood glucose drops substantially at first before increasing slightly or leveling off after a couple of weeks. This is a normal reaction to eating less carbohydrate.

When you're in ketosis, the ideal blood glucose concentration is 3.0 to 3.5 mmol/L (55 to 65 md/dL), which is about half the amount that's conventionally considered "good" or "normal." Remember, that guideline is based on fueling your body on glucose—you won't have levels that high when you're in nutritional ketosis.

We test glucose levels through the blood—a little poke, a drop of blood, and off you go. It can seem intimidating, but it's actually easy. I remember the first time I tested my blood for glucose, I was so nervous that I wasted about ten strips before I got it right! Thankfully, glucose test strips are far less expensive than ketone test strips.

I recommend testing blood glucose three times per day:

- Two hours after you get up, on an empty stomach and before physical exercise, to see what your fasting glucose is

- Two hours after physical exercise, to see how your body settles after physical exertion

- Two hours after your final meal, to see how it compares to your fasting glucose. When your last number of the day matches or is lower than your first number of the day, you'll know that the food, activities, and lifestyle factors you chose that day helped to maintain steady blood glucose, or lowered it even further.

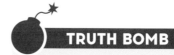

TRUTH BOMB

I use the side of my palm, the meaty place, to draw blood. It's a lot less painful than the finger and yields a consistent blood sample (although it's a personal choice for everyone!).

- Urine ketone test strips are cheap but not very accurate over the long term.

- Blood ketone meters are the most accurate way of determining your ketone level and have a reasonable introductory cost, but they can cost a lot if you're testing frequently.

- Breath ketone testing is much more accurate than urine test strips, and while it's not as accurate as a blood meter, it's a very close second.

- Test your ketones in the evening if you want to know how the day's diet and activity have affected your level.

- Test your ketones in the morning if you want to see how your body is responding to keto overall.

- Ketone production is often increased by dehydration and decreased by stress.

- Using any testing method, it can take upwards of two weeks after you start eating a ketogenic diet to register any ketones.

- While there is a relationship between blood sugar and ketone levels—as blood sugar goes down, ketone levels should go up—slightly elevated blood sugar will not prevent ketones from registering in your blood.

- You may notice that your blood sugar increases slightly when you start eating keto. If you're "doing everything right," this could be a natural response to a low-carbohydrate diet known as physiological insulin resistance, in which your body leaves additional glucose in the bloodstream for the organs that require it instead of shuttling the fuel to storage. Your level should decrease over time; this is not cause for alarm.

- After a carb-up (see page 186), if you've eaten just enough carbs for your body to burn carbs throughout the night, you should be back in ketosis by the next morning. When you test in the evening, your ketone level should be generally the same as in the morning.

- When you're testing, take note of which foods boost your ketones and which lower them.

- For ketones and glucose alike, how you test, what you use, and the approach you take is entirely up to you!

Feedback from Your Body

You could spend your money on testing, or you could gauge where you're at by running through the list below. If you are experiencing three or more of these changes, it's likely that your body is preparing for the metabolic switch!

 You're starting to be able to skip some meals without getting angry.

 There are days when it's easy to go 3, 4, or 5 hours without a snack.

 Most of the time, you're not ravenous or craving carbs 2 to 3 hours after dinner.

 You've been opting for high-fat foods instead of high-carb foods.

 You haven't been fighting the midafternoon slump as much.

 Your clothes are a touch looser than before.

 Your belly bloat as gone down.

 It's consistently easier to think, remember things, and stay on top of your game all day long.

 Your mood is a bit better than usual.

If you're having trouble getting into ketosis, it could be for one of these three reasons.

You're training too hard: High-intensity interval training (HIIT) and a ketogenic diet may not always mix well. If you're doing high-intensity workouts three or more days a week, it can definitely mess up your hormones. If this is the case for you, consider what your goals are. If you want to gain muscle mass or improve your athletic performance, high-intensity training is what you need to do. If you'd like to decrease inflammation in your body, lose weight, live longer, and prevent disease, then a ketogenic diet is the way to go. It can be damaging to try to maintain both of these, so it's important to really consider which is right for you. When you first start eating a keto diet, it can take a while for your body to adjust. During this period, take it easy on the exercise, and slowly ramp up as you feel more comfortable doing so.

You're restricting calories too much: If your body simply isn't getting enough calories, it can mess up your hormones. On a keto diet, people often don't feel as hungry as they used to and don't experience cravings, so they end up eating fewer calories overall. Truthfully, it can be tough to make sure you're eating enough on a keto diet, so it's important to track how many calories you're consuming. You might be surprised to see that you're undereating. Calculate how many calories you should be consuming every day (see page 127 for help with those calculations), and as much as you may be tempted, don't eat less than that. Eating less than your body needs can put your body into starvation mode and will ultimately mess with your hormones.

You had hormone problems to begin with: If you've always had irregular periods or unexplained chronic headaches or backaches, you may have had a hormonal imbalance to begin with. This needs to be diagnosed and treated by a health-care professional.

Introduction to **Macros**

Macro is short for *macronutrient*. Macronutrients are protein, fats, and carbohydrates, and the correct balance of these is all-important when you're trying to get into (and maintain) nutritional ketosis. Don't stress, though—it's a lot simpler than it sounds. And once you know what your ideal macro ratio is, maintaining a state of ketosis becomes easy!

For the most part, nutritional ketosis is best achieved when protein intake is moderate, carbohydrate intake is relatively low, and fat intake is high—much higher than you've likely ever had it before. (*Ever!*)

The way I see it, there are two ways of looking at macronutrient consumption:

- **Percentage intake.** This looks at the percent of total daily calories that comes from each macronutrient. You would say, for instance, "My macronutrient consumption today was 12 percent carbs, 73 percent fat, and 15 percent protein." This approach is great when you're just getting started and you're trying to understand how adjusting a macro changes the amount of food you eat while it all still adds up to 100 percent.

- **Gram intake.** This looks at the actual amount of each macro you consume each day. You would say, for instance, "My macronutrient consumption was 150 grams of fat, 55 grams of carbs, and 70 grams of protein." This approach is best once you already know the exact balance of macros you do best with. Then it's just a matter of hitting the same amount of each macro in grams every day.

You're conveying the same information with either approach—just from different viewpoints.

The Macros That Fit Most People

If you like the idea of eating with macro percentages in mind, a great ratio to shoot for is 70% fat, 20% protein, and 10% carbohydrate. Another good option is 75% fat, 20% protein, and 5% carbohydrate.

Your Relationship to Tracking

In the coming pages, I'll share some suggestions for how much fat, carbs, and protein to aim for each day. These suggestions are great starting points, but remember: my body is different from your body. What you experience will quite likely be different from what I did. These calculations are meant as a resource to set the stage for you and give you the tools you need to figure out what works for you.

Although I've maintained a ketogenic state for years now, I abandoned all forms of counting or tracking percentages after the first six months. Once I was in nutritional ketosis, I started to sense that my body knew where it wanted to go. Weight loss came easily—I ate when I was hungry, I stopped when I was full, and my body naturally did the rest. Calories held minimal significance for me, and still do. Some days I eat lots; other days I do not.

If this kind of body awareness does not come easily to you, yet tracking and counting is overwhelming or triggers you, please do not feel that you have to get super technical—or even count anything at all.

Calculating Your Macros

If the idea of counting or tracking resonates with you, the guidelines in the following pages will help you make sense of it all, from how to calculate your caloric requirements (and how to adjust them if you want to lose or gain weight) to how to determine how much protein you need.

All of the following calculations will give you kick-off points to get you started, but they shouldn't be set in stone. No calculator truly knows what's best for your body. But it's never a bad thing to have numbers to shoot for until you can adjust things as necessary!

Step 1: Calculate Your Calorie Requirements

In order to figure out your target macros, you need to determine how many calories you need each day. These formulas are suitable whether you're already in ketosis or just getting started, but they do assume that you are active for at least thirty minutes three to five times a week.

Women: Current weight in pounds x 15 = Daily Caloric Needs (DCN)

Men: Current weight in pounds x 16 = Daily Caloric Needs (DCN)

Example: A woman who weighs 150 lbs (68 kg) needs 2,250 calories a day (150 x 15).

Once you know your Daily Caloric Needs (DCN), you can calculate the calories you need if you're looking to gain or lose weight with these formulas:

To Lose Weight: DCN – (DCN x 20%) = Weight-Loss DCN

To Gain Weight: DCN + (DCN x 20%) = Weight-Gain DCN

Per our example above, if that same woman with a DCN of 2,250 wanted to lose weight, she would calculate it as:

2,250 x 20% = 450
2,250 – 450 = 1,800

So her weight-loss DCN works out to 1,800: 450 calories less than her base DCN.

If she wanted to gain weight, it would look like this:

2,250 x 20% = 450
2,250 + 450 = 2,700

Her weight-gain DCN would be 2,700: 450 calories more than her base DCN.

To determine your macro requirements, you will need to use your base, weight-loss, or weight-gain DCN in the macro calculations that follow.

Step 2: Calculate Your Protein Goal

Factors such as how your body processes protein, your physical activity, and your basal metabolic rate (the rate at which your metabolism uses fuel just for ordinary bodily functions) all play a role in determining how much protein is right for your body. The practice of moderating protein intake is what differentiates keto from the popular Atkins diet, which has a high-fat, high-protein approach.

A good way to determine how much protein your body needs is to begin with **1.25 grams of protein for every 2.25 pounds (1 kilogram)** that you weigh. If you find that this amount of protein is too much for you—say, you're vegan and eating that much protein is out of the question, or you've tried that amount for a couple of days and you feel sick or off—cut back to **1 gram of protein per 2.25 pounds (1 kilogram)** of body weight.

Based on the two calculations above, the table on the facing page shows roughly how much protein to eat (in grams) based on your body weight—your Total Protein Grams (TPG).

Body Weight (lbs)	Body Weight (kg)	PROTEIN INTAKE (G)	
		1.25 g protein per 2.25 lbs (1 kg) body weight	1 g protein per 2.25 lbs (1 kg) body weight
100	45	57	45
110	50	62	50
120	54	68	54
130	59	74	59
140	64	79	64
150	68	85	68
160	73	91	73
170	77	96	77
180	82	102	82
190	86	108	86
200	91	113	91
210	95	119	95
220	100	125	100
230	104	130	104
240	109	136	109
250	113	142	113
260	118	147	118
270	122	153	122
280	127	159	127
290	132	164	132
300	136	170	136
310	141	176	141
320	145	181	145
330	150	187	150
340	154	193	154
350	159	198	159
360	163	204	163
370	168	210	168
380	172	215	172
390	177	221	177
400	181	227	181

Once you've determined your TPG, you can easily calculate the number of calories you'll be getting from protein:

TPG x 4 calories per gram of protein = Total Protein Calories (TPC)

How can you determine what amount works best for you? If you enjoy measuring, you can track the effect of varying amounts of protein on your ketone levels. At the risk of sounding like a broken record, though, a cheaper and more important way to tell is to just see how you feel. Try 15 percent for week 1 and see how you feel. Bump it up to 20 percent for week 2, and so on. It's a good idea to keep detailed notes about your observations with each increase.

Everyone's body is different, and it might be hard to tell how much protein your body wants or is able to handle, so here are a few signs to look for to determine whether you are eating too much or too little protein.

! SIGNS YOU NEED MORE PROTEIN

Your blood test results show low albumin.

You are preparing for or recovering from surgery.

You feel like you are aging faster than you should be.

You have joint pain.

You feel fatigued.

Wounds heal slowly. (This can also be caused by excess sugar or carbs, however.)

You feel hungry all the time and can't seem to stop overeating.

You're moody.

You're having trouble losing weight.

Your skin, hair, or nails are weak or fragile.

Your hormones are dysregulated.

Your digestion is slow.

Your metabolism is slow.

You're having trouble building muscle mass.

It's difficult to concentrate.

Your blood sugar fluctuates. 8.5

! SIGNS YOU'RE EATING TOO MUCH PROTEIN

You feel dehydrated all the time despite drinking plenty of water.

You're having trouble getting into ketosis.

(In this case, most likely you're not getting enough fat—you need to rebalance your amounts of both fat and protein.)

You're unable to stay in ketosis or lose weight despite adhering to the diet. In fact, you might be gaining weight.

You have signs of poor kidney function, which could include sleep problems, changes in how much you urinate, decreased mental sharpness, muscle twitches, muscle cramps, swelling of your feet and ankles, or chronically low GFR (glomerular filtration rate) or elevated creatinine on blood tests.

You have osteopenia (weakened bones) or osteoporosis. While excess protein is only one factor, it can create a situation where calcium is pulled from bones to help correct the acid-alkaline balance in the body.

Here are a few ways you can boost your protein intake on the ketogenic diet.

Have some protein at breakfast, lunch, and dinner

I've found that the simplest, most effective strategy is to have a relatively good amount of protein in the morning (think about 40 percent of your daily goal), followed by a smaller amount in the afternoon (about 20 percent of your daily goal), and then another amount similar to your breakfast intake at dinnertime. If you feel like you need more protein, eat more at lunch.

Add protein if you're eating twice a day

If you're eating twice a day, at both meals you should aim for roughly the same amount of protein—a portion just a bit larger than the size of your palm.

Fire up your intake with a boosted fatty coffee

You could have a fatty coffee with just fats, or you could boost your fatty coffee with protein. Add collagen peptides, hulled hemp seeds, protein powder, or your favorite nut or seed butter to your fatty coffee to turn it into a Rocket Fuel Latte—get the full recipe on page 144. This little change will add 10 grams of protein to your day!

Take it with your tea

If you enjoy tea or iced tea throughout your day, just add 1 to 2 scoops of collagen peptides. Collagen is packed with a surprising amount of protein, so on days when you've added a couple of scoops of collagen to your tea, it'll be easier for you to hit your protein macro.

Step 3: Calculate Your Carbohydrate Goal

To know your goal for daily carb consumption, you need to figure out how many grams of carbohydrates (Total Grams Carbohydrate, or TGC) your body needs, likes, and wants. This can vary a great deal from person to person, but as a rule of thumb, a reasonable range is somewhere between 20 and 80 TGC per day.

Unfortunately, I can't tell you with full certainty what amount is best for you. A good place to start if you're unsure is 20 TGC per day. You can work your way up or down from there as needed. Calories are calculated based on your total carbohydrate intake, so if you choose to track using net carbohydrates (see page 133), you can calculate your fiber goal afterward.

Adjusting Your Total Carbohydrate Goal

There are certain circumstances in which the most important aspect of your ketogenic diet is your carbohydrate intake, and how much fiber you're eating doesn't matter as much. If you're dealing with the following situations, try to stick to the recommended amount of total carbs:

- Metabolic damage, 20 TGC

- Cancer, 20 TGC

- Neurological imbalances, 20 TGC

- Unstable blood sugar, 30 TGC

For advice on eating right for the stage of life you're in, head to step 3 (page 173).

Once you've identified your body's preferred amount of carbs, you can determine your target number of calories from carbohydrates:

TGC x 4 calories per gram = Total Carbohydrate Calories (TCC)

Step 4: Calculate Your Fat Goal

For weight maintenance, you'll need to find the balance between the amount of dietary fat your body needs for energy and the amount of dietary fat you need to fuel ketone development. For weight loss, you'll need to take in the right quantity of dietary fat so that both body fat *and* dietary fat are burned for energy.

Once you know your target daily calories, calories from protein, and calories from carbohydrate, it's a simple matter of subtraction to figure out your target amount of fat—it's whatever number of calories remain after you account for protein and carbs:

DCN or weight loss/gain DCN – TPC – TCC = Total Fat Calories (TFC)

Once you've determined your target number of calories from fat, you can determine how many grams that works out to by using this calculation:

TFC / 9 calories per gram = Total Fat Grams (TFG)

Net or Total Carbs?

There are two different ways to look at carbohydrate intake. Neither is right or wrong, although each has its own benefits and drawbacks, and you may find that some days you prefer to use one method and some days you prefer to use the other. The approach you end up subscribing to is ultimately up to you.

Option 1: Total Carbohydrates. The sum of all the carbohydrates consumed throughout the day. You may find that this option helps you to maintain better control over your ketone production and blood sugar levels.

Option 2: Net Carbohydrates. The amount of carbohydrates consumed after fiber has been subtracted from total carbohydrates. You may find that this option allows you to eat more non-starchy vegetables and feel full longer. If you're not insulin resistant and don't have huge amounts of metabolic healing to do, you should be able to count net carbohydrates with no negative effect to your overall results.

Example: Leanne eats 50 grams of total carbohydrates in a day, and 20 grams of that amount is fiber. Therefore, Leanne consumes 30 grams of **net carbohydrates** (50 grams − 20 grams = 30 grams).

I find that the best number to select as your fiber intake per day is 30 grams, which is relatively easy to hit while still giving you the benefits of fiber.

Remember, fiber counts when it comes to calories, so whether you usually look at net or total carbs, make sure you use total carbs in your macro calculations.

You're likely wondering, "How the heck am I supposed to eat all that fat?!" (Don't worry—I remember asking the exact same thing.) Here are some tips!

- Eat the whole egg.
- Go for chicken thighs with skin.
- Choose salmon instead of white fish.
- Opt for regular ground beef instead of extra lean.
- Blend tea or coffee with a tablespoon of coconut oil, coconut milk, and/or MCT oil.
- Slather steamed vegetables in coconut oil.
- Double up on the fat in salad dressing! Whatever the recipe calls for, just double it.
- Add your favorite dried herbs and spices, like paprika, basil, oregano, or dried French onion soup mix to homemade mayonnaise and use it as a savory dip or spread with your meals.
- Whip up a batch of fat bombs as an afternoon snack. (If you need help with recipe ideas, go to healthfulpursuit.com/recipes.)
- Cook everything in more fat! Add coconut oil, avocado oil, ghee, tallow, or lard to the pan before preparing any recipe.

Step 5: Calculate Your Macro Percentages

That was a lot of "L, M, N, O, P," right? Okay, let's break it down:

DCN (Daily Caloric Needs) ....The amount of calories you need per day

TPG (Total Protein Grams).....................The amount of protein you need per day, in grams

TPC (Total Protein Calories) ....The amount of protein you need per day, in calories

TCG (Total Carbohydrate Grams) ....The amount of carbohydrate you consume per day, in grams

TCC (Total Carbohydrate Calories).......The amount of carbohydrate you consume per day, in calories

TFG (Total Fat Grams)...........................The amount of fat you consume per day, in grams

TFC (Total Fat Calories)........................The amount of fat you consume per day, in calories

Using these numbers, you can determine the percentage of fat, protein, and carbs in your diet:

(TPC/DCN or weight loss/gain DCN) x 100 = Protein percentage
(TCC/DCN or weight loss/gain DCN) x 100 = Carbohydrate percentage
(TFC/DCN or weight loss/gain DCN) x 100 = Fat percentage

And just one final bit of math: when you add up these three percentages, you should get 100. If you don't, something's gone awry.

Case Study: Bringing It All Together

Let's go through an example with all of the calculations so you can really wrap your head around it all.

Susan is 160 pounds and wants to lose 10 pounds. She's been struggling with unstable blood sugar and can't seem to lose weight.

Step 1: Calorie Goal
Determine DCN: 160 x 15 = 2,400
Determine Weight-Loss DCN: 2,400 – (2,400 x 20%) = 1,920

Step 2: Protein Intake
Determine TPG: 91 grams (1.25 grams of protein per 2.25 lbs/1 kg body weight)
Determine TPC: 91 x 4 = 364

Step 3: Carbohydrate Intake
Determine TCG: 30 (because she has unstable blood sugar; see box on page 132)
Determine TCC: 30 x 4 = 120

Step 4: Fat Intake
Determine TFC: 1,920 – 364 – 120 = 1,436
Determine TFG: 1,436 / 9 = 160

Step 5: Macro Percentages
(364/1,920) x 100 = 19% protein
(120/1,920) x 100 = 6% carbs
(1,436/1,920) x 100 = 75% fat

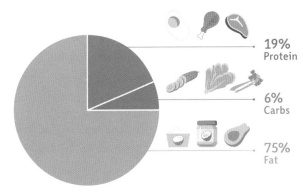

19%
Protein

6%
Carbs

75%
Fat

Tracking Your Macros

Now that you know how much carb, protein, and fat you're aiming for, you're probably wondering how to convert that 15 grams of carbs, 50 grams of protein, or 120 grams of fat into actual food.

The easiest way is to track everything you eat with an app such as MyFitnessPal. But if you want to get a sense of intake without an app—and given all the data entry involved, I don't blame you!—keep reading.

Macro Intakes: Grams to Actual Food

The table on the facing page shows how your macro goals in grams translate to actual quantities of broccoli (for carbs), coconut oil (for fat), and skinless chicken thighs (for protein).

For example, if you want to eat 1,300 calories per day with 5 percent carbs, 20 percent protein, and 75 percent fat, that would translate to:

- 16 grams of carbs, which is equal to approximately 2.7 cups of chopped broccoli

- 65 grams of protein, which is equal to approximately 2.3 chicken thighs

- 108 grams of fat, which is equal to approximately 7.7 tablespoons of coconut oil

Of course I'm not suggesting that you live on broccoli, chicken thighs, and coconut oil! But this example should give you a rough idea of the volume of food to consume on a daily basis.

Yes, there are holes in this approach. The protein from the broccoli and the fat from the chicken thighs are not captured in the table. But I hope this gives you a glimpse of how your macro intake connects with actual food intake.

(In case you're wondering, 1 cup chopped broccoli is 91 grams and an average chicken thigh weighs 116 grams.)

Mindfulness Instead of Tracking

In my years on keto, I've come to see that we really don't need to count our macros in order to reach success. In fact, I have seen time and time again that counting, tracking, and weighing your food can in fact be highly detrimental to your health goals.

Think back to step 1, where you figured out what to eat and how to make it. If you followed this step fully and completely, there wasn't a lot of tracking, just a general sense of eating less carb and more fat, according to the Fat Fueled Food Pyramid. You set the intention to feel good and focus on quality food. Setting this intention is often enough for people—really. Yes, you can learn more and adjust things here and there, but when it comes right down to it, tracking isn't for everybody.

Your body knows what it needs, how much it needs, and what it doesn't need. When I was tracking my macros, I'd often get to the end of the day and still have

		1300		1500		1700		1900		2100		2300		2500	
CARBS	5%	16g	2.7	19g	3.2	21g	3.5	24g	4.0	26g	4.3	29g	4.8	31g	5.2
	10%	33g	5.5	38g	6.3	43g	7.2	48g	8.0	53g	8.8	58g	9.7	63g	10.5
	15%	49g	8.2	56g	9.3	64g	10.7	71g	11.8	79g	13.2	86g	14.3	94g	15.7
	20%	65g	10.8	75g	12.5	85g	14.2	95g	15.8	105g	17.5	115g	19.2	125g	20.8
PROTEIN	10%	33g	1.2	38g	1.4	43g	1.5	48g	1.7	53g	1.9	58g	2.1	63g	2.3
	15%	49g	1.8	56g	2.0	64g	2.3	71g	2.5	79g	2.8	86g	3.1	94g	3.4
	20%	65g	2.3	75g	2.7	85g	3.0	95g	3.4	105g	3.8	115g	4.1	125g	4.5
	25%	81g	2.9	94g	3.4	106g	3.8	119g	4.3	131g	4.7	144g	5.1	156g	5.6
	30%	98g	3.5	113g	4.0	128g	4.6	143g	5.1	158g	5.6	173g	6.2	188g	6.7
	35%	114g	4.1	131g	4.7	149g	5.3	166g	5.9	184g	6.6	201g	7.2	219g	7.8
FAT	55%	79g	5.6	92g	6.6	104g	7.4	116g	8.3	128g	9.1	141g	10.1	153g	10.9
	60%	87g	6.2	100g	7.1	113g	8.1	127g	9.1	140g	10	153g	10.9	167g	11.9
	65%	94g	6.7	108g	7.7	123g	8.8	137g	9.8	152g	10.9	166g	11.9	181g	12.9
	70%	101g	7.2	117g	8.4	132g	9.4	148g	10.6	163g	11.6	179g	12.8	191g	13.9
	75%	108g	7.7	125g	8.9	142g	10.1	158g	11.3	175g	12.5	192g	13.7	208g	14.9
	80%	116g	8.3	133g	9.5	151g	10.8	169g	12.1	187g	13.4	204g	14.6	222g	15.9
	85%	123g	8.8	142g	10.1	161g	11.5	179g	12.6	198g	14.1	217g	15.5	236g	16.9

cups of chopped broccoli   *boneless, skinless chicken thighs*   *tablespoons of coconut oil*

200 calories left to go, so I'd eat just because I felt I could, or out of fear of being hungry the next day if I didn't get the recommended amount of calories in when I had them available. On the opposite side of things, there are days when you just need more food, period, in which case not nourishing yourself can cause more harm than good.

Please don't feel like you need to count every macro that enters your body in order to succeed. In fact, more often than not, people do better on keto when they're *not* counting their macros! If you're really nervous about the idea of not tracking at all but you know it'd be best for your mental well-being, the following step-by-step plan may help you hit your goals without the need to incessantly track every morsel. (I know, sounds intriguing, right?)

Waiting for the Magic to Happen

From the time you realize you're in a solid state of ketosis, it can take another 2 to 4 weeks to become fully fat adapted, sometimes longer. It takes time for your body to get here, and that's okay! You're not missing out on anything by working toward becoming fat adapted.

1. Calculate your target macros, as described on pages 127 to 135.

2. If you're unfamiliar with what constitutes a carbohydrate, fat, or protein, get familiar with this by tracking your last meal of the day *only*. This will help you get a sense of what foods contribute to which macros and how it all adds up without getting too deep into counting and tracking.

3. Now that you have a good sense of the portions that contribute to you hitting your macro goals, stop tracking that last meal of the day.

4. Pick one meal a week to track so you can check in with your macros and portion sizes to see if anything needs adjusting.

Bringing **Fasting** into It

The word *fast* used to make me cringe because, as a sugar-burner, going long periods of time without food was absolute torture. If you feel the same, you're in luck! As a fat-burner, fasting takes on a whole new meaning. It's easy, it's beneficial, and you actually feel good doing it. If you're still not convinced, think of intermittent fasting (IF) as intermittent eating instead. (Sounds much more bearable, doesn't it?)

During step 2, as your body transitions to being fat adapted, you may notice that your hunger levels change. All of a sudden you may not be interested in having breakfast, or perhaps you've skipped a dinner here or there, or lunch just doesn't have the same magic it once did. A lot of us don't know how to handle this energy. After all, as women we're told to fight against our appetite, that it is a force to be reckoned with—but after a couple of weeks eating lower-carb, it dissipates without a fight.

Now, this may not be your experience. You may be hungrier than ever. This is normal, too. If you're hungrier, eat more fat. Continue to eat fat until you feel satiated, and repeat. Your hunger will dissipate as you get nearer to fat adaptation. Play around with different fat types, switching from saturated to monounsaturated and back again. See what feels right and what satiates best, and know that this, too, shall pass.

If you're not hungry, you may be freaking out a little, as I did. Don't worry! It's a natural and expected part of becoming fat adapted. I welcome you to the world of intermittent fasting for women.

How Fasting Works

When we're in a state of glucose-burning, the main reason we're hungry all the time is that our blood sugar is constantly moving up and down. When we eat, our blood sugar rises, and about two or three hours later it drops, we get hungry, and we have to eat to boost our blood sugar again.

In contrast, being in a state of nutritional ketosis naturally regulates hunger: because we can easily get fuel from body fat, not just food, our blood sugar stays steady, keeping hunger at bay and making intermittent fasting so much easier.

Fasting is good for you for a lot of reasons, but there are two primary benefits. First, it effectively boosts ketone levels because you're relying so heavily on stored fat for fuel—as more fat is burned, more ketone bodies are created. The more ketones that are created, the more concentrated they become in our blood, the higher our ketone level, and the more balanced our blood sugar will be over time. (And remember, most of us have more fat than we know what to do with for the body to use!)

Second, intermittent fasting increases autophagy, the normal physiological process of cleaning out damaged cells, toxins, and proteins to regenerate newer, healthier cells. Think of it as your body's process of "self-eating" (the literal translation of the word "autophagy"), a detox or cleanse that your body undergoes to clean out damaged cells and generate new ones.

High autophagy rates are seen in young organisms and slowly drop as the organism ages, which allows cellular damage to accumulate. Aging just is the accumulation of damage. As we age, we can no longer repair damage as readily or recycle damaged cell components. Because autophagy does both, its benefits range from cancer prevention and reduced markers of aging to the maintenance of lean muscle mass and improved cardiovascular health—all made possible because old, less efficient cells are replaced by new, optimally functioning cells.

Think of your body as a dream craft room (I'm super into crafting). After making a beautiful birthday photo album for your niece, you clean up your craft table, seal the washi tape, recycle the paper pieces, sort your stamps, and wipe down the table. You now have a perfectly clean crafting room! This is autophagy doing its job for your body, cleaning up all the scraps and getting everything back in order.

Now, think of the same scenario, but this time you ask your less detail-oriented partner to clean up your craft room. They leave the scraps on the table and stack the stamps up randomly on the side; some recyclables land in the bin, the others end up on the floor. Maybe the damage isn't too bad after that one photo album, but the more and more projects you complete, the more waste starts to build up

---

Amp Up Autophagy!

- Pair your ketogenic diet with intermittent fasting.
- Practice high-intensity interval training.
- Drink Earl Grey tea in the morning (its bergamot oil increases autophagy).
- When you fast, stick to water and tea only.
- Work out in a fasted state.
- Get a restorative sleep.
- Do a protein fast (more on page 183).
- Vary your daily calories—eat less on some days, more on others.

and the more unorganized everything becomes. This is what happens when autophagy is not able to do its job well.

When autophagy is activated, the aging process is slowed down, neurodegenerative diseases are prevented or delayed, inflammation is reduced because the dead stuff that's causing issues is eliminated, and immunity is strengthened.

By fasting intermittently, varying calorie input, eating a ketogenic diet, and exercising, you can reset autophagy rates to those of a younger person.

Fasting is probably the best way to increase autophagy. But fasting can be a challenge when you're not on a ketogenic diet. Autophagy is suppressed in the presence of insulin resistance and hyperinsulinemia (high insulin levels). So if you're fasting on a sugar-burner's diet while experiencing these imbalances, it can make increasing autophagy much more challenging.

Taking a Healthful Approach to Fasting

There's a lot of misinformation out there about fasting, just about as much as there is about keto for women! So before we get into the details of fasting, how to do it, and how often, it's important that I set the tone on how to do fasting safely.

Fasting can mean different things to different people. Fasting can mean not eating food for a period of time, only drinking water for a period of time, only drinking diet sodas for a period of time, only drinking broth, only drinking coffee, just focusing on tea... You get the idea.

Fasting triggers a natural caloric deficiency, so you should not count calories *and* fast as a way to lose weight. No matter how much weight you have to lose or how much progress you think you have to make, forcefully limiting your calorie intake on top of forcefully fasting every day will not help you. In fact, it can be very dangerous. Fasting encourages your body to eat less, naturally. When you forcefully restrict calories on top of this natural reduction, you are going against what your body needs. You will likely find it challenging to overcome weight plateaus, and you could even harm your hormones and overall health in the long term.

You do not need to fast every day to realize the benefits. Many people don't need to fast every day to realize the benefits of fasting. Instead of planning to fast every day, just set the intention of not eating, but be open to eating if you feel you need to. If you wake up hungry, eat. If you don't, fast!

Women generally require more eating periods than men and therefore respond better to shorter periods of fasting. We need different fasting strategies depending on what our hormones are doing as a whole. If your sex hormones are running high (think: PCOS), you may find you're able to fast longer than a girlfriend whose sex hormones are low (think: amenorrhea).

Fasting should not be a painful experience. I never, ever force myself to fast. I do not starve myself or go for hours feeling hungry and struggling to get by. Fasting is not about that. It should come naturally, with grace and ease, as a natural progression and part of ketosis. Play around, have fun, and know that there are multiple ways to approach this. There is no right or wrong.

Fatty coffees and bone broth can extend your fast. There are two core goals in fasting: increased autophagy, which reduces overall inflammation, and stable blood sugar. Increased autophagy is best achieved by fasting with only water, but if your primary goal is stable blood sugar, you can include things like fatty coffees (just what it sounds like: coffee with added fat), small fat bombs (treats that are super high in fat), and bone broth—all of which can help you extend the fast. Neither option is better than the other; it just depends on your goal. And you don't even need to decide on one goal over the other! You can practice water-only fasting sometimes and fatty coffee / bone broth fasting other times. (There's much more about using fatty coffees during your fast on page 143.)

Okay, now that we've gotten that out of the way, let's look at how you can use intermittent fasting to balance your keto body.

Why I Love Intermittent Fasting

Supported by nutritional ketosis and IF, I've been freed to:

- Stop obsessing about food every waking moment
- Go for a day trip without stressing about packing snacks with me
- Step away from a strict and restrictive eating schedule
- Go without breakfast (and even lunch!) without any threat of violence to myself or others
- Work out in a fasted state with loads of energy
- Effortlessly maintain a calorie deficiency (with the awareness that a slight variance in calories is the key to balanced health)
- Reduce evening food cravings. (I would say they've been eliminated entirely, but I do get the odd craving now and again during times of stress, or when I let my emotions get the better of me.)

SIGNS THAT INTERMITTENT FASTING ISN'T RIGHT FOR YOU

Particularly if you're a woman, intermittent fasting may not be right for you—like, at all. Here are the signs to watch for.

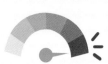 During fasting, do you experience a "high" or an energetic feeling of "I can accomplish anything, I can do everything, I'm invincible"? It could be your adrenals running on overdrive or cortisol pumping through your body, causing a hot mess behind the scenes.

 You have an eating disorder, a history of disordered eating, or get crazy around food (I mean that in the most loving, concerned, caring way possible).

You're pregnant.

You've lost your appetite.

You're breastfeeding.

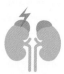
You have adrenal dysfunction.

You tend to feel overwhelmed easily and/or suffer from anxiety and/or depression.

You experience hypothyroid symptoms (cold and clammy hands, hair loss).

You have a hard time sleeping.

You have imbalanced hormones (specifically amenorrhea or PCOS).

IF YOU'VE DETERMINED THAT INTERMITTENT FASTING ISN'T RIGHT FOR YOU, HERE ARE SOME SUGGESTIONS:

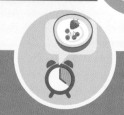

Keep your eating window—the interval between your first meal and your last—to around 12 to 14 hours. Or just listen to your body and eat when you're hungry.

MONDAY
☑ Breakfast
☑ Lunch
☑ Dinner

Plan around 3 meals a day instead of 2—the standard breakfast, lunch, and dinner works well.

Eat every 4 hours or so and make the meals a bit smaller to accommodate for a longer eating window.

The "eating window" is the interval between your first meal of your day and your last.

How to Tell If You're Ready

It can't get any easier: if you're naturally able to effortlessly last anywhere between twelve and twenty-four hours without food—sleeping time counts—then congratulations! You're ready to practice intermittent fasting.

Fatty Coffees and Fasting

Think of intermittent fasting as a tool to heal your body that has two settings: it can increase autophagy and balance blood sugar, or it can just balance blood sugar. Which setting you choose is up to you, and you can rotate between settings. Perhaps on Monday, you choose autophagy and blood sugar, and on Tuesday you choose to just balance blood sugar.

If you focus on just blood sugar, you aren't limited to water-only intermittent fasting. Instead, you're able to consume some drinks or snacks to help extend your fast. These items could be things like bone broth, fat bombs, or the beloved fatty coffee. By eating fat during your fast, you maintain balanced blood sugar levels and keep insulin low, and your body is able to stay in fat-burning mode, uninterrupted by actual food.

Let's focus on coffee, because most of us are familiar with...the *butter coffee.* The classic blend includes (obviously) butter, which you may be sensitive to without knowing it. I've found that consuming one butter coffee a day can lead to cravings, low blood sugar, shakiness, inflammation, and hormone fluctuations.

So in 2015, I adjusted the original recipe to work better for those who experience issues with the classic butter coffee. My recipe, called the Rocket Fuel Latte (RFL), keeps you in a fat-burning state, maintains your morning fast, regulates hormones, and doesn't use butter.

RFLs incorporate all three macronutrients to encourage your body to "fast" while also providing it with energy:

1. Unlimited fat

2. 10 grams of protein or less

3. 3 grams of carbs or less

By following these guidelines, you'll be able to enjoy a touch of fatty goodness in the morning while staying in fasting mode and keeping your insulin low.

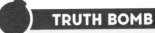

TRUTH BOMB

If you drink decaffeinated butter coffees or RFLs and experience mild jitters afterward, this could be a sign of insulin resistance (see page 41) or adrenal dysfunction (see page 378).

ROCKET FUEL LATTE

MAKES: **one 16-ounce (475-ml) serving or two 8-ounce (240-ml) servings**

This creamy latte has a hint of white chocolate flavor, but the variations are endless. If you don't have a high-powered blender to pulverize the hulled hemp seeds, substitute your favorite low-carb nut or seed butter.

1¾ cups (415 ml) hot brewed coffee (regular or decaf) or tea

1 tablespoon MCT oil or coconut oil

1 tablespoon cacao butter

1 tablespoon hulled hemp seeds

2 to 4 drops liquid stevia (optional)

¼ teaspoon vanilla extract or powder

Pinch of finely ground Himalayan rock salt (optional)

1 tablespoon collagen peptides or protein powder or 1½ teaspoons unflavored gelatin

Pinch of ground cinnamon, for garnish

1. Place the hot coffee, oil, cacao butter, hemp seeds, stevia (if using), vanilla, and salt in a high-powered blender (see note above). Blend on high speed for 1 minute, or until the hemp seeds are pulverized.

2. During the last 10 seconds, add the collagen and continue to blend.

3. Transfer to a mug, sprinkle with cinnamon, and enjoy.

STORE IT: *Keep in an airtight container in the fridge for up to 3 days.*

REHEAT IT: *Pour the RFL into a saucepan and place over medium heat, stirring often, until it comes to a light simmer. Or you can use the microwave, heating until the desired temperature is reached.*

PREP AHEAD: *Brew the coffee or tea, let it cool, and store it in the fridge for up to 3 days. When ready to prepare the RFL, reheat the coffee or tea on the stovetop or in the microwave, then follow the instructions above.*

MAKE IT VEGAN: *Replace the collagen with an additional 2 tablespoons of hulled hemp seeds.*

VARIATION: HOT CACAO. *Combine 1¾ cups (415 ml) hot brewed coffee or tea (peppermint tea is awesome in this version!), 1 tablespoon cacao butter, 1 tablespoon of MCT oil or coconut oil, 1 tablespoon chia seeds, 1 tablespoon cacao powder, 2 to 4 drops liquid stevia (optional), a pinch of finely ground Himalayan rock salt (optional), and 1 tablespoon collagen peptides or protein powder or 1½ teaspoons unflavored gelatin.*

VARIATION: COCONUT PARTY. *Combine 1¾ cups (415 ml) hot brewed coffee or tea, 1 tablespoon coconut oil, 1 tablespoon MCT oil, 1 tablespoon melted coconut butter, ¼ teaspoon vanilla extract or powder, 2 to 4 drops liquid stevia (optional), a pinch of finely ground Himalayan rock salt (optional), and 1 tablespoon collagen peptides or protein powder or 1½ teaspoons unflavored gelatin.*

VARIATION: GREEN TEA LATTE. *Combine 1¾ cups (415 ml) hot water, 2 tablespoons coconut oil, 2 tablespoons full-fat coconut milk, 2 teaspoons matcha powder, 2 to 4 drops liquid stevia (optional), and 1 tablespoon collagen peptides or protein powder or 1½ teaspoons unflavored gelatin.*

VARIATION: EGGNOG. *Combine 1¾ cups (415 ml) hot brewed coffee or tea, 2 tablespoons full-fat coconut milk, 1 tablespoon MCT oil, ½ teaspoon ground cinnamon, ¼ teaspoon ground nutmeg, 2 to 4 drops liquid stevia (optional), and 1 tablespoon collagen peptides or protein powder or 1½ teaspoons unflavored gelatin.*

VARIATION: AYURVEDIC. *Combine 1¾ cups (415 ml) hot brewed coffee or tea, 1 tablespoon coconut oil, 1 tablespoon MCT oil, 1 tablespoon tahini, ½ teaspoon turmeric powder, ¼ teaspoon ground cardamom, ¼ teaspoon ginger powder, 2 to 4 drops liquid stevia (optional), a pinch of finely ground Himalayan rock salt (optional), and 1 tablespoon collagen peptides or protein powder or 1½ teaspoons unflavored gelatin.*

NUTRIENT INFORMATION (PER 16-OZ/475-ML SERVING):

calories: 339 | calories from fat: 301 | total fat: 33.4g | saturated fat: 24.9g | cholesterol: 0mg

sodium: 192mg | carbs: 1g | dietary fiber: 1g | net carbs: 0g | sugars: 0g | protein: 8.5g

RATIOS:

fat:	carbs:	protein:
89%	1%	10%

Coffee
Caffeine per serving of RFL **164**

Yerba mate tea
Caffeine per serving of RFL **141**

Espresso
2 shots (1.5 fl. oz. each)
Caffeine per serving of RFL **140**

Matcha tea powder
1½ teaspoons
Caffeine per serving of RFL **116**

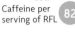
Black tea
Caffeine per serving of RFL **82**

Four Sigma Foods mushroom coffee with cordyceps
2 packets
Caffeine per serving of RFL **79**

White tea
Caffeine per serving of RFL **46**

Green tea
Caffeine per serving of RFL **42**

Raw cacao powder
1 tablespoon
Caffeine per serving of RFL **12**

Decaf black tea
Caffeine per serving of RFL **0** to **20**

Decaf green tea
Caffeine per serving of RFL **0** to **3**

Swiss Water decaf coffee*
Caffeine per serving of RFL **<1**

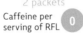
Decaf espresso
2 shots (1.5 fl. oz. each)
Caffeine per serving of RFL **20**

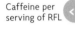
Four Sigma Foods chaga mushroom elixir
2 packets
Caffeine per serving of RFL **0**

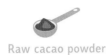
Herbal tea
Caffeine per serving of RFL **0**

Rooibos tea
Caffeine per serving of RFL **0**

Hot water
Caffeine per serving of RFL **0**

Swiss Water coffee is 100 percent chemical-free; water, coffee, time, and temperature are the only elements Swiss Water uses to remove caffeine.

All caffeine levels are measured in mg.

For tea, the caffeine amount is based on a 3-minute steep time. Steep time affects the caffeine content: a change from 1 minute to 5 minutes can increase the caffeine level by as much as 276 percent.

SIGNS IT'S TIME TO LOWER YOUR CAFFEINE INTAKE: You can't go a day without it. You're slightly panicked, nervous, or anxious most days. Your sleep sucks. You experience rambling and random thoughts. You're thirstier than normal. You need that cuppa joe to get started in the morning or as a pick-me-up in the afternoon. If any of these sound familiar, transform your Rocket Fuel Latte into a less-stimulating version by replacing the coffee with lower-caffeine alternatives.

NOTE: *Caffeine levels in tea vary by brand. If you are concerned about your caffeine intake, it may be best to choose one of the 0 mg items.*

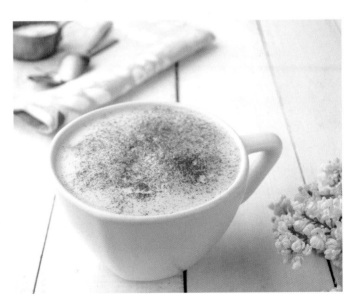

Get creative! Make your own flavor, take a picture, and tag it with #rocketfuellatte. A good amount of fat to start with is 2 tablespoons. I'd love to see what you create!

Answers to Your RFL Questions

Are they suitable for everyone?

No, and the reason is really, really simple—anyone who is healing needs nutrients, and RFLs (as magically awesome as they are) won't provide as many nutrients as a plate full of greens, grass-fed beef, and coconut oil will. They just won't. So if your body needs to balance itself out—whether as a result of adrenal dysfunction, thyroid imbalances, hormone irregularities, or childbirth—it needs a maximized load of nutrients to do it.

This doesn't mean that you can never enjoy an RFL, just that you may benefit from more nutrient-dense food on a regular basis.

Do I have to follow the recipes or variations perfectly in order for this to work?

No! Have fun with it. Here are some ways that you can sub out the ingredients in the recipe on page 144 with items you have on hand:

- Instead of coffee: tea, decaf coffee, hot water, hot milk

- Instead of MCT oil or coconut oil: avocado oil, red palm oil, ghee or butter (if tolerated)

- Instead of cacao butter: MCT oil, coconut oil, red palm oil, ghee or butter (if tolerated), avocado oil, 100% dark chocolate

- Instead of hemp hearts: chia seeds, almond butter, sunflower seed butter, cashew butter, tahini, coconut butter

- Instead of alcohol-free stevia: monk fruit sweetener, erythritol, xylitol

- Instead of collagen: 3 tablespoons of hemp hearts or nut/seed butter, gelatin, your favorite low-carb protein powder, egg yolk(s)

When should you drink RFLs?

- *Is pre- or post-workout okay?* If you're lifting heavy things, drinking an RFL pre-workout is a great idea. In fact, having caffeine and fat beforehand will likely do wonders for your results. If you're engaging in aerobic exercise, you may find that the caffeine sets you off before a workout, but if you switch to a caffeine-free option, you may have luck with that. As for post-workout, you'll do better sticking to a keto meal or protein shake with a small amount of carbs for anaerobic training, and a high-fat meal for aerobic training.

- *Is it better to have it in the evening or morning?* You can have it anytime. If you're drinking an RFL in the evening, caffeine-free might be best.

- *Can you have it as a snack?* You bet!

- *Does it replace a meal or is it better with a meal?* Eat when you're hungry—sometimes I have an RFL with a meal, sometimes I don't!

- *Can you have more than one in a day?* You bet!

Intermittent Fasting Strategies and Schedules

Current research shows that certain benefits of IF might only be realized after longer periods of fasting—as in around twenty to twenty-four hours, depending on your activity level. But these studies are based on glucose-fueled individuals who have a very different metabolism than someone who is eating a ketogenic diet. Someone who is already in ketosis can experience the same benefits in a much shorter fasting period. In other words, it's very possible that sixteen to eighteen hours is long enough to fast for the keto adapted. If you're generating ketones, you're already reaping awesome benefits.

It all comes down to how your body responds to fasting and what works best for your schedule. The IF strategy that you choose will be different from mine or anyone else's, and that's okay!

Combining Intermittent Fasting with Exercise

Many researchers have concluded that combining the benefits of exercise with IF makes a perfect anti-aging, detoxifying, energy-boosting, weight-loss-promoting health elixir, each enhancing the benefits of the other. Find out more about fasting and workouts on page 208.

Daily-ish Intermittent Fasting Options

 Fast When You Feel Like It

Practice Frequency: Whenever you feel like it

Level of Difficulty: 1

Format: Let your body be your guide. When you're not hungry, don't eat. Break your fast when you're ready. Don't bother counting hours; just listen to your body.

Notes: This method brings success only when you don't overthink it. Just eat when you're hungry, stop when you're full, and fast when you wake up and food isn't on your mind. Trust in the process.

Natural Calorie Reduction: Aligned purely and completely with what your body needs in the moment.

Tips: You can have fatty coffee or bone broth while you're fasting.

This fast is great as a daily practice and really easy to implement, with no effort required.

 16-Hour Fast

Practice Frequency: 3 to 5 days per week

Level of Difficulty: 2

Format: Fast for 16 hours, eat for 8 hours. Example:
- Day 1: Stop eating at 9 p.m.
- Day 2: Start eating at 1 p.m.

Notes: This approach may not limit calories significantly, but it does give your body the time needed to increase ketones and also gives the digestive system a nice break.

Natural Calorie Reduction: May be observed by comparing your daily intakes. Eat when you're hungry during the 8-hour eating window and don't worry too much about how many calories you're consuming.

Tips: You can have fatty coffee or bone broth while you're fasting.

This fast is great as a daily practice and really easy to implement with little effort.

 24-Hour Fast

Practice Frequency: 2 to 3 days per week

Level of Difficulty: 3

Format: Fast for 24 hours. Example:
- Day 1: Stop eating at 5 p.m.
- Day 2: Start eating at 5 p.m.

Notes: Because the fast starts in the evening, it reduces overall caloric intake without making you feel like you're going a full day without a meal.

Natural Calorie Reduction: Can be observed by looking at your overall weekly intake. Eat when you're hungry during your eating window and don't worry too much about how many calories you're consuming.

Tips: You can have fatty coffee or bone broth while you're fasting.

It's tempting to break this fast with an all-out gorge, but don't do it!

 Caveman

Practice Frequency: 3 to 5 days per week

Level of Difficulty: 2

Notes: Fasting during the day boosts energy and stimulates fat-burning when practiced on a regular basis. Eating in the evening lays the groundwork for overnight tissue repair and growth. This fasting style reduces the meal count to reduce the time you need to dedicate to meal prep, without making you feel deprived.

Natural Calorie Reduction: Can be observed by comparing your daily intakes. During your single meal, eat until you're full and don't worry too much about how many calories you're consuming.

Format: Fast all day and eat one large meal in the evening.

Tips: You can have fatty coffee or bone broth while you're fasting.

It's tempting to break this fast with an all-out gorge, but don't do it!

Breaking your fast with a carb-up meal (see page 194) is an awesome strategy for a lot of people.

If having just one meal in the day sets you up for failure, approach the meal as a two-part feast—two to four hours after your first meal in the eating window, have a second meal. This strategy can be particularly helpful in place of a carb-up meal if having carbs after a long fast doesn't feel good in your body.

Protein-Sparing Modified Fasting

There is another fasting method that I didn't include with the others on the facing page because I don't see it as a daily or even weekly or monthly strategy, making it less of an intermittent fasting protocol and more of a fasting protocol all on its own. It's called a protein-sparing modified fast (it's known as PSMF on the keto block), and it's designed to kick-start weight loss *for people who are severely obese.*

PSMF reduces calories to the lowest possible amount while keeping protein high enough that lean tissue mass is preserved and maintaining enough micronutrients to avoid malnutrition.

I have some concerns about this strategy:

- Many women remain on it longer than they should.

- Many women who are not severely obese pick it up as a strategy for weight loss when they could benefit instead from a different approach to their ketogenic diet.

- Many women trying this approach have been on restrictive diets for years... and they haven't worked. So going on yet another severely strict diet may only affect the metabolism further and throw women even further out of touch with their bodies.

- Micronutrient deficiencies don't just happen overnight. The fact that the strategy is designed to avoid micronutrient deficiencies tells me that the practice should only be done for short periods. However, when something works for us ladies, we have a hard time not doing more of it. My concern here is that when we've found something that works, we will naturally want to do more of it, and in this case, doing more could be detrimental.

- All the studies I was able to locate on PSMF recommend that it be done under the constant supervision of medical professionals.

If you're interested in PSMF and think you'd be a great candidate, I highly urge you to locate a medical professional in your area to guide you through a medically supervised version of this approach.

Keto **Weight Loss**

If you've followed step 1 through to this section of step 2, you've probably already lost water weight, or you're well on your way to it. If weight loss is your goal with keto, this is about the point in your process where it becomes beneficial to understand what can help you succeed and the roadblocks standing in your way.

You may not need to adjust anything on your ketogenic diet in order to reach your goal weight. Many women simply eat keto, get in the groove of what feels good in their bodies, and don't need to adjust much after that. Even if that's you, it can be helpful to know how to adjust things should you be met with frustrations later on. And if that's not you, don't worry! It doesn't necessarily mean you're doing anything wrong—but there are some tricks and tools that can help.

Know Your Body

To better understand hunger, your metabolism, and why eating less food isn't always best for your health or for weight loss, flip back to page 28. You'll find the reason why it's so hard to lose weight when you eat less and answers to other thorny metabolic questions, so that you can unlock lasting weight loss.

Tools to Help You Lose

Following a standard ketogenic diet isn't always enough to lose excess weight. I know, I know, a lot of people out there say it is, but for us ladies, adjustments are often needed. If you've been dieting for a while, you may think of adjustments as things like eating less, working out more, going hungry, fasting longer, and so on. But these aren't generally the ways to success. Think about it: if they'd worked in the past, then you wouldn't be jonesing to lose weight right now, right?

Thankfully, the necessary adjustments aren't overly complicated, and they're all laid out for you below! Making these small healthful shifts in the way you approach keto may help you shed excess weight that just isn't serving you anymore.

Increase One Kind of Body Fat

We all have different types of fat, or adipose tissue, in our bodies. When most people think of fat, they're really thinking of white adipose tissue (WAT)—the fat that tends to be stored around the waist, hips, and butt.

However, we also have brown adipose tissue (BAT). This kind of fat actually raises the basal metabolic rate—the rate at which we burn energy simply to exist—by converting the food we eat into heat rather than usable energy.

BAT cells have a high level of uncoupling proteins, and these little proteins make it more difficult for the cell to create the energy that's required for just about everything we do. Because the cell has to work harder to produce energy, more calories are burned, which ramps up our metabolism.

So increasing the amount of BAT aids in weight loss because it means we need to burn more calories to create the same amount of energy. But how do we increase BAT?

Overeating increases BAT, whereas restricting calories decreases BAT. Because of the health concerns associated with overeating day in and day out, let's not go with that option. This is where ketones come in: just the mere presence of ketones in your body will increase BAT. If you're the type of person who doesn't generate loads of ketones, exogenous ketones can be a big help. You may remember from chapter 3 that exogenous ketones are ketones that come from outside your body. Supplementing with exogenous ketones increases the amount of BAT in your body, leading to an increased metabolic rate. My favorite exogenous ketone supplement is by Perfect Keto.

Support Detoxification

Did you know? Toxins are stored in fat, so as you lose weight and your body fat is burned for fuel, those toxins are released into your body. You need to flush out those toxins—otherwise, they can affect your ability to lose weight and, worse, cause health imbalances.

A ketogenic diet is naturally detoxifying because it limits sugar and grains, and by eliminating these items, you (1) make more space in your diet for nutrient-dense foods; (2) heal leaky gut, which can cause inflammation and make it more challenging to detoxify; and (3) often drink more water. But there are additional things you can do to assist detoxification. If weight loss is your biggest goal, ensuring that toxins are released safely should be of the utmost importance to you!

Now, you may be thinking, *Detox...detox...like a cleanse? A juice cleanse or tea cleanse?* No, it doesn't need to come to that, and in fact, those kinds of cleanses may not be the best way to support detoxification. All we need to do to detoxify is support the organs most involved with detoxification: the kidneys, liver, and gut. We can do this by eating supportive foods that have the following components:

- Flavonoids, molecules found in plant foods that eliminate oxidative stress and support the digestive system

- Bitters (made from aromatic herbs, bark, roots, and/or fruit), which balance the gut and support liver and kidney detoxification

- Amino acids, which combine with oxidized chemicals freed during the process of detoxification to be excreted through the bile

- Methionine, an amino acid that's particularly important for the excretion of oxidized chemicals

- Sulfur, which is needed for the production of glutathione, an antioxidant

- Choline, which supports the liver

- Magnesium, which plays a role in the removal of toxins and heavy metals from the body

- Vitamin C, which plays a role in heavy-metal detoxification

Emphasizing some of these nutrients at different times, as described in the illustration on the facing page, will help support different stages of detoxification. (You'll also find more information about supporting detoxification on page 303.)

ACTIVATE YOUR DETOX PATHWAYS

Shifting some of your food choices (while staying on keto) can help support detoxification. You could run through this cycle monthly, for ten days a month.

- ● Flavonoids
- ○ Bitter foods
- ● Amino acids
- ● Methionine
- ● Sulfur
- ● Choline
- ● Magnesium
- ● Vitamin C

FIRST, EAT MORE OF THESE FOODS FOR 5 DAYS:

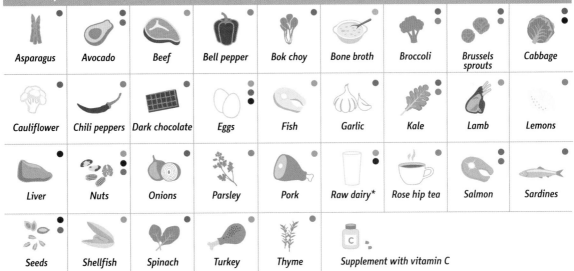

Artichoke	Arugula	Blueberries	Broccoli	Brussels sprouts	Cabbage	Chocolate	Dandelion	Eggplant

Ginger	Kale	Onions	Radicchio	Strawberries	Supplement with B complex, glutathione, milk thistle

THEN, FOR AT LEAST 5 MORE DAYS, ADD THE FOLLOWING:

Asparagus	Avocado	Beef	Bell pepper	Bok choy	Bone broth	Broccoli	Brussels sprouts	Cabbage

Cauliflower	Chili peppers	Dark chocolate	Eggs	Fish	Garlic	Kale	Lamb	Lemons

Liver	Nuts	Onions	Parsley	Pork	Raw dairy*	Rose hip tea	Salmon	Sardines

Seeds	Shellfish	Spinach	Turkey	Thyme	Supplement with vitamin C

*Dairy is rich in compounds you require, but I don't recommend it, for the reasons outlined on page 99. If you do choose to consume dairy, opt for grass-fed and grass-finished sources.

Swap Saturated Fats

Trade saturated fats, like coconut oil, meat, and dairy foods, for monounsaturated fats, like fatty fish, avocado, olives, and olive oil. You should see an improvement in weight loss in a week or two.

Check Your Nuts

Nuts are really easy to overeat, especially if you keep a whole jar of them handy at your desk for all-day snacking. Eating nuts is okay, but eating nuts on autopilot while engrossed in your work and not being mindful of what you're eating isn't.

   If you're going to snack throughout your workday, take five minutes to sit with those nuts and fully immerse yourself in enjoying your snack—the smell, the taste, and the quiet time you're creating in your day. Pay attention to your body's cues telling you when you've had enough (often just a handful will do the trick), and move on with your day.

Avoid Refined Oils and Dairy

Both of these foods can cause inflammation in the body, which leads to more weight gain. When it comes to foods made with processed oils, the goal is to make sure they're made with the safe oils outlined on page 97—think mayonnaise that's made with avocado oil instead of canola oil.

Ditch the Butter Coffee

Many women don't do well on traditional butter coffee, due to its high amounts of caffeine and fat (which may be the wrong fats for their bodies), its lack of protein and carbs, its ability to encourage fasting (which may not work for them), and a number of other reasons. If the traditional butter coffee isn't serving you, swap it for an actual keto breakfast, fast until lunch, or try a Rocket Fuel Latte (page 144) instead.

Lower Your Carbs

If you're postmenopausal, you may benefit from lowering your carbohydrate intake even further, to as low as 20 total carbohydrates or 20 net carbohydrates (assuming you stick to about 30 grams of fiber). You may thrive on fewer carbohydrates than you did during your reproductive years.

Try Fasted Workouts and Fed Workouts

Some people thrive on fasted workouts while others don't. I find that fasted high-intensity interval workouts are okay, but a full-on spin class, running session, or any pedal-to-the-metal workout that lasts for at least thirty minutes requires a bit of fueling-up in advance. You'll find information about how to fuel properly before and after your movement sessions on page 209.

Add Supportive Supplements

Incorporating the following early on in your keto journey can encourage healthful weight loss:

- Vitamin D

- Green tea

- At least 40 grams of fiber per day (focus on whole-food sources, as outlined in the Fat Fueled Food Pyramid on page 103)

- MCT oil or powder

Check Your Fat Intake

You may think that you're eating a lot of fat—after all, not long ago you cooked your vegetables in water and now you cook everything in bacon grease—but surprisingly, many people still fear the fat after eating keto for months! Going from a lifetime of low-fat to a high-fat diet is a paradigm shift that isn't always easy to achieve. The only way to get over the hump is to trust the keto process and enjoy the fat wholeheartedly. Because of the unique biochemical responses your body has to dietary fat, it's highly improbable that you can eat too much of it. So rest assured, you'll likely stop before you eat too much!

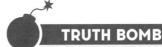

TRUTH BOMB

If your fat intake is under 60% of your total calories, it may not be high enough for you to experience the benefits of a ketogenic diet.

Signs That You May Not Be Eating Enough Fat

If you experience any of these symptoms after being keto for more than 30 days, try eating more fat:

- You get shaky following a meal.
- Your experience with PMS gets worse.
- You've recently tested your progesterone, estrogen, DHEA, or cortisol levels and they're lower than they should be.
- You're always hungry, even 30 to 60 minutes after eating.
- You're tired all the time.
- You suffer from anxiety or feel overwhelmed.
- You're always cold.
- You've hit a weight-loss plateau.
- You're low in vitamins A, D, E, or K.
- Your memory is horrible.
- Your joints hurt.
- Your HDL cholesterol is low.

Signs That You May Be Eating Too Much Fat

If you experience any of these symptoms after being keto for more than 30 days, try cutting back on your fat intake:

- You've hit a weight plateau and none of the tips in this chapter are working.
- You eat a *lot* of nuts and seeds.
- You enjoy feeling almost uncomfortably full after each meal.
- You've been known to add 4+ tablespoons of butter, ghee, or coconut oil to your fatty coffee.
- You're experiencing candida flare-ups.

If you need to increase or decrease your fat intake, adjust it by 5 percent for seven days. If you're still experiencing symptoms, adjust it by another 5 percent for another seven days. Repeat if necessary.

It's always best to make changes slowly so you give your body time to catch up! You can use the chart on the facing page to match what you're currently consuming for your fat macro to the adjustment you'll make either up or down.

Customizing Fat Intake for Optimal Weight Loss

Current Fat Intake (g)	INCREASE			DECREASE		
	5%	10%	15%	5%	10%	15%
	Increase Your Fat Intake To (g)			Decrease Your Fat Intake To (g)		
80	84	88	92	76	72	68
85	89	94	98	81	77	72
90	95	99	104	86	81	77
95	100	105	109	90	86	81
100	105	110	115	95	90	85
105	110	116	121	100	95	89
110	116	121	127	105	99	94
115	121	127	132	109	104	98
120	126	132	138	114	108	102
125	131	138	144	119	113	106
130	137	143	150	124	117	111
135	142	149	155	128	122	115
140	147	154	161	133	126	119
145	152	160	167	138	131	123
150	158	165	173	143	135	128
155	163	171	178	147	140	132
160	168	176	184	152	144	136
165	173	182	190	157	149	140
170	179	187	196	162	153	145
175	184	193	201	166	158	149
180	189	198	207	171	162	153
185	194	204	213	176	167	157
190	200	209	219	181	171	162
195	205	215	224	185	176	166
200	210	220	230	190	180	170
205	215	226	236	195	185	174
210	221	231	242	200	189	179
215	226	237	247	204	194	183
220	231	242	253	209	198	187
225	236	248	259	214	203	191

Your Plateau Is Not Caused by Calories

Please pay attention here—I really want this information to change your perception of weight loss and help you see your body for what it truly is. Calories are only one small piece of the big picture. Restrictive keto protocols such as fat fasting, egg fasting, or restricting your food intake to the bare minimum will likely not provide the solution you need to lose weight.

If you are not losing weight, nine times out of ten it has absolutely *nothing* to do with the quantity of calories you are consuming and everything to do with the amount of calories you are *not* consuming.

Below are thirteen possible reasons why you're unable to lose weight—proof of just how complex our bodies are. In the end, your weight-loss success boils down to pumping as many health-promoting nutrients into your body as possible so that you can lose weight with a healthy body, and keep the weight off for life.

Many of these concerns are covered in more detail in chapters 8 and 9.

TRUTH BOMB

Weight loss should be your lowest priority whenever your body has any underlying health imbalances. Until you heal your body, you're not likely to be successful in losing weight or maintaining a new lower weight.

Hypothyroidism

Your thyroid is the master of your metabolism, and hypothyroidism—low thyroid function—is very common. Many resources point to the soy in our foods, low-fat foods, and a lack of iodine in our diets as the key causes of low thyroid function, but I'd like to spotlight stress as the most likely cause of thyroid imbalance.

Your adrenal glands are closely connected to your thyroid. When you're stressed, your adrenals wreak havoc on your thyroid, leading to imbalances in your ability to process thyroid hormones efficiently. Create self-care rituals that help you stay positive, balanced, and loving (for some examples, see page 165), and review the thyroid information on page 367.

Underlying Inflammation

Inflammation is the silent player in many of the health issues that plague modern society, such as cancer, heart disease, diabetes, Alzheimer's disease, and even depression. The standard American diet—full of sugar, artificial sweeteners, highly processed oils, and processed foods—lack of exercise and sleep, and overabundance of stress all increase systemic inflammation. Inflammation running rampant in your body forces your body to constantly devote resources to managing it instead of managing your actual health. Inflammation is the first thing that has to be addressed before your body can heal. Simply eating a keto diet will go a long way toward that—just make sure to follow the Fat Fueled Food Pyramid (page 85). And, if you want to go even deeper into resolving inflammation, there are oodles of tips beginning on page 251.

Unknown Food Sensitivities

A food allergy or sensitivity can stand in the way of your weight-loss goal, primarily because it can cause inflammation. Although you may not even realize you have a sensitivity, every time you eat a food that you're sensitive to, an inflammatory response is triggered, forcing your body to focus on healing the damaged and inflamed areas instead of on managing your weight. For information on how to get support for potential food sensitivities, see page 274.

Wonky Hormones

Insulin, leptin, estrogen, testosterone, glucagon, ghrelin, progesterone, DHEA, and HGH are all pieces of a puzzle that need to fit together perfectly. When your hormones are all balanced, you feel energized, free of cravings, and ready to take on the world. When they're imbalanced, you feel tired, out of control, and weighed down.

Eating keto will naturally balance your insulin, leptin, glucagon, and ghrelin right off the bat, but your sex hormones can be a bit more finicky. For more sex hormone support, head to page 333.

Imbalanced Digestive Tract

Many of us are dealing with impaired gut function due to excessive carbohydrate and sugar consumption, stress, lack of sleep, and the use of antibiotics and other prescription drugs. Never doubt that your gut is the seat of your health—really, it is. You want the healthiest, most balanced gut you can achieve as the foundation of your health, so you can achieve balanced, mood-stabilizing hormones, eliminate cravings, and allow nutrients to be fully absorbed. You can be eating "perfectly," but if your gut isn't healthy, you're not getting all the nutrients you need. Tools and tips for healing gut imbalances start on page 256.

Lack of Sleep

When it comes to sleep, I imagine that my body is like my iPhone. My iPhone can only handle so much activity until it needs to be charged, and until it's plugged into the wall, it will just continue being drained. And there's no way to speed up the charging process—it must be plugged in for a specific period of time in order to charge. Sleep is the same way—there is no way around it, and you have to do it for long enough to yield benefits.

If you're trying to decide between sleeping in and waking up early to go to the gym, it's a no-brainer—sleep! Waking up early to work out messes up your hormonal balance, which is critical for weight loss. The bottom line is that losing sleep just to hit the gym is counterproductive.

The reason that a lack of sleep can take such a toll on your body is that it messes with your internal clock and circadian rhythms. Your organs are set to operate at different levels depending on the time, which is informed by your internal clock. If you mess with your sleep schedule, they won't operate at their optimum levels and maximum fat loss simply can't be achieved.

And then there's hormone regulation, including the hormones that control your hunger. More specifically, two hunger hormones are negatively impacted by a lack of sleep. The first is ghrelin, which is the hormone that makes you feel hungry. Ghrelin levels are increased when you don't get enough sleep. The second is leptin, which is the hormone that makes you feel full. Leptin levels are decreased when there is a lack of sleep. This combination leads to a struggle with overeating and weight loss.

Aim for a minimum of eight hours of sleep and shuffle things around as needed to make this work. I know it's not easy, but it's imperative to help you move forward with your goals. If creating a defined sleeping schedule helps, do it. Personally, I find it a bit too limiting to promise myself that "I will be in bed by 9 p.m. every night." Instead, I arrange my schedule so that, no matter what time I go to bed, I can sleep until I wake up naturally.

TRUTH BOMB

If you work late at night or are constantly exposed to artificial light after the sun has set, get yourself a pair of blue-light-blocking glasses. They can help with melatonin production, promoting a healthful, restful sleep.

Vitamin D Deficiency

Vitamin D plays a role in so much more than just bone health. It supports positive moods, strong immune function, healthy metabolism, and more. If your vitamin D is below normal, you're likely to have a slow, sluggish metabolism.

Supplement with 2,000 to 5,000 IU of vitamin D_3 every morning. If you're like me and can't take vitamin D supplements due to an uptake issue (I get crazy headaches, lethargy, and face pain), getting out in the sun works just as well! Twenty to thirty minutes of sun exposure per day usually does the trick.

Chronic Stress

High stress can often lead to issues with weight loss because of cortisol. This stress hormone is released when your body is under stress or in fight-or-flight mode and pushes your body to store fat around your stomach, so when there is excess cortisol, your body will struggle with weight loss.

Additionally, cortisol pushes glucose to the muscles instead of the brain, so it can prevent the brain from getting the energy it needs. Cortisol can also lead to acne. Bummer, right?

Now, don't go thinking cortisol is evil. I know, I've painted that picture, but we *do* need it to survive, to stay alert, motivated, and awake. The good news is that when your stress is under control, cortisol gets to do what it was meant to do: regulate your sleeping cycles, boost motivation, and be your friend throughout the day. It's only when the hormone is overproduced that weight loss is hindered.

And the even better news is that on keto, your hormones are more regulated. Keto-friendly foods have anti-inflammatory properties that help to reduce cortisol levels and improve your sleep. This means that you can better manage stress and keep your cortisol levels in check while following a ketogenic diet.

The less stress you put on your body, the better it is for your overall health and your ketone levels. Counting and monitoring everything you eat as part of your effort to achieve a certain weight can actually hold you back from achieving your goals. The hormones released when you're under stress can even trigger a spike in blood sugar, without glucose ever being consumed. This is undesirable for anyone looking to lose weight because an increase in glucose can lead to more cravings and an increase in insulin, which accompanies a spike in blood sugar, means an end to fat-burning.

Schedule five minutes a couple of times throughout your day to practice meditation. If you're not sure how to meditate, the CALM meditation app is great.

Any and All Artificial Sweeteners

We want to eat as many whole foods as we can in order to heal, and our cup just doesn't have space for anything artificial, especially sweeteners. This includes xylitol, stevia, monk fruit, and erythritol—while better choices than most sweeteners, if you're struggling with weight and can't pinpoint the problem, it's worth removing them for a while to see if conditions improve.

Current research shows that artificial sweeteners are anything but okay for our health. As much as three hundred times sweeter than regular sugar, they confuse our metabolism, some raise our blood sugar, and some impact the healthy bacteria in our gut.

Follow the Fat Fueled Food Pyramid (page 85) and you'll be just fine!

Alcohol Consumption

No matter what kind of alcohol you drink, it will have a noticeable effect on your ketone levels, blood sugar levels, and food choices. Studies show that it can also interfere with your ability to have a sound night's sleep. Your liver's job is to metabolize fat, but if it's busy metabolizing alcohol from the night before, what do you think your liver is *not* doing?

I'll leave this one to you. Check out the information on page 87 to help you decide whether drinking or not drinking alcohol is the best choice for you.

Hidden Carbohydrates

In order to stay in ketosis, you need to avoid copious amounts of carbs. I know you're thinking, *Leanne, tell me something I don't know.*

A lot of women are just eating the wrong kind of carbs, which increases their total carbohydrate intake unnecessarily. Carbohydrates in your favorite low-carb protein bar are very different from the carbohydrates in your favorite low-carb vegetables, like broccoli, cauliflower, and spinach.

Your best bet? Opt for low-carb whole foods whenever possible and avoid all the processed "low-carb" foods that are not so low-carb at all.

Excessive Exercise

As the saying goes, everything in moderation—including exercise.

Don't get me wrong, exercise is one of the best things you can do for your body. It has been proven in study after study to improve your health in many different ways. Plus, it makes us all feel good. But there is a limit.

There are two reasons overdoing exercise can be harmful. The first is related to inflammation. While all forms of quality exercise will lead to some temporary acute inflammation, excessive exercise often leads to both oxidative stress and systemic inflammation.

The second reason excessive exercise isn't a great idea is that if you're overdoing exercise, it's likely with cardio, or aerobic training. The problem with overdoing aerobic training is that it burns so many calories, making your body feel deprived and increasing your appetite. In the end, you'll overeat to restore the calories your body burned—your willpower just can't overpower your biology.

Leptin Resistance

Leptin is the hormone that helps to control fat stores. Essentially, it sends a message to your brain when enough fat cells are present so that your brain knows it's time to stop eating. The hormone itself is produced by fat cells, and it plays a big role in calorie intake, calorie-burning, and the amount of fat you store on your body.

When you become resistant to leptin, your brain no longer receives the message that there are enough fat cells. And when that happens, you won't know when you're full. Leptin resistance is a big reason that people with obesity struggle to lose weight—they have plenty of leptin, but their brains aren't able to process the signal, so they never feel satiated. Reasons for leptin resistance include having poor sleep patterns, being in starvation mode, eating a diet high in processed foods, restricting calories, overeating, and being under stress.

Following a ketogenic diet should slowly aid in the balance of leptin and your body's ability to use it properly.

Step 2 **Problems** and **Solutions**

There are some common problems that many people encounter on this stage of the keto journey. You may not experience any of them, but in case you do, here are my best tips for handling these issues. Be sure to also review the common problems in step 1, listed on page 109.

Stress Is Stopping You from Being Awesome

Most of the stress we feel is a reaction to our perception of the world around us. Through our own reactions, we unintentionally give people and situations the power to take charge of our lives and our health. By learning to change our perceptions, we can be in a much better place.

Of course, problems with work, family, and finances can all be huge contributors to stress, but we often don't take into account the health-related stress we place on ourselves. The pressure we subject ourselves to around food, weight, health, and nutrition choices can be a serious drain on our energy, time, and money. Even as we strive to make our bodies as healthy and balanced as possible, we are often working against ourselves by being so uptight about it all—constantly thinking about our next meal, stressing about healthy food choices while traveling, worrying that we'll feel like the odd person out at our next work function, or fearing that we'll eat too much and spike our macros for the day. No matter how it manifests for you, dietary stress is a real thing, and it can happen on any kind of diet, including the ketogenic diet.

So how can we flip this situation upside down? I've learned that we have to condition ourselves to see our health and nutrition choices as just that: *choices*. You are *choosing* to eat this way, because it makes you feel good. And by eating this way, you are providing your body with the nutrients it needs to thrive. It's as simple as that. If you deviate from the template, it doesn't mean that you are no longer following a keto diet. As long as you know what makes you light up and feel good, that's half the battle.

Next time you have a dinner outing planned, don't look at the menu ahead of time—go to the restaurant completely blind and make choices in the moment. This will help you connect to what your body feels like eating, eliminate stress leading up to the event, and make you less likely to overeat while you're there.

Does the thought of doing that make you nervous or anxious? If so, you may want to ask yourself why. What rules have you set for yourself that you're fearful of breaking, and what's going on behind that?

I'm confident that once you've introduced your body to eating a ton of fat (and lowered your carbohydrate intake as a result), your brain will work better, your moods will normalize, and all the heavy stuff you're fearful of dealing with head-on will become a lot easier to manage.

Create a list of ten things you've been wanting to do for yourself—like painting your nails, listening to music outside, dancing around your house, or taking an Epsom salt bath. Complete one of these things every single day for the next ten days.

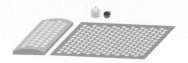

Grab yourself a Yantra acupressure mat and make it a priority to spend time on it as soon as you get home from work, both as a mental recalibration and as a buffer between your work day and your home life.

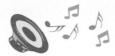

Blast the tunes in your car and sing along as loudly as possible.

Start the morning with a walk, or head out for a five-to-ten-minute walk if you feel overwhelmed during the day.

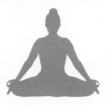

Begin your day with a five-minute meditation before getting out of bed.

Remove social media apps from your phone for one week. Alternatively, don't connect to social media before 3 p.m. every day.

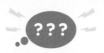

Whether you're stressed about a thought or feeling that you're having, a person you're interacting with, or a project you're working on, ask yourself throughout the day, "Is this enriching my life?"

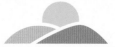

Create a morning practice that feeds your soul and creates inspiration outside of your job. For me, this means taking an untimed, untracked walk with my dogs in the summer (followed by a drink on my patio) and cuddling up by the fireplace in the winter.

Hair Loss

So you've been losing hair in small chunks, and you're terrified that one day very soon, you'll wake up as bald as Captain Jean-Luc Picard.

My guess is that you've been following a ketogenic eating style for some time without much of a focus on periodically increasing your carbs, as described on page 181, or else you've been doing carb-ups every five to ten days, thinking that the longer you go between them, the more powerful your ketogenic state will be. If I've hit it right on the money, continue reading. If you've always dealt with hair loss or thin hair regardless of your eating style, this section is not so much intended for you.

Many of the keto resources out there will tell you that a low-carb ketogenic diet can't possibly be the cause of any hair loss you're experiencing. But I'm here to tell you that, from my personal experience, a strict ketogenic diet can, without a doubt, be entirely to blame for your hair loss. There are two main reasons why this is so.

A lack of carbs: Your thyroid needs carbohydrates to convert hormones that are used to maintain its balance and health. Without enough carbohydrates, it can't convert these hormones and won't stay balanced, and the result can be hair loss—simple as that.

An increase in dietary stress: When your body is experiencing stress, including dietary stress, your adrenal glands go into overdrive, which in turn throws your thyroid out of whack. Imagine the hormone balance in your body as a three-legged stool. Each leg represents a hormone group: one is your adrenal-based hormones, one is your thyroid-based hormones, and one is your sex hormones. When one leg collapses, the stool falls over.

On a strict keto diet, dietary stress can be caused by the heavy consumption of the following:

- Foods you're sensitive to

- Inflammatory foods, such as conventional meat and processed "keto" food

- Vegetable oils, such as canola, safflower, and grapeseed

- Excess caffeine

All forms of intermittent fasting can also cause dietary stress.

By eliminating these things or consuming or practicing them in moderation, you can eliminate or reduce your dietary stress and any associated symptoms, including hair loss.

Weird Poops

Maybe the consistency, frequency, or scent of your fecal matter has changed and you're concerned about it. And hey, if you've never checked out your poop, now's the time! Here are a couple of circumstances to watch for and what to do if they occur. If you're concerned about the consistency of your stools, there's no harm in making an appointment with your health-care provider to make sure all is well.

Floating poop is usually due to nutrient malabsorption or excess gas. Be sure to take your time while eating, and ensure you're eating the foods right for your body (for information on detecting food sensitivities, see page 274).

Strong-smelling or greasy-looking stool could be due to a viral or bacterial infection, lack of enzymes, lack of stomach acid, imbalanced gut bacteria, or the use of stool softeners (including an excess of magnesium).

- Put the brakes on your magnesium supplementation. The food you eat today should be eliminated by your body twenty-four to forty-eight hours from now. If what you're eating for breakfast is showing up in the toilet in the evening, it's a sure sign that things are moving a bit too fast!

- Grab a good digestive enzyme paired with HCl to assist your body in breaking down and assimilating your meals efficiently.

Gas and digestive discomfort are usually the result of consuming things like dairy, cabbage, and sugar-free candies. Excessive gas and/or any mucus surrounding your floating stools could also be a sign of an underlying food allergy or sensitivity.

- Remove dairy, cabbage, and sugar-free items to see if your situation improves.

- Overeating can cause gas, so be mindful of the portions on your plate.

- Turn to page 274 for help with identifying potential food allergies and healing your body from their effects.

Muscle Aches and Pains

Aches and pains are often a sign of keto flu. Rewind to page 109 for keto flu info and relief strategies.

Nervousness and Anxiety

If you have a history of anxiety, nervousness, and/or depression that has been in remission but all of a sudden rears its ugly head while you're on keto, it could be a sign that you're not consuming enough carbohydrates.

Acne!

If you don't have a history of acne but have experienced a bout or two since starting keto, a hormonal imbalance is likely to blame. By eating a keto diet, we are helping our bodies balance our hormones, but on the way to recovery, it's likely that our hormones will do some wacky things, including possibly causing a bit of acne (which I think is a small price to pay for becoming more awesome).

These are some of the things I've identified that can aggravate *my* skin:

- Carbonated drinks (including fermented drinks, sugar-free drinks, mineral water—anything that's fizzy)

- Face washes containing honey, coconut oil, or minerals

- Foods high in FODMAPs (especially high-fructose fruits)—see page 284 for more

- Dairy foods, as well as any supplements or prescriptions that contain dairy

- All nuts

- Hormonal changes related to my cycle (especially before ovulation and before starting my period)

Insomnia

Chronic insomnia is a serious condition that, if left unaddressed, could affect all organ systems, body functions, and intellectual performance. The quantity and quality of your sleep has a sweeping impact on your health and quality of life.

Insomnia is typically described as poor sleep or the inability to fall asleep and/or stay asleep. It can be either acute or chronic. Acute insomnia is usually related to a trauma, traveling, or changes in life circumstances, like having a baby, and will generally pass without treatment once the body adjusts. With chronic insomnia, the sleep disruption lasts more than a month, at which point it's likely to start impairing life functions.

Difficulty sleeping is a serious matter, especially if it persists for more than four weeks. Quality sleep contributes to so much more than just keeping you beautiful. Your body works hard to protect you, and it deserves rest!

SYMPTOMS OF SLEEP-QUALITY ISSUES

- Cognitive slowing, including poor memory and brain fog
- Emotional dysregulation, including depression and anxiety
- Depressed immune function
- Fatigue
- Decreased ability to perform daily tasks
- Increased pain
- Reduced quality of life in general

Get Your Beauty Rest!

The human body needs at least seven and a half hours of sleep nightly to adequately detoxify the body and repair the brain. Insomnia is such a worrisome condition because it is associated with so many diseases, including high blood pressure, cardiovascular disease, stroke, weakened immune system, increased inflammation, obesity, and diabetes. Lack of sleep can also lead to anxiety, higher perceived stress, and, eventually, adrenal dysfunction.

There are also newer studies showing that insomnia might be a causative factor in the development of depression and anxiety, not a symptom of those states, as was originally thought. Also, we now know insomnia leads to increased risk of chronic disease and is a significant risk factor for developing Alzheimer's disease.

Insomnia is a major contributing factor to almost every chronic disease! By resolving it, you can not only reduce risk of disease but also take an incredible step toward a healthier, happier body.

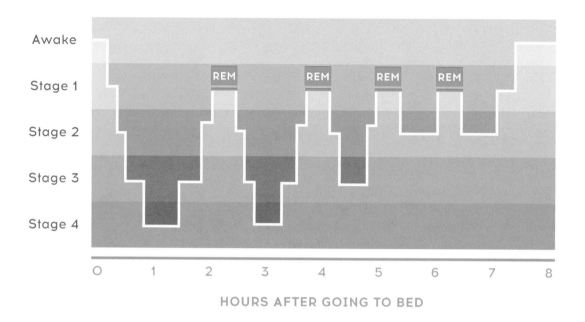

A Typical Full Night's Sleep

HOURS AFTER GOING TO BED

Let's break down what a normal sleep cycle looks like. Each sleep cycle lasts ninety minutes and includes five stages. If we are lucky, over the course of a night we repeat the cycle five times without interruption. That equates to about seven and a half hours of sleep, the minimum most adults need for good health.

During the first four stages, sleep becomes deeper and deeper. The last stage is when we experience REM sleep—rapid eye movement—and most dreaming occurs. The final two and a half hours are the most important because that is when a lot of memories get moved from short-term to long-term storage, so waking up too early increases the risk of cognitive impairment by interfering with the ability to form new memories.

Causes of Insomnia

1 This one's probably intuitive, but overstimulation during the day can make it harder to fall asleep at night. There's a scientific reason for this: overstimulation results in higher levels of adrenaline, which has all kinds of physiological effects that make you feel alert and ready for action—and which impede good sleep. Stimulation also increases cortisol, which usually rises in the morning to help us wake up—so having high cortisol before bed makes it almost impossible to sleep.

2 Watching violent or disturbing TV, whether movies or news, right before bed can make it difficult to relax enough to fall asleep.

3 Light, especially the blue light emitted from electronic screens, decreases your body's melatonin production, a hormone necessary for falling and staying asleep. Avoid looking at screens for at least one hour before going to bed—that means computer monitors, TVs, and smartphones! If this is not an option for you, blue-light-blocking glasses are a great alternative.

4 Shift work also affects melatonin production. Try taking a small dose—0.5 mg—of melatonin about one and a half hours before bed. Also make sure you have blackout curtains and cover all light sources in your room.

5 Medical conditions such as chronic pain, sinus congestion, restless leg syndrome, poorly regulated diabetes, and heartburn can make it hard to get a good night's sleep. Talk to your health-care provider about treatment options that can help you rest.

6 Hormonal imbalances, such as an adrenal or cortisol imbalance from high stress or hyperthyroid disease, and a blood sugar imbalance work against your body when it's time to sleep. The keto diet should help remedy both problems.

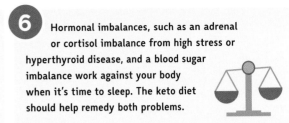

7 Hormonal changes and fluctuations that come with the menstrual cycle or menopause can affect sleep. For example, the sudden drop in progesterone and estrogen before your period can lead to insomnia in some women. The best approach here is to work to balance your hormones step by step, using the guidelines starting on page 335.

8 Medications, especially those taken for allergies, asthma, autoimmune diseases, high blood pressure, thyroid disorders, and heart disease, can affect sleep quality. Talk to your health-care provider if you're taking medication and having trouble sleeping.

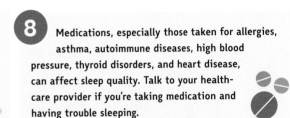

9 Sleep apnea, in which you stop breathing during sleep, is a serious condition and can lead to brain cell degeneration, among many other health problems. If you or your partner experience big snores followed by a brief pause before the next snore, it is likely sleep apnea. Talk to your doctor—a CPAP machine can make all the difference.

10 Recent research has shown that psychiatric disorders both cause and are caused by insomnia. Again, talk with your health-care provider about possible remedies.

Tips for Better Sleep

Say Yes To

GOOD SLEEP HYGEINE

That means sleeping in the dark, maintaining a regular sleep schedule, and avoiding caffeine, sugar, and alcohol before bed. (But your keto diet already has you managing these well, right?) Avoid exercise right before bedtime, but try to exercise daily. Avoid naps, and avoid screens that emit blue light an hour before bed.

ADRENAL ASSISTANCE

Balance your adrenal and cortisol levels by managing stress (see page 165).

HELPING YOUR THYROID

Just adopting a ketogenic diet is a mega step in a positive direction for you, your body, and your sleep cycle. If thyroid health is a particular concern, see page 367.

MANAGING YOUR PRESCRIPTIONS

Make sure you understand the side effects of each medication you're taking. If one of them may be causing issues with your sleep quality, chatting with your physician or pharmacist about options is a great first step. They may be able to help you switch to an different medication.

Say No To

BLUE LIGHT EXPOSURE

To block stimulating blue light after the sun sets, avoid watching TV, keep your house lights to a minimum, and install an app like f.lux on your computer and cell phone. If for any reason you're simply unable to follow these suggestions, you can always wear blue-light-blocking glasses.

RESTLESS LEG SYNDROME

Take magnesium and rule out low ferritin levels.

6

STEP 3: CUSTOMIZE YOUR FAT FUELED LIFE

Congratulations! You've made it to step 3 and are a thriving fat-burner! Up until now you've been following a very one-size-fits-all approach to getting your body into ketosis. You've learned how to feed yourself with whole foods to encourage ketosis, you've focused on how your body responds when you calculate and adhere to macronutrient goals with the aim of generating ketones...and perhaps you've become a bit frustrated.

Maybe the boundless energy you were promised hasn't happened yet, or you've lost faith in your body's ability to generate ketones, or if you hear one more person say, "I lost 20 pounds my first week on keto!" you may hit the roof.

In all of these situations, the knee-jerk reaction is to push harder to make the diet that seems to work for everyone else work for you.

But here's another idea: instead of feeling like your body needs to change to meet the demands of your diet, adjust the diet to meet your body where it's at right now.

That's what step 3 is all about. It's time to play with food amounts, types, and timing to make the diet yours.

Sometimes standard keto doesn't work for women. In fact, most women struggle with something that they wish the keto diet had solved. In actuality, all they need to do to realize the full potential of keto is adjust a small factor of their diet. By doing this, they get into alignment, keto starts working for them, and voilà!

After you've adjusted keto to work for *your* body, you should experience:

- An easing of inflammatory symptoms such as food sensitivities, gut irritability, painful joints, and headaches

- Less hunger

- Balanced hormones and a reduction in hormonal symptoms such as painful breasts, hot flashes, and painful periods

- Good digestive function, from regular healthy bowel movements to virtually no bloating

- Sustained, even energy

- The elimination of specific food cravings

Think of This Step as
Keto Rehab

There's a lot of stuff that other people don't know about you and your body. This includes doctors on the internet, keto social media influencers, even your favorite YouTuber. They don't know you, and they can't possibly have all the answers to your keto prayers. When we accept information blindly, without pausing to think critically about it or consider that the information we've received may not be right for our bodies, we run the risk of never reaching our goals and potentially doing something that's dangerous.

Damaging Dogma

There are many, many ways to eat keto—some good and some not so good. It all starts with the food we choose to eat.

The main feature of a poor keto protocol is that it doesn't honor individuality. If you're currently struggling with a keto plan that does not promote adjusting the protocol to suit your needs or doesn't mention individuality, and you're being told to push harder and do more, not to take a step back and ask yourself what's working and what's not, then the protocol is likely the problem, not your body.

There's no one-size-fits-all way to do keto successfully. So if anyone in the keto space has told you that it's either their way or no way at all, you may want to look elsewhere for nutrition support.

Below are the four most common recurring myths you may see in the ketogenic space. These ideas demand that everyone follow the same keto template and therefore deny women the ability to shape their diets to suit their own needs.

Myth: You have to eat less than 20 grams of carbs per day, regardless of your hormone profile or activity level.

Truth: How many carbohydrates you can consume without it affecting your glucose or ketones depends on your metabolism, as well as other factors (see the box below).

Your Carbohydrate Tolerance

Your carbohydrate tolerance may vary from day to day. Factors that affect it include the following:

- Where you're at in your cycle—you'll be more carb tolerant during the ovulatory and luteal phases (days 15 to 28 of your cycle)

- Your hormone profile—you'll be more carb tolerant if you have a thyroid imbalance than you would if you have PCOS

- How active you are overall—you'll be more carb tolerant if you work out often

- When you worked out last—you'll be more carb tolerant after working out

- When you choose to eat the carbohydrate—you'll be more carb tolerant in the evening than in the morning

- How much of the particular food you enjoy—the less you eat it, the more tolerant you'll be of the item

- How long you've been ketogenic—you'll be more carb tolerant the longer you eat keto

- How much fat or protein you eat with the carbohydrate—the better the macro balance, the better the carbohydrate tolerance

---

Myth: Avoid eating plants; they have too many carbs and make you bloated.

Truth: Plants contain electrolytes, which are necessary when you're going into a state of ketosis. Many women find that since plant foods contain a lot of fiber, they can count net carbs instead of total carbs and eat more plants without affecting their ketogenic state. Additionally, eating plant foods (fiber specifically) helps feed beneficial gut bacteria. A gut-based reaction to plant-based foods in the form of gas, bloating, constipation, or diarrhea may be a good indication that you need to better support your gut, not avoid plants altogether. (For guidelines on how to support your gut, see page 256.)

Myth: Only macros matter, not micronutrient intake or food quality. Quest bars? Perfect. Coke Zero? It's totally keto.

Truth: You are what you eat. You cannot expect to have thriving health if you're consuming packaged bars, treats, and goodies. Whether or not they're "keto," if the items you're consuming are devoid of nutrients, your body will be devoid of nutrients, too.

Myth: Gluconeogenesis will wreak havoc on your blood sugar levels, so avoid excess protein.

Truth: Most people do not experience glucose spikes in response to protein. More about this on page 65.

How Your Genes Dictate Which Fats You Eat

Consuming high amounts of saturated fat on your ketogenic diet is the best way to stay satiated and happy...except for some people whose genes have a different plan for them. Yes, I said *genes*.

So why do some people negatively react to saturated fat while others thrive? It comes down to how our bodies respond to cholesterol.

As humans, we carry two APOE genes, which act as an instruction manual for our body on how to make apolipoprotein E (APOE). There are three types of APOE genes:

- APOE2—Best suited for a keto diet with ample saturated fats; cholesterol levels are relatively low

- APOE3—Up for anything; cholesterol levels are relatively low

- APOE4—Best suited for a keto diet with ample monounsaturated fats (avoid saturated fat as much as possible); cholesterol levels are generally higher than average

Because we each carry two of these genes, there are six possible combinations—in order, from most common to least: 3/3, 4/3, 2/3, 4/4, 4/2, and 2/2. Someone with two APOE2 genes is best suited for a ketogenic diet rich in saturated fats, which would not affect their cholesterol level. Someone with two APOE4 genes, however, would do best on a ketogenic diet that focuses on monounsaturated and omega-3 fats.

Why does the APOE gene have the potential to affect cholesterol? It signals fats and cholesterol to form lipoproteins, which transport fat and other lipids in the blood. When you increase your dietary fat, you increase your lipoprotein levels, which triggers the body's cholesterol production to increase. That's why, in essence, a high-fat diet is equivalent to a high-cholesterol diet.

Now, before you start freaking out about increasing your cholesterol on keto, if you have two APOE2 genes, you will thrive on a high-fat diet because you have the proper metabolism to handle the high cholesterol output. (Remember, cholesterol isn't the bad guy it's made out to be—see page 59 for more.) And if you have two APOE3 genes, you can do as you like, thriving on saturated fats, monounsaturated fats, and anything in between.

However, studies have shown that people with one or two APOE4 genes are less likely to be able to metabolize cholesterol as well as their APOE2 and APOE3 pals. They are the most affected by high cholesterol, and therefore they are the ones who are told by doctors and health-care professionals to stop eating all the fat.

But going fat-free as an APOE4 carrier may not be the best idea. Here's why:

1. APOE4 carriers are two hundred times more likely to be diagnosed with Alzheimer's.

2. Alzheimer's is, in essence, type 3 diabetes—the brain just isn't able to process glucose as it used to, and that affects the brain's ability to function.

3. By fueling the body with ketones rather than glucose, the ketogenic diet allows those with Alzheimer's a second chance at life.

4. Therefore, APOE4 carriers, with their higher risk of Alzheimer's, will do better when fueled by ketones.

5. APOE4 carriers can thrive on a low-carb diet that emphasizes monounsaturated and omega-3 fats. The best of both worlds!

If you're an APOE4 carrier, think about doing keto Mediterranean style, with loads of fatty fish, avocado, olives, and olive oil.

So if you're on a ketogenic diet, pounding back coconut oil, and wondering why your cholesterol is increasing faster than a dog eats a fresh-cooked ham (this actually happened to us once, during Thanksgiving dinner), it could be because you are a carrier of a certain gene that makes it more challenging for you to metabolize saturated fat! Don't you worry, though; this doesn't mean you can't do the ketogenic diet. With a little switch in your fat choices, you'll be right as rain.

If you're interested in finding out which APOE genes you carry, have your genetic profile run by a genetic testing service. Once you have the results, you can have the raw data analyzed by a doctor who understands genetics, or you can upload the data to a secondary service that will outline which genes you have and interpret the data in much more detail.

Types of Keto Diets

The ketogenic diet is customizable. Figuring out what works best for you is key to your ketogenic success. There are four main variations of the diet, and there are ways to customize each even further depending on your needs.

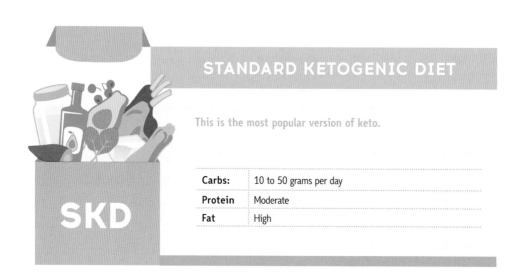

STANDARD KETOGENIC DIET

This is the most popular version of keto.

Carbs:	10 to 50 grams per day
Protein	Moderate
Fat	High

SKD

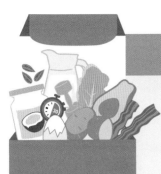

TARGETED KETOGENIC DIET

This version of keto is "targeted" to increase energy during workouts.

Carbs:	25 to 75 grams per day, timed 30 minutes to 1 hour prior to exercise
Protein	Moderate
Fat	High

TKD

CYCLICAL KETOGENIC DIET

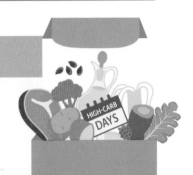

This version of keto increases carbohydrates or proteins cyclically, in many different ways, from adjusting macro amounts every couple of days in the evening to adjusting them for an entire week. How many times this is repeated is up to the individual. This could be practiced one, two, or three times a week for the day-to-day practice, or once every four to eight weeks for the weekly practice.

Carbs:	25 to 50 grams per day as a baseline; on certain days or weeks, 150 grams on average but possibly over 200 grams
Protein	Moderate
Fat	High except on higher-carb days, when fat is decreased

CKD

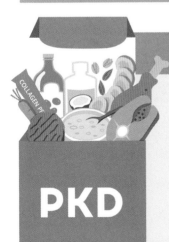

HIGH-PROTEIN KETOGENIC DIET

This version of keto is ideal for elite athletes and as a weight-loss-plateau buster; it's similar to CKD, but instead of increasing carbs, you increase protein to varying degrees—you can even go as far as practicing a carnivore diet, which is a keto-based diet that includes only protein and fat from animal sources.

Carbs:	0 to 20 grams per day
Protein	High
Fat	Moderate to high

PKD

There are ways to personalize these four key options even further while still remaining fat fueled. Here are some ways you might want to refine your keto diet to customize it for your needs.

Customizing Keto

 INCREASE YOUR CARBOHYDRATE INTAKE

A diet of 20 grams of carbohydrates per day may not allow you to get enough nutrient-rich vegetables, which are necessary for your long-term overall health.

 CHOOSE MONOUN-SATURATED FAT

Your genes determine whether saturated fat or monounsaturated fat is best for your body. Most people do well on saturated fats, but not everyone! And standard keto tends to empha-size foods rich in saturated fats, like coconut oil, meat, and lard. You may find that foods rich in monounsat-urated fats, like olive oil, avocado oil, nuts, and seeds, work better for you. Making this small adjustment can make a world of difference on how you experience keto. For more information on how to determine if you'd do better with monounsaturat-ed fats, see page 176.

 AVOID DAIRY

You do not need to include dairy in your keto diet to be successful. If you're experiencing an increase in inflamma-tion (which may manifest as joint pain, gut pain, acne, psoriasis, or eczema, for example), you're having difficulty losing weight, you've started to notice you're reacting to random foods other than dairy (like nuts, seeds, or certain herbs and spices), or you experience digestive upset after meals, dairy could be the culprit. For more on why my approach to keto doesn't include dairy, head over to page 99.

 FOCUS ON FOOD QUALITY

Your body is your cup, and every day you eat to fill it up. Imagine if, at the end of the day, all of the less-nourishing foods were removed from your cup. So instead of being filled to the brim, your cup is now only half full, because half of the food you ate that day was nutritionally less than optimal. Instead of providing your body with a full cup of nutrients, you supplied it with half of what it needs.

Our goal, then, is to fill our cup only with nourishing foods, so that, at the end of the day, nothing is taken away from the cup.

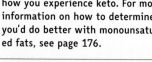 **EAT LESS ANIMAL PROTEIN (OR NONE!)**

You may thrive on more of a plant-based approach to your eating style, and even though some keto "experts" would advise against it, I think you're the best judge of how your body thrives, not a stranger on the internet. If you decide to be a keto vegan, a keto vegetarian, or keto pes-catarian, it's completely doable. The Fat Fueled Food Pyramid (page 85) offers ample plant-based proteins so that you can thrive where you feel best.

ADJUST YOUR MACROS

By adjusting your ratio of fat, carbohydrate, and protein, you'll get a better sense of what your body responds to best. Even a slight variation in protein can mean ending sugar cravings. Increasing your fat intake by as little as 10 grams per day can mean the difference between daily headaches and no headaches at all.

CYCLICALLY INCREASING PROTEIN OR CARBS

Our bodies are built to adapt to changes in our environment, and we can actually thrive in a state of change, even though it may be a bit mentally challenging to embrace. Diet is no different. Keeping our bodies in the same metabolic state day in and day out can be taxing on our mental, physical, emotional, and psychological well-being.

Varying your carbohydrate and/or protein intake can allow you more dietary freedom, make it easier for you to follow a ketogenic protocol, reset your hormone levels to boost fat-burning, and help you to conquer stubborn weight-loss plateaus. We'll cover cycling more in the coming pages.

The ebb and flow of your body demands an ebb and flow to your diet. Making any or all of these changes may lead to success, or it may not. It's up to you to assess and adjust as you see fit. Knowing that there is wiggle room could make all the difference to how you feel on keto.

Cyclical Keto for Ketogenic Women

No one style of keto is better than the rest, and all will lead you to fat-burning if you've chosen the right one for you. Which one you choose is entirely in your power, and that's why we're here: so I can help lead you to the one that'll make you thrive. Now, figuring out what's what can be a little bit of a challenge, and that's why I created Fat Fueled Profiles—keto templates that'll act as jumping-off points and that offer slightly different approaches to keto based on your dietary needs and goals.

But before we get to the individual profiles, there's one aspect of them that you need to understand, and that is the concept of cycling in and out of your ketogenic diet by adjusting your protein or carbohydrate intake.

When you practice cyclical keto, you adjust your carbohydrates or protein in order to do one or more of the following:

1. Completely remove yourself from a ketogenic state

2. Increase autophagy (cell turnover)

3. Reset your hormone levels

4. Balance your appetite

5. Bust through a weight-loss plateau

INCREASE Carbs on Keto? That Can't Be Right

There's no way you can stay in ketosis, reach your full fat-burning potential *and* eat carbs...is there?

While eating too much carbohydrate may be quite damaging to our bodies, strategically consuming small amounts on top of our usual target for carbs can actually aid us on our ketogenic journey. In fact, once you're fat adapted, your metabolism has become more flexible, and you should be able to jump from burning glucose to burning fat and back again without it affecting your fat-burning capabilities.

You see, glucose is necessary for key bodily functions, including converting thyroid hormone to its active form—which in turn is necessary for regulating the metabolism, maintaining energy levels, and keeping digestion regular. Glucose is also fuel for the brain and red blood cells. While it is true that even in ketosis the body can create glucose to meet these needs, the occasional intake of carbs can still be really beneficial.

If you're nervous about the carb angle, don't worry. Having an apple at dinner never hurt anyone. Remember, just because you're eating carbs doesn't mean you're going to stop burning fat. There's a huge difference between burning fat and generating ketones. Yes, your ketones may dip when you eat more carbs, but that doesn't change your metabolic state overnight. Just as it took you time to become fat adapted, it would take time to get out of your fat-burning state. All we're doing here is adjusting your macros for a short period of time and then going right back to your usual targets! So, in a cyclical keto practice where carbohydrates are increased, your body simply burns the glucose you ingest when your carbs go up and then jumps right back into ketosis. How quickly it happens depends entirely upon how many carbs you eat, what types of carbs they are, and the duration of the higher-carb period.

Types of Cyclical Keto

There are six basic approaches to cyclical ketosis: Dipping Out of Ketosis, Carb Backloading, Carb Days, Protein Fasting, Protein-Ups, and Carb-Ups. The one that's best for you depends on your health goals, the current state of your body, and your carbohydrate tolerance. Any one or a combination of these practices will help make your keto lifestyle sustainable for the long term.

Dipping Out of Ketosis: You take your body out of a ketogenic state and stay out for one to two weeks. This process is generally repeated every twelve weeks or so. Since you should be fat adapted at this point, one to two weeks out of ketosis isn't going to undo the work you've done. However, it's still important to try to stick to healthful carbohydrate options (which we'll talk about on page 192).

Macros: 50% fat, 30% protein, 20% carbs

Who it's good for: Nonathletes who require consistent energy output, women of reproductive age, people without sensitive relationships to food

Who it's not good for: Those who have a poor relationship with food or go crazy for things like cheat days or "free weekends"—the more time you spend eating carbs, the further you offset your fat adaptation and the harder it'll be to get back into ketosis. Also stay away from this option if you're insulin resistant or dealing with any other type of blood sugar dysregulation, if you have PCOS, if you are looking to lose weight quickly, or if you want to stay in a constant ketogenic state.

Carb Backloading: You eat low-carb, high-fat until after an extremely heavy lift, at which point you eat a ton of carbs. The idea behind this approach is that it supports significant advances at the gym. The standard approach for carb backloading is to consume junk food to get the best results. But women generally do better focusing on healthful carbohydrate options (we'll talk about those on page 192). Ideally, you want to eat so many carbs during the refeed period that you don't get back into ketosis until the following evening. This is how you know you've had enough during the refeed. For female heavy lifters, I advise using this strategy only twice a week, not every time you lift. Reserve it for the really heavy lifts of the week.

Macros: 10% fat, 20% protein, 70% carbs

(Basically, the heavier you lift, the higher your carbs.)

Who it's good for: Women who have prioritized gym gains over everything else

Who it's not good for: Those who are insulin resistant or dealing with any other type of blood sugar dysregulation, those with PCOS, those who don't lift, those who want to stay in a constant ketogenic state

Carb Days: Every seven to fourteen days, you have one full day of eating whatever you want. You'll know you've had the right amount of carbohydrates when it takes no more than forty-eight hours to get back to the ketone level you had before the carb day.

Macros: Indulge in some carbs, whatever your macros may be.

Who it's good for: Those who have no emotional attachment to the concept of a cheat day, those who aren't doing keto to lose weight, and those who are massively fat adapted

Who it's not good for: Those who are insulin resistant or dealing with any other type of blood sugar dysregulation, those with PCOS, those with disordered eating tendencies, those who want to stay in a constant ketogenic state

Protein Fasting: After doing keto for six days, for one day you eat less than 15 grams of protein while consuming as much fat and carbs as you like. Afterward, you jump back into keto for another six days. The idea behind this approach is that it can reduce inflammation, help you bust through a plateau after you've been doing keto for a while, and increase autophagy (more about that on page 139).

If you try this approach, for best results, I'd suggest breaking up the fast day into two parts, consuming mostly fat for the first half and mostly carbs for the second half. In the morning and afternoon, your macros would be 95 percent fat, 0 percent protein, and 5 percent carbs. In the evening, they'd be 40 percent fat, 0 percent protein, and 60 percent carbs. (Even though you can eat up to 15 grams of protein, it works out to 0 percent because 15 grams of protein isn't a lot.)

Keep in mind that eating under 15 grams of protein for a day is easier said than done. Many foods that you wouldn't think are high in protein—broccoli, for example—actually contain good amounts of protein. Also, the FDA allows companies to label anything with less than 1 gram of protein per serving as having zero grams. So even if you're reading labels closely, you could be consuming enough protein to exceed the 15-gram daily limit.

Macros: The only thing you care about here is eating less than 15 grams of protein (but see my suggestions above).

Who it's good for: Those who are chronically inflamed and those who are using keto for disease prevention

Who it's not good for: Pregnant or breastfeeding women; people who want to stay in a constant ketogenic state. I'd also advise against this strategy if you have any blood sugar dysregulation issues or PCOS, unless you keep your carbs low during the first half of the day, focusing primarily on fats, and then shift to carbohydrates in the evening. However, even this adjustment could make you feel unwell.

Fatty acids are broken down via a process called beta-oxidation (an enzymatic process that gets stronger the longer you eat keto) to form a molecule called acetyl-CoA.

When you follow a ketogenic diet, this acetyl-CoA is used in the Krebs cycle—the process that produces energy within cells—to synthesize ketone bodies. In contrast, when you eat a carbohydrate-rich diet, this same acetyl-CoA needs to be further broken down via the Krebs cycle before it can be used to produce energy.

Deaminated amino acids (imagine these as singular proteins that have been torn apart by the liver and are ready to be utilized) that are ketogenic, such as leucine, also feed the Krebs cycle, forming acetoacetate and acetyl-CoA, and thereby promote ketones, too!

The fact that amino acids are used by the Krebs cycle supports the theory that nutritional ketosis should be practiced in a cyclical action, whereby your protein intake is adjusted to support the production of ketones. So if your usual protein intake is on the low side (determine this using the signs on page 130), a cyclical keto practice that boosts protein can raise your ketone levels.

Protein-Ups: This approach is the opposite of a protein fast: instead of limiting protein for one day, you increase it well beyond your norm, up to 60 percent of your total daily calories. Protein-ups are great when practiced every once in a while to accelerate weight loss or bust through a stubborn plateau. Another name for this approach is a "carnivore diet," which is a keto-based diet that focuses on protein and fat from animal sources only.

The additional protein encourages your body to use more fat for fuel, break through stubborn weight-loss plateaus, and accelerate healing, without relying on carbohydrates. And, because the body has to use more energy to metabolize protein, you effectively burn an extra 25 percent of the calories you ingest that day.

Macros: 40% fat, 60% protein, 0% carbs

Who it's good for: Those who find that the carb-up approach (see the facing page) stimulates intense hunger

Who it's not good for: Vegans and vegetarians may have a difficult time with this one, just because the protein requirements are so high.

Carb-Ups: Carbohydrates are increased and fat is decreased during your last meal of the day. Carb-ups can be practiced every day, every other day, once a week, once a month—whatever you prefer.

How often you boost your ketogenic diet with a carb-up will determine how many carbs you should have in each one. The key to a successful carb-up is to think of your fat intake as inversely proportional to your carb intake. So if you're increasing your carb intake for the evening, then you're also going to reduce your fat intake.

Macros: 10% to 50% fat, 15% protein, and 35% to 75% carbs (depending on how often you carb up—head to page 194 for help in calculating your macros for a carb-up)

Who it's good for: Anyone experiencing ongoing symptoms from keto, such as poor sleep quality, thyroid dysregulation, low body temperature, unstable appetite, hair loss, or imbalanced hormones. Carb-ups are also good for people looking to lose a lot of weight and those who've hit a weight-loss plateau, as carb-ups will shrink fat cells, create more muscle mass, and help you shed more fat and get leaner. Anaerobic athletes whose training has been negatively affected by ketosis will benefit from carb-ups, too.

What's more, carb-ups allow you to enjoy the food you like, such as fruit, without falling off the wagon—making social situations way easier.

And since carb-ups are the only cyclical ketogenic practice that will keep your ketone level steady, they're a great option for someone who wants to remain in a ketogenic state for good.

Who it's not good for: Those who've tried carb-ups and, for whatever reason, just don't like them

I also advise caution if you are insulin-resistant or dealing with any other type of blood sugar dysregulation or if you have PCOS. Carb-ups can work for you, too, but be very careful of the amount of carbs you consume.

Carb-Ups: Made for **Women**

As you can see, there are numerous ways to change up your macros on keto. Some of them will work for you, others won't. Because you're a woman on keto who (I'm assuming) has completed steps 1 and 2 of the process outlined in this book, I'm just about certain that the strategy you'll find most effective is the carb-up. Why? Because it's a perfect balance of adding variation, not going overboard, staying balanced, being in control, having a healthy relationship with carbs, and boosting your nutrient intake.

Benefits of Carb-Ups

Because carb-ups are practiced at the end of the day, they offer a host of unique benefits. An evening carb-up will:

Replenish your systems. When you're fat adapted and consume a touch of carbs in the evening, your body uses the glucose to support your endocrine, muscular, and nervous systems—and then slides back into ketosis by morning. While the metabolism does slow down during sleep, this only applies to fat and protein. Carbohydrate metabolization stays steady and then increases before you wake up. Meaning, your fear of eating carbohydrates before bed is officially *busted*.

Provide better sleep and more serotonin. Eating carbs at night increases the brain's uptake of tryptophan, which is used to produce melatonin, the sleep hormone. Tryptophan also boosts serotonin, which leads to improved sleep, mood, weight loss, fat loss, exercise recovery, and immune health. What's more, better sleep means better insulin and leptin sensitivity. And, speaking of sleep, you'll dream right through the brain fog, blood sugar spike and crash, and cravings that often result from consuming carbs.

Build muscles. If you work out in the evening, a carb-up is the perfect post-workout go-to. Your insulin will send the glucose from the carb-up straight to your muscles to aid in recovery and growth.

Encourage a weight-loss whoosh. When we shed weight, fat is removed from our fat cells and replaced with water. So even though you may have lost inches, your weight can remain unchanged. But carbs bind to water—every gram of carb needs 4 grams of water—and this is where carb-ups come into play. The carbs we eat pull the water from our fat cells, and a couple days later we get a whoosh of weight loss, rocketing us past a plateau.

You're probably beginning to see why I love carb-ups so much.

Good Things About Eating Carbs at Night	Bad Things About Eating Carbs in the Morning
• Avoidance of brain fog, blood sugar spike, and energy crash • Accelerated weight loss • Fewer cravings, which leads to better nutrition choices • Ability to mobilize and burn fat all day long • Improved leptin sensitivity, which means less hunger • Facilitated fat loss and muscle retention • Increased tryptophan uptake in the brain for functional sleep • Boosted serotonin levels for improved sleep duration and quality, increased weight/fat loss, faster post-workout recovery, and improved immune health • Increased insulin sensitivity	• Further increase in already-elevated glucose and insulin levels • Ongoing hunger throughout the day as we ride the blood sugar roller coaster from meal to meal • More incidents of brain fog • Complete halt of the natural morning fat-burning process • Decrease in the body's ability to access fat stores for energy throughout the day • Fatigue and energy crashes as your body continues to crave a quick glucose fix throughout the day • Increased tendency to eat carbs all day

Are You Ready for a Carb-Up?

So, are you ready for a carb-up? Good question.

The answer is different for keto newbies and keto veterans. By now, if you've followed steps 1 and 2, you can consider yourself ready for a carb-up.

But if you're a keener and are reading this whole book before you get started with step 1, please read on to determine whether or not you're ready.

Keep in mind that carb-ups aren't mandatory. Some people do better without them, while others need to carb up one, a few, or even seven days a week. For example, I've found that women need carb-ups more often than men, likely because our hormonal landscape is more complex.

But with all this in mind, you're ready for a carb-up when you can say yes to at least three of the following:

- You test your ketones and they're higher than 1.5 mmol/L for more than five days in a row.
- You can skip meals without getting angry.
- It's easy to go three, four, or five hours without a snack.
- You don't get ravenous or crave carbs two to three hours after your last meal.
- You crave high-fat foods over high-carb foods.
- You don't need carbs to push through exercise plateaus.
- You experience steady energy throughout the day, without afternoon crashes.
- Your thoughts seem clearer and more focused.
- You no longer experience keto flu.
- You've been practicing strict keto (low-carb, high-fat intake) for more than four weeks.
- You have been low-carb for more than four weeks and have developed bingeing tendencies.
- You are a woman.
- Your hair is falling out on strict keto.
- You've been practicing keto for a little while and find that you're never hungry.
- You have hit a weight-loss plateau.
- You've been having a hard time sleeping since adopting strict keto.
- You lift weights one or more times per week (regardless of the duration of your workouts).
- You enjoy going out for dinner with friends.
- You have adrenal dysfunction.
- You have a thyroid imbalance (specifically hypothyroidism).
- You are looking to heal and balance your hormones (estrogen, progesterone, testosterone, HGH, DHEA).

Your exercise regimen can tell you a lot as well. If you're not getting the results you want, can't seem to put on muscle, or can't maintain even a moderate intensity while training, it's time for a carb-up.

What to Eat and How to Make It, Carb-Up Style

When you move from strict keto to incorporating carb-ups, what you eat changes slightly, and that affects how you prepare a dish. So let's revisit the guidelines from chapter 4 to see what's different!

Adjusting the Fat Fueled Food Pyramid

Remember the Fat Fueled Food Pyramid on page 85? Incorporating carb-ups into your keto life changes the pyramid—new foods are added, and the amounts change somewhat.

It can be helpful to think of two pyramids, one for days where carb-ups are practiced and one for the week as a whole, so you can see the big picture.

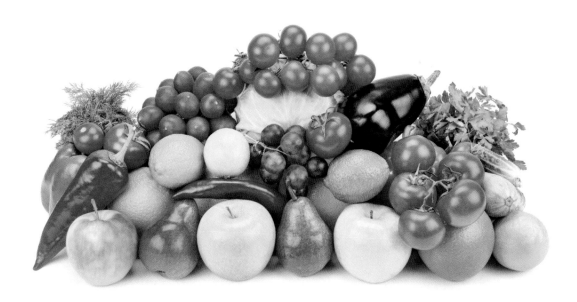

Fat Fueled Food Pyramid: On the Day You Carb Up

On days when you have a carb-up in the evening, this is what your full day of eating would look like.

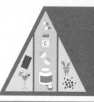

THE EXTRAS

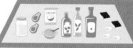

HEALTHY FATS

PROTEIN

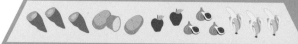

NON-STARCHY VEGETABLES

STARCHES AND FRUITS

WATER

THE EXTRAS

- **Indulgences:** alcohol, dark chocolate, sweeteners, whole-food keto treats
- **Supportive supplements:** multivitamins, omega-3s, probiotics, superfood powders
- **Dried herbs and spices:** basil, oregano, red pepper flakes
- **Fresh herbs:** cilantro, parsley
- **Condiments:** apple cider vinegar, ketchup, mustard

STARCHES AND FRUITS

- Apples, bananas, figs, plantains, potatoes, sweet potatoes

PROTEIN

- **Plant-based:** natto, nuts, seeds, tempeh
- **Animal-based:** bone broth, collagen, eggs, fatty fish, free-range chicken, grass-fed beef, organ meats, pasture-raised pork

NON-STARCHY VEGETABLES

- Broccoli, Brussels sprouts, cabbage, cauliflower, greens, onions

HEALTHY FATS

- **Plant-based:** avocado oil, avocados, coconut cream, coconut oil, olive oil
- **Animal-based:** duck fat, ghee (if you're not sensitive to dairy), lard, tallow

WATER

Fat Fueled Food Pyramid: Weekly Snapshot

If you're incorporating carb-ups two to three times per week, here's what the pyramid looks like as an overall summary of your week.

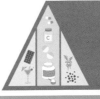
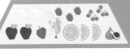
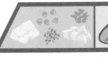

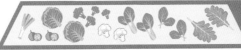
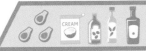
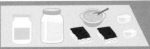

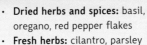

THE EXTRAS

STARCHES AND FRUITS

PROTEIN

NON-STARCHY VEGETABLES

HEALTHY FATS

WATER

THE EXTRAS

- **Indulgences:** alcohol, dark chocolate, sweeteners, whole-food keto treats
- **Supportive supplements:** multivitamins, omega-3s, probiotics, superfood powders
- **Dried herbs and spices:** basil, oregano, red pepper flakes
- **Fresh herbs:** cilantro, parsley
- **Condiments:** apple cider vinegar, ketchup, mustard

STARCHES AND FRUITS

- **Daily:** berries, grapefruit, lemons, limes
- **Carb-ups:** apples, bananas, figs, plantains, potatoes, sweet potatoes

PROTEIN

- **Plant-based:** natto, nuts, seeds, tempeh
- **Animal-based:** bone broth, collagen, eggs, fatty fish, free-range chicken, grass-fed beef, organ meats, pasture-raised pork

NON-STARCHY VEGETABLES

- Broccoli, Brussels sprouts, cabbage, cauliflower, greens, onions

HEALTHY FATS

- **Plant-based:** avocado oil, avocados, coconut cream, coconut oil, olive oil
- **Animal-based:** duck fat, ghee (if you're not sensitive to dairy), lard, tallow

WATER

FOR YOUR CARB-UP, PICK FROM THESE HEALTHY HIGHER-CARB OPTIONS

STARCHES

Acorn squash
Arrowroot
Cassava flour
Cassava/yucca root/manioc
Delicata squash
Green banana flour
Green plantains
Kabocha squash
Parsnips
Potatoes
Sweet potatoes
Tapioca starch
White rice*
Yams

FRUITS

Apples
Apricots
Bananas
Cherries
Dates
Figs
Grapes
Kiwi
Melons
Oranges
Pears

SWEETENERS

Coconut sugar
Pure maple syrup
Raw honey
Yacón syrup

Grains don't work well for everyone.

REVISITING HOW TO MAKE IT

Think of a carb-up as one of the following three meal choices, enjoyed in the evening:

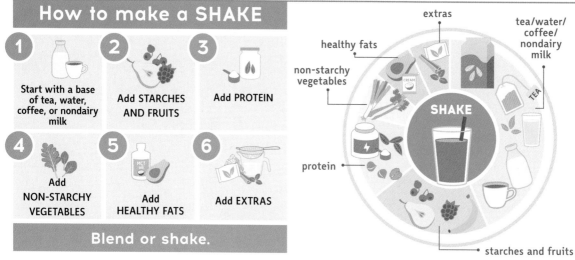

How to make a SHAKE

1 Start with a base of tea, water, coffee, or nondairy milk

2 Add STARCHES AND FRUITS

3 Add PROTEIN

4 Add NON-STARCHY VEGETABLES

5 Add HEALTHY FATS

6 Add EXTRAS

Blend or shake.

Examples	Bananarama Smoothie	
	Base	Almond milk
	Starches and Fruits	Banana
	Protein	Collagen
	Non-starchy Veg.	Spinach
	Healthy Fats	None
	Extras	Ground cinnamon, pure maple syrup

Creamy Perfection Shake	
Base	Lite coconut milk
Starches and Fruits	Dates
Protein	Walnuts
Non-starchy Veg.	None
Healthy Fats	None
Extras	Pure vanilla extract

Sweet Tea Smoothie	
Base	Chilled herbal tea
Starches and Fruits	Grapes, banana
Protein	Hemp seeds
Non-starchy Veg.	None
Healthy Fats	Yogurt
Extras	None

How to make a HOT MEAL

1 Choose **STARCHES & FRUITS**

2 Choose **PROTEIN**

3 Choose **NON-STARCHY VEGETABLES**

4 Choose **HEALTHY FATS**

5 Choose **EXTRAS**

Heat the healthy fat in a pan. Add the starches and protein, and cook until fork-tender and cooked through. Add any fruits, non-starchy vegetables, and extras and sauté for a couple moments longer. You can also approach these options as soups or stews, or cook items separately for better presentation.

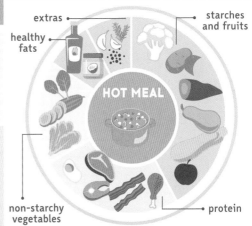

extras
healthy fats
HOT MEAL
starches and fruits
non-starchy vegetables
protein

Examples

Cassava and Pork Chops with Spiced Veggies

Starches & Fruits	Steamed cassava
Protein	Pork chop
Non-starchy Veg.	Bell peppers, cabbage
Healthy Fats	Coconut oil
Extras	Paprika, garlic, salt

Rosemary Chicken and Sweet Potato

Starches & Fruits	Sweet potato
Protein	Chicken
Non-starchy Veg.	Kale
Healthy Fats	Avocado oil
Extras	Rosemary, salt

Sweet Sausages and Squash

Starches & Fruits	Delicata squash
Protein	Pork sausages
Non-starchy Veg.	Bok choy
Healthy Fats	None
Extras	Coconut aminos, pure maple syrup

How to make a COLD MEAL

1 Choose **STARCHES & FRUITS**

2 Choose **PROTEIN**

3 Choose **NON-STARCHY VEGETABLES**

4 Choose **HEALTHY FATS**

5 Choose **EXTRAS**

Combine the liquid ingredients in a large salad bowl. Stir to combine, then add the remaining ingredients and toss to coat.

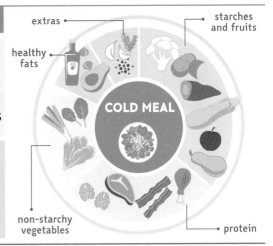

extras
healthy fats
COLD MEAL
starches and fruits
non-starchy vegetables
protein

Examples

Balsamic Sprouts and Chicken Bowl

Starches & Fruits	Cooked & cooled white rice, pears
Protein	Chicken
Non-starchy Veg.	Brussels sprouts
Healthy Fats	Olive oil
Extras	Balsamic vinegar, oregano, salt, pepper

Triple Green Salad

Starches & Fruits	Cooked & cooled acorn squash, apple
Protein	Walnuts
Non-starchy Veg.	Lettuce, celery, steamed and cooled broccoli
Healthy Fats	Avocados
Extras	None

Sweet Potato & Fig Spinach Salad

Starches & Fruits	Cooked & cooled sweet potatoes, figs
Protein	None
Non-starchy Veg.	Spinach, shallots
Healthy Fats	Olive oil, macadamia nuts
Extras	Fresh thyme, salt

The Nitty-Gritty: How to Carb Up

If you decide that cyclical ketosis has a role in your ketogenic diet and you want to give carb-ups a try, here is a helpful chart for determining how many carbs to consume *during your carb-up*. These carbohydrates aren't to be distributed throughout the day—they're for your carb-up meal *only*.

Calculating Carb-Ups

The easiest way to go about incorporating carb-ups into your life is to just eat keto at breakfast and lunch, as you have been up to this point, and at dinner, remove most of the fat from your meal and replace it with the amount of carbs that match your weight and carb-up frequency in the chart on the facing page. Easy.

To use the chart, first decide how many times per week or per month you want to carb up, then find the column in the chart that's closest to that frequency. Then find your body weight in the left-hand column and slide along the row until you find the carb-up amount that aligns with the number of times you'll be carbing up.

The Fat Fueled Profiles (page 198) include guidelines for how often to carb up. If you want to try carbing up on your own, without following a profile, a simple rule of thumb is to carb up every one to four days.

But if you want to get *complicated*, and you love precision, let me show you how you could calculate the macros and calories for your carb-up. This practice is really helpful if you use a tracking app and the very thought of having different macros during the day and at night is making your head spin. Basically, you want to know how to combine your daytime macros and goals with your carb-up macros and goals.

The best way to show you how to calculate macros for carb-ups is to provide an example:

Let's say you weigh 150 pounds and you have decided that you're going to carb up two to three times a week. According to the chart, you will need 75 grams of carbs in your carb-up. (Remember, that's *just* for your carb-up, not for the day as a whole.)

Let's also say your target macros are 80 percent fat, 15 percent protein, and 5 percent carbohydrate. Assuming you eat 1,800 calories per day, you generally eat about 160 grams of fat, 68 grams of protein, and 22 grams of carbohydrates when you are *not* having a carb-up.

Because you are doing a carb-up, let's figure out how many calories you'll need to set aside for the carb-up. There are 4 calories in every gram of carbohydrate, so the 75 grams of carb in your carb-up equals 300 calories.

		How Many Carbs to Include in Your Carb-Up			
		when carbing up **EVERY DAY**	when carbing up **2 TO 3 TIMES A WEEK**	when carbing up **ONCE A WEEK**	when carbing up **ONCE EVERY 2 WEEKS**
Body Weight (lbs)	**Body Weight (kg)**	**1/4 g carb** per 1 lb (0.45 kg)	**1/2 g carb** per 1 lb (0.45 kg)	**3/4 g carb** per 1 lb (0.45 kg)	**1 g carb** per 1 lb (0.45 kg)
120	54	30 g	60 g	90 g	120 g
125	57	31 g	63 g	94 g	125 g
130	59	33 g	65 g	98 g	130 g
135	61	34 g	68 g	101 g	135 g
140	64	35 g	70 g	105 g	140 g
145	66	36 g	73 g	109 g	145 g
150	68	38 g	75 g	113 g	150 g
155	70	39 g	78 g	116 g	155 g
160	73	40 g	80 g	120 g	160 g
165	75	41 g	83 g	124 g	165 g
170	77	43 g	85 g	128 g	170 g
175	79	44 g	88 g	131 g	175 g
180	82	45 g	90 g	135 g	180 g
185	84	46 g	93 g	139 g	185 g
190	86	48 g	95 g	143 g	190 g
195	88	49 g	98 g	146 g	195 g
200	91	50 g	100 g	150 g	200 g
205	93	51 g	103 g	154 g	205 g
210	95	53 g	105 g	158 g	210 g
215	98	54 g	108 g	161 g	215 g
220	100	55 g	110 g	165 g	220 g
225	102	56 g	113 g	169 g	225 g
230	104	58 g	115 g	173 g	230 g
235	107	59 g	118 g	176 g	235 g
240	109	60 g	120 g	180 g	240 g
245	111	61 g	123 g	184 g	245 g
250	113	63 g	125 g	188 g	250 g
255	116	64 g	128 g	191 g	255 g
260	118	65 g	130 g	195 g	260 g
265	120	66 g	133 g	199 g	265 g
270	122	68 g	135 g	203 g	270 g
275	125	69 g	138 g	206 g	275 g
280	127	70 g	140 g	210 g	280 g
285	129	71 g	143 g	214 g	285 g
290	132	73 g	145 g	218 g	290 g
295	134	74 g	148 g	221 g	295 g
300	136	75 g	150 g	225 g	300 g

Of course, you're going to be eating protein and fat at your carb-up meal, too. **No matter how many grams of carbs you have in your carb-up, for most people, an acceptable starting-off point for fat and protein during a carb-up meal is 15 grams of fat (135 calories) and 30 grams of protein (120 calories).** You may find that these amounts fluctuate, but for the purpose of calculating for your first couple of carb-ups, these are the numbers you can use.

So you will need 300 calories of carb in your carb-up, plus 135 calories of fat, plus 120 calories of protein. That's 555 calories needed for your carb-up meal.

Going back to your daily calorie goal of 1,800: subtract 555 (the calories needed for your carb-up meal) from 1,800, and you get 1,245 calories left for the rest of the day. So your breakfast and lunch will have a macro goal of 80 percent fat, 15 percent protein, and 5 percent carbohydrates, with a calorie goal of 1,245.

If you're using an app to track your macros, punch 1,245 calories into your app for the day and try to hit that for breakfast and lunch with your macro goal of 80 percent fat, 15 percent protein, and 5 percent carbohydrates. Once lunch is done, go back into the app and add 75 grams of carbohydrates, 15 grams of fat, and 30 grams of protein to the day's goal. Voilà, you have your carb-up goals and macros in your app!

Another way to do this is to treat your carb-up dinner as a separate day, tracking your breakfast and lunch as day 1 and your dinner as day 2. This way, your macros will be separated and you can clearly see the separation.

Here are the calculations you can use to determine the above with your own numbers:

1. _____ (A) = how many carbohydrate grams you will consume in your carb-up (see the chart on page 195)

2. (A) x 4 = _____ (B) = how many carbohydrate calories you will consume in your carb-up

3. _____ (C) = how many total calories you aim to eat in a day

4. (C) – (B) – 135 – 120 = (D) = how many calories you aim to eat for breakfast and lunch before your carb-up

5. (B) + 135 + 120 = (E) = how many calories total you'll aim to eat for your carb-up

Plan Not to Plan

If you're coming from a diet mentality, it's likely that you have become really good at creating lists of everything you can and cannot have, and I'm guessing that having these buckets of "good" and "bad" foods has led to occasional bingeing in the past. For example, you go on a diet for two weeks and do really well, but then you find yourself face-deep in a carton of ice cream and swear that tomorrow will be the start of something awesome. But four days later, you once again find yourself face-deep in that same ice cream carton.

If I've just described the last five years of your life, you need to really pay attention, because *what I'm about to tell you is very, very important*:

Do not plan your carb-ups. Do not pick a day when you intend to carb up, do not create a list of all the foods you're going to eat for your carb-up, do not mentally or physically plan for your carb-up and then look forward to it every waking moment until the time has finally arrived.

By planning when you're going to eat carbs, you're sending a signal to your brain that you're currently in "restriction mode" and there will be a big feast soon. In my own experience, beginning from a place of restriction and then opening the floodgates and allowing myself to pound the carbs for one day a week led me down a dark path of emotional eating. I was able to regain control before it got out of hand, but it's definitely not a path I want you to go down yourself.

Take Action to Avoid Binge-like Carb-Ups!

If you find yourself planning and looking forward to carb-ups, making lists of the carbs you're going to eat, or feeling restricted day to day, try these tips.

Check in with yourself. Ask yourself what you're feeling and what planning your carb-ups means to you—anticipating freedom from restriction, feeling in control, finding an outlet for or distraction from other things going on in your life....

Make your carb-up a night out with friends. Eating carbs around friends keeps us feeling "normal" and helps eliminate a feeling of restriction, which can otherwise lead to emotional eating and bingeing. When your emotional needs are being met in the company of good friends, you're more likely to lose yourself in the moment and less likely to have an emotional response to eating.

Go with the flow. You don't have to have a carb-up on the same day every week. Perhaps you've aimed for a carb-up every three days, but on day 3 you're not feeling it. In that case, hold out until day 4 to see how you feel. And vice versa—if you're only at day 2 but desperately feel like you need carbs, have some carbs.

And if the concept of carbing up a few times a week is stressing you out, have carb-ups less often or cut them out completely for a while.

Welcome to
Fat Fueled Profiles

So now that you understand what cyclical ketosis is and how carb-ups can play a role in your ketogenic diet, it's time to decide on a Fat Fueled Profile.

There are multiple ways to approach keto, and none of them are wrong. Fat Fueled Profiles (FFPs) are five unique templates that I've developed over the years to show you the different ways your keto diet could look. Finding a profile that you resonate with and adjusting it to suit your needs can make a world of difference for you, but it isn't required. If you already have a good handle on how to eat keto and what works well for your body, carry on! FFPs are just here to make your life easier.

Signs an FFP Could Be Right for You

✓ You like being told exactly what you need to do.

✓ You enjoy following a template.

✓ You're not fully confident that you'll be able to listen to your body, and you'd prefer having a clear path to follow.

✓ You're tired of what you're doing now.

✓ What you're doing now isn't working: you still have goals to hit, and you have no idea how you'll hit them.

✓ You like adding variety to your diet.

✓ You have a specific health imbalance and hope keto will improve your symptoms, but you need to be extra careful about your macros.

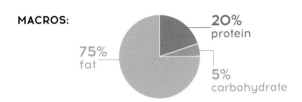

CLASSIC KETO

MACROS:

- 20% protein
- 5% carbohydrate
- 75% fat

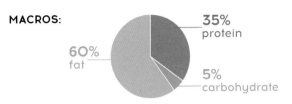

PUMPED KETO

MACROS:

- 35% protein
- 5% carbohydrate
- 60% fat

This low-carbohydrate, moderate-protein, high-fat approach is a strict keto diet—and the foundation of the rest of the Fat Fueled Profiles.

Who It's Good For:

- Those who are in the process of becoming fat adapted
- Sedentary or less-active individuals
- Those seeking weight loss
- Those without hormonal imbalances
- Menopausal and postmenopausal women
- Aerobic athletes
- Anyone whose health-care team has recommended a strict ketogenic approach

Changing FFPs: If you begin to feel like you need more carbs, switch over to the Full Keto profile. If you begin to feel like you need more protein, switch over to the Pumped Keto profile.

This profile includes more protein and less fat than Classic Keto. This is a fabulous option for those who are not interested in doing carb-ups but don't feel quite right on Classic Keto.

If you don't want to commit to this eating style full-time, you can treat it as a "protein-up" plan. Instead of following it full-time, aim for the Pumped Keto macros in just one meal or over the course of a single day. (See page 184 for more on protein-ups.)

Who It's Good For:

- Hypoglycemic individuals
- Those who experience dysregulated blood sugar or cortisol imbalances on Classic Keto after becoming fat adapted
- Those who don't feel quite right on Classic Keto but are not interested in doing carb-ups
- Those who experience constant hunger on Classic Keto
- Those who are struggling to break through weight-loss plateaus

Changing FFPs: If you begin to feel like you need more carbs, switch over to the Full Keto profile. If you find you can't eat this much protein or feel like it's standing in the way of your success, switch over to the Classic Keto profile.

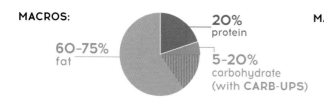

fk) FULL KETO

MACROS:

60–75% fat

20% protein

5–20% carbohydrate (with **CARB-UPS**)

afb) ADAPTED FAT BURNER

MACROS:

60–75% fat

20% protein

5–20% carbohydrate (with **CARB-UPS**)

With Full Keto, carb-ups happen weekly. You can time your carb-ups to correspond with anaerobic workouts if you like.

This profile is great if you're already fat adapted. If you're not yet fat adapted, start with Classic Keto or Pumped Keto. Once adapted, c'mon over to Full Keto!

Who It's Good For:

- Those with no health imbalances who engage in anaerobic activity one to three times per week

- Those who are sedentary

- Those who are interested in pairing weight loss with physical training

- Those trying to break through a weight-loss plateau

- Those with dysregulated blood sugar or insulin resistance

Carbing Up: Once you're fat adapted, start carbing up once a week, preferably at night—see the chart on page 195 for how many carbs to eat in your carb-up. If you feel like you need carb-ups two to three times a week, shift to the Adapted Fat Burner profile (at right). If you feel like you need carb-ups more than three times a week, shift to the Daily Fat Burner profile (page 201).

With the Adapted Fat Burner profile, carb-ups happen two to three times per week. You can time your carb-ups to correspond with anaerobic workouts if you like.

This profile is great if you're already fat adapted. If you're not yet fat adapted, start with Classic Keto or Pumped Keto. Once adapted, c'mon over to Adapted Fat Burner!

Who It's Good For:

- Those with minimal health imbalances who engage in anaerobic activity three to seven times per week

- Those interested in pairing weight loss with physical training

- Those with minor health imbalances that don't influence hormone levels, such as minor inflammation, energy inconsistencies, or digestive complications like IBS

If you have minor health imbalances but are not active, Classic Keto or Full Keto may be the best options for you.

Carbing Up: Once you're fat adapted, start carbing up two to three times a week, always at night—see the chart on page 195 for how many carbs to eat in your carb-up. If you feel like you need carb-ups more than three times a week, shift to the Daily Fat Burner profile (page 201).

The Full Keto, Adapted Fat Burner, and Daily Fat Burner profiles all pair very well with intermittent fasting (see page 138). Combining carb-ups with fasting helps you maintain high ketone levels while eating foods that make you feel good.

If you're practicing carb-ups for weight loss and you're following the Adapted Fat Burner or Full Keto profile, you may gain a little water weight after a carb-up, but sticking with this practice should enable you to break through a weight-loss plateau and keep losing weight. Just wait until you've dropped below your plateau weight before you do another carb-up.

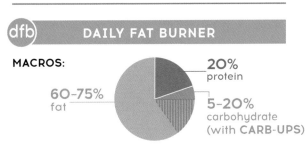

dfb   DAILY FAT BURNER

MACROS:

60-75% fat

20% protein

5-20% carbohydrate (with **CARB-UPS**)

With this profile, you'll start with evening carb-ups right away rather than waiting until you're fully fat adapted. You likely will not experience a ketogenic state in the traditional sense. Although you will be priming your body for fat-burning, you may not register ketones in the first couple of weeks, or ever. But fat adaptation should take hold as you lower the amount of carbohydrates in your carb-ups over time. You can time your carb-ups to correspond with anaerobic workouts if you like.

Who It's Good For:

- Those with health imbalances (for example, thyroid imbalances or adrenal dysfunction)

- Children

- Those who feel extremely restricted on the other profiles

- Vegans

- Those with candida (too much fat may cause a flare-up, so this offers an in-between option)

- Those interested in pairing weight loss with body healing

- Those who enjoy taking things day by day

Carbing Up: As soon as you switch over to the keto diet, start carbing up every night. As long as you feel like having carbs, do it up! See the chart on page 195 for how many carbs you should start with in your carb-ups. As your body becomes better at fat-burning, you may find you don't need as many carbs as when you first started, so you would slowly decrease the frequency or intensity of your carb-ups as you go. If you go more than three or four days without carb-ups at night, shift to the Adapted Fat Burner profile.

There are three Fat Fueled Profiles that incorporate carb-ups: Full Keto, Adapted Fat Burner, and Daily Fat Burner. Here's what makes these profiles different:

- *When you start carbing up once you start eating keto*

- *How often you carb up*

- *How many carbs you eat on a carb-up*

The best time to do a carb-up is after a heavy workout. The ideal scenario is working out in the afternoon and then having a carb-up dinner that swaps carbs for the usual fat.

Which FFP Is Right for Me?

I'm sure you're wondering how to figure out which Fat Fueled Profile you should choose. The goal is to find what works best for you. This will take some trial and error, and that's okay.

Whether you're menopausal, at risk for dementia, have issues with inflammation, or are dealing with another health concern, the questionnaire on the following pages will give you an idea of which FFP may be best for you.

If you have multiple concerns, decide which is the most important to you and start there. Once you have things under control, you can move on to the next concern and the profile recommended for it.

Which profile you do best on depends completely on your body. And once you've decided on an FFP, you can customize your diet and eating style further so they're ideal for you. We'll talk about that in chapters 8 and 9. In the end, you'll have an eating style that works perfectly for you and doesn't require pushing, prodding, and stuffing yourself into a box that doesn't fit your life or your body.

If you've decided that following an FFP feels right for you, there are several ways that you can get started.

1. **Jump right in:** Start with Classic Keto. If that doesn't feel right, play around with increasing protein through Pumped Keto or adding carb-ups through Full Keto. If you go with Full Keto and things still aren't feeling optimal, try switching to Adapted Fat Burner and increasing the number of times you engage in a carb-up every week. If this still doesn't feel great, move to Daily Fat Burner. See which one feels best and run with it for a while.

2. **Be noncommittal:** Start with one FFP, move to another, go back to the first one again. Decide which you'll follow according to how your body feels on any given day. Gradually, through trial and error, you can find a custom combination that works for you and your body.

3. **Keep your health in mind:** If you have a health imbalance, condition, disease, or any other health concern that you're interested in supporting with your Fat Fueled lifestyle, chances are there's a specific FFP that'll work better for you than the others. Review the summaries on pages 199 to 201 to see what profiles are recommended for different concerns.

4. **Take the quiz!** The quiz on the next page may help you determine which approach could be best for you.

Here's how to use the following questionnaire to get a sense of which Fat Fueled Profile would be best for you:

1. If you answer yes to a question, place a check mark in all the blank boxes beside that question.

2. Add up the check marks in each column and enter the result in the row marked "TOTAL."

3. Take the total of each column and multiply as instructed. Weighing your scores helps you prioritize in the event of a tie; your score on Health Status, for instance, should trump your score on Hormone Status, even if you have the same number of check marks for both.

At the end of the questionnaire, you'll have a score for each FFP in each category. Focus on the category with the highest score first. Once you have mastered one category with a particular FFP, it's time to move on to the next.

HEALTH STATUS

	ck	pk	fk	afb	dfb
Are you in cancer recovery?					
Have you been a chronic dieter, eating 1,200 calories off and on for years?					
Did your health-care provider recommend that you go keto?					
Are you breastfeeding?					
Do you have digestive issues such as IBS, sensitivity to FODMAPs, or SIBO?					
Do you have a history of anxiety or depression?					
Do you have a history of, or are you currently suffering from, candida?					
Do you have an autoimmune condition such as Hashimoto's, arthritis, or lupus (not including autoimmune conditions that can make you incredibly tired or type 1 diabetes)?					
Do you have an autoimmune condition that can make you incredibly tired, such as MS, fibromyalgia, or chronic fatigue syndrome?					
Do you have heart health concerns such as high cholesterol and high blood pressure?					
Do you have neurological health concerns such as Alzheimer's disease or Parkinson's disease?					
Do you suffer from blood sugar irregularities such as dysglycemia, hypoglycemia, type 1 or type 2 diabetes, or insulin resistance?					
Has your gallbladder been removed? Or do you have fat absorption issues?					
TOTAL					
multiply the total by 5 for your category score					

RELATIONSHIP WITH FOOD	ck	pk	fk	afb	dfb
Are you easily triggered by weighing or measuring food?	●	●	●	●	
Do you have a history of an eating disorder?	●	●	●	●	
If you have yo-yo dieted, has it led to binges?	●	●	●	●	
TOTAL					
multiply the total by 4 for your category score					

HORMONE STATUS	ck	pk	fk	afb	dfb
Do you have adrenal dysfunction?	●		●	●	●
Are you in menopause or postmenopausal?		●	●	●	●
Are you of reproductive age with no hormone concerns?	●	●		●	●
Are you of reproductive age with hormone concerns such as amenorrhea (lack of period), high estrogen, low progesterone, low DHEA, or low libido (everything except PCOS)?	●	●	●	●	●
Do you have PCOS?	●	●	●	●	●
Do you have Hashimoto's (treated or untreated)?	●	●	●	●	●
Do you have hyperthyroidism (treated or untreated)?	●	●	●	●	●
Do you have hypothyroidism (treated or untreated)?	●	●	●		●
TOTAL					
multiply the total by 3 for your category score					

DIETARY PREFERENCES	ck	pk	fk	afb	dfb
Does eating too many carbs from the Fat Fueled Food Pyramid make you feel weird?	●				
Do you feel better eating more carbs from the Fat Fueled Food Pyramid than protein?	●		●		
Do you feel better eating protein over fat or carbs?	●		●		
If you've tried keto before or you're currently keto, have you felt / do you feel awful even after a couple of weeks?	●		●		
If you've tried keto before or you're currently keto, have you felt / do you feel amazing?	●				
Do you want to start slow, steadily reducing carb consumption day by day?	●				
Are you vegan or vegetarian?	●				
TOTAL					
multiply the total by 2 for your category score					

PHYSICAL ACTIVITY	ck	pk	fk	afb	dfb
If you are already fat adapted, do you primarily practice aerobic activities?		●	●	●	●
If you are already fat adapted, do you primarily practice anaerobic* activities?		●	●	●	●
If this is your first attempt at keto, do you primarily practice aerobic activities?			●	●	●
If this is your first attempt at keto, do you primarily practice anaerobic* activities?	●		●	●	●
Are you pretty sedentary?		●	●	●	●
TOTAL					

*Anaerobic activity is high-intensity training such as HIIT, sprints, heavy weight training, or CrossFit.

Bringing **Movement** into It

There is definitely an argument to be made for fat adaptation in athletes.

The fat-adapted athlete who weighs 150 pounds (68 kilograms) and has 10 percent body fat has the equivalent of 15 pounds of pure fat on their body, which translates to 52,500 calories of available energy.

The glucose-burning athlete who weighs 150 pounds (68 kilograms) and has 10 percent body fat can store around 600 grams of glycogen, which translates to 2,400 calories of available energy.

Let's compare: that's 52,500 available calories in the keto-adapted body versus 2,400 available calories in the sugar-burning body! I'm pretty sure the keto-adapted athlete comes out on top with this one.

However, the benefits of being fat adapted may vary depending on the kind of training you're doing. Aerobic training (also known as cardio), where endurance is required, includes activities like swimming, rowing, boxing, running, or walking. Anaerobic training, where short bursts of energy are required, includes activities like power lifting, resistance band exercises, body weight exercises, and high-intensity interval training (HIIT).

In ketosis, the body finds it easy to access fat for fuel during aerobic training, but it's a bit more challenging during anaerobic training. With anaerobic training, a certain amount of muscle glycogen—glucose stored in the muscles—is *required*. Some ketogenic anaerobic athletes experience no issues whatsoever with their performance, whereas others find they need to increase their intake of carbohydrates whenever they're engaging in anaerobic activities.

I've experienced this personally. As my body composition goals have shifted over the course of my ketogenic journey, some maneuvering of macronutrients has been necessary in order to achieve results. For instance, when I wanted to bulk up muscle, I practiced daily carb loading after workouts, whereas when I wanted to lean out, I switched to plenty of aerobic training with no carb loading at all.

As always, I encourage you to do what feels best and most natural to your body.

The Less-Is-More Approach

When I was glucose fueled, I had to work out really hard (and eat a lot) to get the results I wanted in the gym, and I dealt with loads of inflammation, cravings, weight gain, and hormone imbalance because of it. I was pushing myself too hard and had everything backwards. Little did I know that there was a way that I could have it all—I could feel great, move my body in a way that felt good, look great, and not have to spend hours and hours and hours in the gym.

Don't get me wrong, I love going to the gym and really enjoy being active, but being a slave to my workout regimen, feeding the more-is-more mentality, and living in fear of not going to the gym...it just wasn't working for me.

For this reason, the whole concept of "enduring (and hating every moment of) working out so I can obtain a hot body" doesn't appeal to me anymore. But it wasn't an overnight change of heart. Becoming fat adapted and using fat as your primary fuel source takes time, but it encourages the body to use food differently. The process is efficient, creates energy, involves the entire body, and allows us the opportunity to see our workouts from a less-is-more perspective, as opposed to the more-is-more approach that we're all used to.

Yet another reason why I love nutritional ketosis—I spend less time working out and more time living.

There are three kinds of workouts that I enjoy in a ketogenic state:

Movement: Recommended Daily
A brisk walk or calming yoga practice session each day inspires lasting change by reinforcing healthy choices and encouraging strong bones, a light spirit, and a happy mind. Whether you choose to set a steps-per-day goal or just get out in nature and enjoy yourself, the point is to move! Blast some tunes or find a favorite podcast and get your blood flowing.

Strength Building: Recommended 2 to 3 times per week
When we think of strength building, we often think of going to the gym and lifting weights. But it can also mean engaging in a fun activity like power yoga, golfing, dancing, racquet sports, tennis, archery, or paddle boarding. I find that the more you enjoy an activity, the more you'll naturally and effortlessly want to do it.

High-Intensity: Recommended 1 to 2 times per week
High-intensity workouts help balance hormones, flush the system of toxins, boost metabolic rate, and clear the mind. Go pedal-to-the-metal for a couple of minutes during your strength-building sessions, or find a HIIT program to follow online. Keep in mind that high-intensity training can be as short as five minutes (I find it easiest to wedge it in before my morning shower), and you only need to do it once or twice a week.

Keto and Performance

No matter what your activity or exercise of choice may be, there's a lot to be gained by incorporating a ketogenic diet into the mix. Having said that, if you have a big competition, event, or race coming up, or if you're immersed in beast training mode for any other reason, it would be best to hold off on switching nutritional gears until you've resumed your normal level of training or activity.

When you are ready, let's take a look at some of the adjustments you could consider making to improve your performance while on a ketogenic diet.

The absolute best exercise to pair with keto is aerobic exercise, which requires the output of a steady level of energy with limited (or no) bursts of intense activity. One example of this is running a marathon. Aerobic athletes can be fueled exclusively on fat. These athletes do not need to practice carb-ups while training for or participating in an event—in fact, they usually perform better without carb-ups.

Anaerobic exercise, in which athletes engage in short bursts of intensity followed by rest, is trickier to pair with keto. CrossFit and HIIT are two examples of anaerobic exercise. Anaerobic athletes require some form of glycogen or glucose in order to be successful. While the liver can make glucose through gluconeogenesis, that doesn't necessarily happen during activity or in sufficient quantities to fuel the activity. For this reason, anaerobic athletes on a ketogenic diet will almost always be able to perform better, harder, and faster with the addition of carb-ups. Which carb-up practice is most effective depends on activity level, intensity, goals, and fat-adaptation ability.

A great way to determine which Fat Fueled Profile to choose for your activity is to ask yourself these two questions:

How often do I work out?

- Once or twice a week: Full Keto

- Three or four times a week: Adapted Fat Burner with two carb-ups

- Five or more times a week: Adapted Fat Burner with two or three carb-ups

How many really heavy lifts/sessions do I have per week?

- One: Full Keto

- Two: Adapted Fat Burner with two carb-ups

- Three: Adapted Fat Burner with three carb-ups

During the fat-adaptation process, the body is full of glycogen just waiting to be burned off. Because glycogen is required for any anaerobic exercise, a few HIIT sessions will help you deplete those glycogen stores so your body becomes fat adapted quicker. You'll experience immense energy and a quicker adaptation process!

HIIT sessions usually last anywhere from five to twenty minutes, and each session alternates between periods of intense activity, where you're going as hard as possible, and periods of rest. Generally, this pattern is repeated for the entire duration of the HIIT session.

Here are a few suggestions to help you hit the ground running with HIIT:

- Google "elliptical HIIT," "stairs HIIT," "bike HIIT," or "running HIIT" for free workout ideas.

- Follow fitness coach Zuzka Light (zuzkalight.com) for mini workouts.

- If CrossFit is your thing, have at it!

Fasted Cardio

If you enjoy waking up and working out before you do anything else (even flossing your teeth), you're going to love this! I remember in my previous life, when I was a long-distance runner and cyclist, I needed to fuel up before, during, and after my training sessions—no ifs, ands, or buts. Now here I am, a couple of years later, recommending that you try fasted cardio on your ketogenic diet. Have I lost my mind? Not even close.

Fasted cardio is exactly what it sounds like: you wake up, strap on those running shoes, and hit the pavement on a completely empty stomach. This is beneficial because it increases autophagy, generates higher ketones, extends your fast, and generally means a boost in energy during your session.

If the idea of running on empty doesn't tickle your fancy, you're probably not ready for fasted cardio, and that's okay. If you have hormonal imbalances, I'd avoid trying fasted cardio until balance is restored. But when you become interested in getting your heart pumping without consuming anything beforehand, give it a try and see how you feel!

I never, ever, ever recommend continuing to fast after a workout, even if you feel you could go six more hours without food. It is important to eat after a workout to fuel your body properly and assist with building muscle. Don't think that you're doing yourself a favor by skipping the post-workout meal. Trust me—I did this for months because I was curious about what would happen (and, you know, because Dwayne Johnson was doing it, so why couldn't I?). But I'm sad to report that it was a big mistake. It affected my ability to generate ketones, spiked my cravings, affected my muscle composition, and extended my recovery time.

Suggested Timing for Exercise and Eating

The following are if-then scenarios for timing your snacks and meals in relation to your exercise preferences. Some include carb-ups; others suggest using carbs in small doses to boost performance.

All of these suggestions are based on my personal experiences and/or those of people I've encountered. This isn't intended as the be-all, end-all of solutions—it's more of a starting point to help you define a strategy that works best for your body.

If you're not yet fat adapted, you may find that the process of becoming fat adapted will affect your training and/or increase your appetite. Follow the steps on page 110 for overcoming keto flu, and eat more fat until your body fully adjusts to the new fuel source.

Morning Exercise, Aerobic
Pre-workout
Option 1: Stay fasted.
Option 2: If you need something in your belly, have your first meal before working out and skip the post-workout meal.

Post-workout
Option 1: Enjoy your first keto meal 30 to 45 minutes after the activity.
Option 2: If you ate before your workout, skip the post-workout meal and wait until you get hungry to enjoy a balanced keto meal.

Morning Exercise, Anaerobic

Pre-workout
Option 1: Stay fasted.
Option 2: Have a Rocket Fuel Latte (page 144) 1 hour before your activity.
*Option 3: Have a small quantity of carbs (about 20 to 40 grams) 15 to 30 minutes before the activity. This is not considered a carb-up—it's just to supply your body with enough glucose to get going.

Post-workout
Option 1: Enjoy your first keto meal 30 to 45 minutes after the activity.
*Option 2: Enjoy a carb-and-protein snack 30 to 45 minutes after the activity. This is not considered a carb-up—it's just to supply your body with enough glucose to replenish muscles.

Afternoon Exercise, Aerobic

Pre-workout
Follow your Fat Fueled Profile all morning. Exercise on an empty stomach (2 to 4 hours after eating).

Post-workout
Have a Fat Fueled snack, or wait to eat until your next meal.

Afternoon Exercise, Anaerobic

Pre-workout
Option 1: Exercise on an empty stomach (2 to 4 hours after eating).
*Option 2: Have a small quantity of carbs (about 20 to 40 grams) 15 to 30 minutes prior to the activity. This is not considered a carb-up—it's just to supply your body with enough glucose to get going. It's not helpful for all (some athletes perform worse) but is beneficial for some, and it's an option you can play with.

Post-workout
Option 1: Enjoy your second meal 30 to 45 minutes after the activity.
*Option 2: Enjoy a carb-and-protein snack 30 to 45 minutes after the activity. This is not considered a carb-up—it's just to supply your body with enough glucose to replenish muscles.
*Option 3: Potentially a good time for a carb-up.

TRUTH BOMB

Afternoon workouts (anytime between about 2:30 p.m. and 5:00 p.m.) are the most beneficial for hormones, weight management, sleep quality, and mood stabilization.

Evening Exercise, Aerobic

Pre-workout

Option 1: Enjoy your last keto meal of the day, then head to the gym at least 30 minutes after eating.

Option 2: Exercise on an empty stomach (4 to 6 hours after your last meal).

Post-workout

Option 1: Give your dog, husband, children, and/or other loved ones a little snuggle and get ready for bed.

Option 2: Enjoy your last keto meal of the day.

Evening Exercise, Anaerobic

Pre-workout

Option 1: Exercise on an empty stomach (4 to 6 hours after your last meal).

*Option 2: Have a small quantity of carbs (about 20 to 40 grams) 15 to 30 minutes prior to the activity.

Post-workout

Option 1: Enjoy your last keto meal of the day 30 to 45 minutes after the activity.

*Option 2: Potential opportunity for a carb-up 30 to 45 minutes after the activity.

Only an option if you're following the Daily Fat Burner profile, or if you're already fat adapted and are following the Full Keto profile or Adapted Fat Burner profile.

Suggested Workouts

Because I have seen the power of HIIT on my own body, on the following pages I've outlined a couple of HIIT workouts that don't require equipment—you can even do them when you're traveling. All you need is a clear space where you have some room to move.

If you're not familiar with any of these movements, a quick Google search will do the trick.

CORE EXERCISES #1

30 seconds each, repeat set 4 times, rest 10 seconds between movements

1. Front Plank
2. Side Plank (right)
3. Side Plank (left)
4. Back Plank

CORE EXERCISES #2

25 seconds each, repeat set 4 times, rest 5 seconds between movements

1. High Knees
2. Crunches
3. Front Plank
4. Knee Tucks
5. Superman Planks

ARM EXERCISES

30 seconds each, repeat set 4 times, rest 10 seconds between movements

1. Jumping Jacks
2. Push-ups
3. Triceps Dips
4. V Push-ups

LEG EXERCISES

30 seconds each, repeat set 3 times, rest 10 seconds between movements

1. High Knees
2. Tuck Jumps
3. High Knees
4. Squats
5. High Knees
6. Wall Sit
7. High Knees
8. Jump Lunges

FULL-BODY EXERCISES

3 sets

1. High Knees — 75 (left and right combined count as 1)
2. Push-ups — 15
3. Squats — 20
4. Triceps Dips — 20
5. Tuck Jumps — 5
6. Inchworms — 5
7. High Knees — 75 (left and right combined count as 1)
8. V Push-ups — 15

Overcoming Exercise Hurdles on Keto

I'm crashing during my workouts. What can I do?

If you're a few weeks into the fat-adapting process and you're still having issues with energy and performance, try these suggestions.:

1 Move your workouts to the afternoon. If that doesn't help, move them to the evening.

2 If you're following Full Keto, work out the day after a carb-up, then have a carb-and-protein snack after the workout.

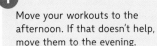

3 For all Fat Fueled Profiles, increase the amount of carbs you consume in the evening or during a carb-up. Start with a 10-gram increase per sitting, working up to as much as 30 grams (which I think would be an optimal amount).

4 Do not fast before your workouts. Try having an RFL (page 144) or a full breakfast 45 to 60 minutes before the activity.

5 Try a different Fat Fueled Profile.

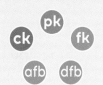

This just doesn't seem to be working.

You might be going at things a little too hard, or you could be hung up with the whole keto concept because you believe it won't actually make a difference in your performance. Try following the steps under "What's the best exercise combo?" below and see how things go.

How much carbohydrate should my carb-and-protein snacks contain?

An overripe banana works best, because it has more glucose than anything else. Start off with half a medium banana. If you seem to need more, have a full one. If you can't do bananas, any glucose-rich carbohydrate will do, such as white rice blended into your protein shake, a handful of grapes, or Medjool dates.

What's the best exercise combo?

I've seen many people experience the most success in reaching their weight-loss and muscle-building goals with this specific combination:

- Morning walks seven days a week (getting out in the morning light helps with circadian rhythms)
- HIIT sessions two to three days per week in the late afternoon / early evening, right before your last meal (so that the carbs you have with dinner become your post-workout fuel)
- If you're still not seeing results after a couple of weeks, try reducing the amount of fat you consume in the evening after your workout. It's okay to still have a tablespoon or so, but try to cut out the rest and see how you do!

Won't eating extra carbs (whether in carb-ups or another kind of cyclical keto) sabotage my keto quest?

Once you've become fat adapted, eating a small quantity of carbohydrates following your morning or afternoon workout shouldn't affect your fat-burning power. If you stick to 20 to 40 grams, it should be just the right amount of carbs needed to refuel your muscles.

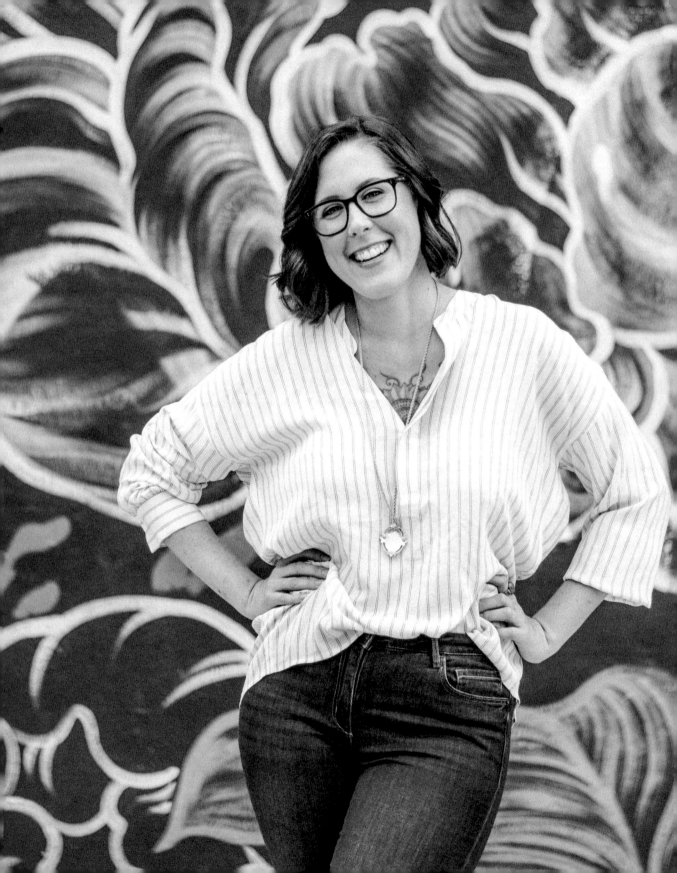

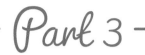

Part 3

HEALING
YOUR BODY

You've graduated the three steps to fat-fueled freedom, you're a fat-burner, you've found a Fat Fueled Profile that fits well for the space you're in right now, and maybe you've even played around with cyclical strategies to make living a keto lifestyle that much easier.

Since starting *Keto for Women*, you've done a lot of healing, too. Even if you didn't realize it, the moves you've made up to this point have positively affected imbalances in your body, even just slight ones. You're in a wonderful place now to start addressing larger imbalances that may be keeping you stuck in an endless loop and that, until now, no diet has been able to solve.

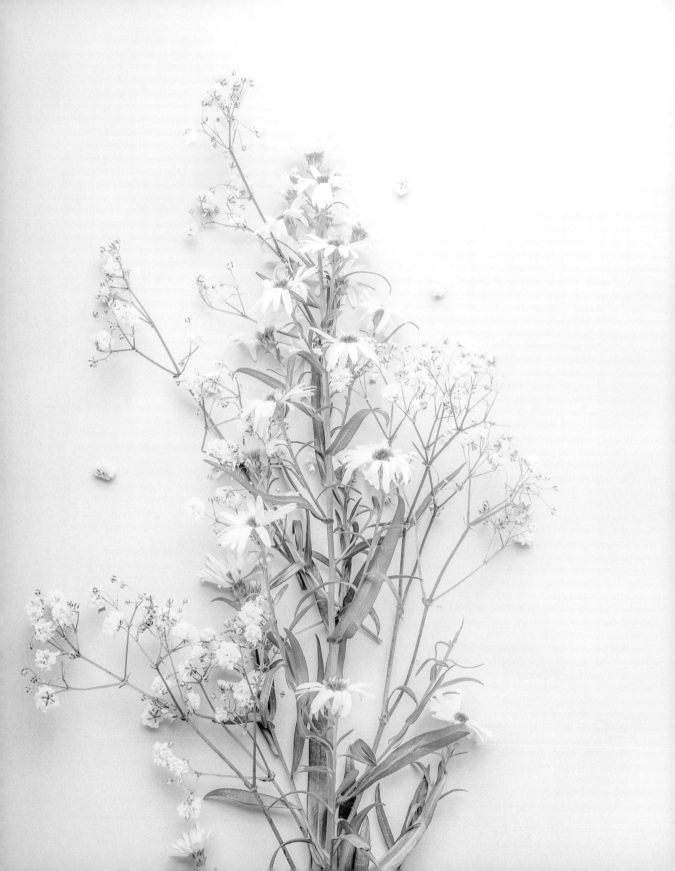

7

REPAIRING YOUR RELATIONSHIP WITH YOUR BODY

You know "that woman" we'd all like to be? Confident, fierce, unapologetic—that woman who walks into a room and it instantly lights up.

Notice I didn't say anything about her body.

That woman who loves getting dressed in the morning and jumps in front of photo ops. That woman who's too busy dying with laughter, flirting with the cute bartender, and hitting the dance floor with her friends to think about her body, how she looks, or what others may think of her.

Notice I didn't say anything about her jeans size, Fitbit points, or body fat percentage.

You *are* that woman. Deep down inside you, there's a radiant goddess who doesn't let a number on a scale dictate her self-worth. Your journey to find her begins now.

Newsflash: diet alone is not a magic ticket to health. It never will be. Healing your body begins with healing your relationship with your body, learning to respect and accept your body, and then forging ahead with your fresh perspective to make adjustments to your diet and lifestyle with grace.

Maybe you think all of this is baloney. I did too. I thought I was just one macro adjustment or another twenty minutes in the gym away from pure happiness. As if happiness were a destination that, if I worked hard enough on looking my best, I would reach, and all my dreams would come true. This logic is flawed. Life is messy and our bodies keep us guessing. The only constant is change itself. And when you learn to embrace change in a body you accept and respect, everything is different.

Your relationship with your partner massively improves.

Confidence becomes your best quality.

You care less about what people think.

You look at others with love.

You eat to live, not live to eat.

Moving your body starts to feel good instead of being something you obsess over or feel obligated to do.

Your mood improves.

You find more things you're passionate about.

So this last part of *Keto for Women* is dedicated to helping you learn to respect and appreciate your body and showing you how to tweak diet and lifestyle factors to support both body and mind. Regardless of where you're currently at in your physical journey, you absolutely must form a new relationship with your body. And that has nothing to do with your macros, ketone levels, or body composition.

It has to do with your mindset.

It Starts with **Kindness**

Most of us learn how to be kind to one another early on in life—to share our toys, say hello to our friends, and be mindful of others' feelings. Kindness is about being friendly, generous, and considerate, all qualities we work so hard on in our relationships with others and yet so often lack in our relationship with ourselves.

Think about passing the kindness you show everyone else on to your body. Be friendly, generous, and considerate to your body in how you treat it and how you connect to it. With body kindness, you accept yourself just as you are right now. With body kindness, you can slowly let go of that negative internal voice and treat yourself with compassion instead of shame. With body kindness, you'll put your energy into boosting positive motivation for creating a better life in a way that works for you.

You're probably thinking, *But if I accept my body the way it is, then I won't be able to change it. I'm here to change my body.*

I hear you. Acceptance is certainly counterintuitive, going against everything we've been conditioned to believe will lead to a healthy and happy life. But let me ask you this: How have your past approaches to weight loss worked out?

With body kindness, you finally put your body first, honoring it, trusting it, and taking care of it. And I have a sneaking suspicion that the body kindness practices I recommend are much better for your mind and body than anything you may have tried in the past to lose weight.

There are no rules for developing body kindness. That's because body kindness should, ultimately, be a habit, and rules don't create habits—choices do. By learning how to make the best choices for yourself, you'll effortlessly build a solid framework of self-love that will positively change your life.

Here are the three pillars of body kindness:

1. **Love:** Make all choices from a place of love and acceptance.

2. **Connect:** Check in with your body and respond to its needs. Maybe it's asking for sleep, food, a deep breath, a good laugh, or a mind-blowing orgasm.

3. **Care:** Fully commit to your self-care rituals, no matter what. Maybe that means going for a daily walk with your favorite music, running a bubble bath for yourself on Tuesdays, going to your favorite yoga class every Sunday, or spending extra time brushing your hair every morning. Pick one self-care ritual that excites you and commit to it. Make it your number one priority, and don't let your schedule or other people get in the way of completing it. As you practice, it'll become easier and easier to make time for yourself and your self-care.

Your current weight has nothing to do with your ability to practice body kindness. Numbers are just that—numbers. They'll change over time for a myriad of reasons. The more you let go of trying to control them, the freer you will become and the less fear will consume you. Promise!

When you practice the three pillars of body kindness, you invite into your life self-acceptance, self-compassion, and positive motivation to pursue your deepest desires for a healthy mind and happy body.

Signs You're Ready for a Different Approach

There are some common signs that it's time to build a different relationship with your body. Read the list below and count how many of these statements apply to you.

I sometimes say,

"I don't trust myself around [insert food here]."

Thinking about food preparation and accessibility while traveling makes me anxious.

I beat myself up over things I did or didn't do—when I go off track, I feel shame and guilt and judge myself harshly.

I believe there is a specific and predetermined track that I should not stray from.

I try to control all my food choices. Everything I eat is tracked and monitored as a means to help me reach my goal. And sometimes I fail at this miserably, sending me off the deep end.

I experience lots of gas and can't pinpoint what foods may be causing it.

I feel anxious about the possibility of missing a workout.

I sometimes say,

"To hell with it. I screwed up. I'll start again tomorrow."

I get stressed out in new eating situations. Going out to dinner with friends means checking the menu beforehand and figuring out what I can have, what I can't, and what questions I'll ask the server. This process puts me in defensive mode, makes me anxious, or has me canceling at the last minute.

I have a long, long list of food rules.

I have a love-hate relationship with healthy eating.

I intentionally eat alone.

I judge the way other people dress, how they move, how they look, etc.

I jump on the scale every morning.

I am constantly thinking about which foods I can and cannot have.

I am dealing with ongoing inflammatory issues and stress.

I have said,

"When my weight (or body shape) changes, life will be better."

I am envious of people who can just eat what they want. How do they do that? I don't get it.

I am overwhelmingly fearful of weight gain.

My cycle is off. Missed periods, crazy PMS...you name it.

My relationships have become unhealthy, in part because I find myself constantly talking about food, weight, and dieting choices with my friends.

My weight seems to constantly fluctuate.

Your Score

(1) Of these twenty-two statements, how many apply to you? _____

(2) Write a little note to yourself about which of these attitudes you hope to transform the most during the next 30 days, and set a reminder in your calendar to come back to this page in 30 days' time.

(3) Continue on with step 3 for a solid 30 days before going through all the questions again.

Now, how many statements apply to you? _____

How I Learned to Stop Worrying and **Love My Body**

I share a lot on my website and on social media, and I get negative comments about my videos, my body, and the information I share all the time. I don't see all comments, and when a negative one pops up, I don't normally engage with the negative conversation. But once I received a very pointed comment that stuck with me for so, so many reasons. The man said, "Who would trust a woman who has love handles for dieting advice?"

I send the guy love. Maybe he was having a bad day, or maybe he had nothing better to do with his time. Maybe he was displacing his feelings about his own body onto me. I know that these kinds of comments have little to do with me. But they still hurt. I'm sure you've been hurt like this before. While making negative body-focused comments is a jerk thing to do, it's part of the world we live in.

Here's what the world tells me: if I share health advice and I'm not dressed up in a bikini showing off my six-pack abs and talking about how lean and toned I am, then I can't possibly be knowledgeable about being healthy. And this isn't just an issue in the fitness and health community. Regardless of how you put yourself out there, if you aren't the perfect model of success, then somehow you're made to feel unworthy. And it's unfair.

The way that your body looks should not dictate your worth in society. The gifts you have to give the world have nothing to do with the way you look. Your body shouldn't dictate how you provide information to others, how you support others, or how you choose to live your life.

Here's the good news: as much as the criticism sucks, you don't have to give it any importance in your life. Your health is a lot more important than the number on the scale. All you have to do is make a decision that taking care of this temple—your body—is more important to you than reaching a specific body weight, no matter what the haters say. That doesn't mean the two can't coexist. It doesn't mean that you can't pursue optimal health while also trying to reach your ideal body weight. The "ideal" may just be different than what you had in mind.

I've learned over time that it's not possible for my body to be thin and healthy at the same time. It's just not. When I was 131 pounds, I wanted so desperately to get down to 125. Those 6 pounds were all that I cared about. I busted it out at the gym and restricted foods like crazy. I did everything and anything I could to lose them. And finally, I got to that 125. I'll never forget that day because I jumped on the scale and started dancing and singing, "Yeah, yeah. I'm awesome. My life is so good."

That night, I had a square of dark chocolate, one little square. When I woke up the next day, I was 132 pounds.

One square of chocolate, and my dream was ruined. I berated myself, regretted the treat, and thought I was weak for the indulgence. All that mattered to me was that stupid number on the scale. When it was up, I felt powerless, and when it was down, I felt unstoppable.

Now I know what it takes for my body to get down to 125 pounds. But I also know that my body cannot be 125 pounds unless I do a lot of unhealthy things to make that happen. And when I do all of those things, it restricts my ability to be healthy.

I'm sure there are people out there that can be thin and healthy at the same time. Me, I'm not that girl. And the definition of *thin* is so broad and very much self-defined.

When I'm pushing to be thin beyond what my body wants, I'm letting the number on the scale dictate my worth and define who I am. I'm restricting and counting food. Instead of engaging in conversation with my husband, I'm counting calories in my head and stressing about dinner taking me over my fat macros. I'm going to the gym and pushing myself much further than I would normally. The whole time, I'm thinking about how much of a failure I am, how I need to push harder, go longer, and do better than before. These are all unhealthy behaviors for me.

As soon as I started eating when I was hungry, stopped restricting food, and stopped pairing restriction with fasting—and I was eating a healthy keto diet— my body started healing and my health began to improve. My hormones became balanced, I stopped feeling anxious, my ADHD and constipation disappeared. At the same time, my weight crept back up. For me, 125 pounds wasn't healthy—it wasn't where my body wanted to be, and the things I needed to do to reach that weight were damaging to my overall well-being.

Health cannot exist without ample positive behaviors sprinkled throughout the day. For me, these are things like waking up and having a shower first thing, doing my hair, brushing it out, meditating, and engaging in movement that makes me feel good, such as yoga or walking. These activities allow me to stay in close contact with what my body needs, whether that's busting through a mountain of work or taking a break to eat. While I may be heavier than 125 pounds when I practice these things, I'm not in shackles. I'm not restricted. I refuse to be a victim of society's demand that I look a certain way regardless of how I feel or what my body's telling me it needs.

Where does the ketogenic diet fit in all of this? For me, personally, it set me free. I get to eat when I want to. My hormones are bang-on. My fertility is fabulous. My carb-up practice allows me to enjoy time out with friends, without stress. When I'm at home, I eat a ton of fat, and I feel so much happier than I did when I was restricting. I have developed solid healthy behaviors, in part because when I eat enough fat, my brain feels stabilized, my mood is good, and it's easier for me to make healthful decisions than when I'm carb-crazy and shaking.

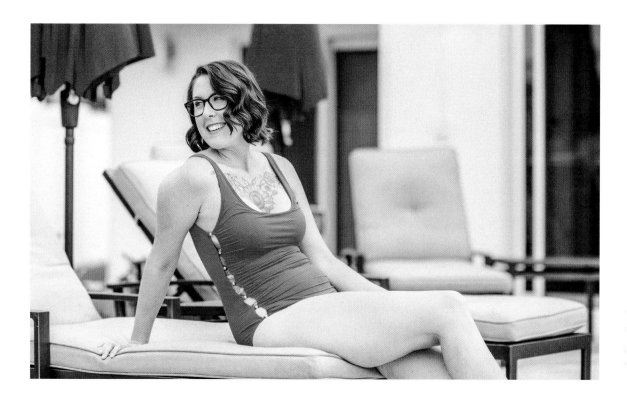

It works in the reverse, too: eating keto helps me feel good, and when I feel good, it's easier to get into ketosis. When you're stressed, obsessed, and controlling, ketosis becomes harder to catch than a Heffalump (please tell me you like Winnie the Pooh).

So whether your life goal is to be a nutrition coach, a lawyer, a PR rep, a stay-at-home mom, an administrative assistant, a teacher, a poet, or a motivational speaker, don't think for a second that your body dictates your success. In my experience, if you let your body goals run the show, you will never truly feel successful, and you'll have wasted a great deal of time, energy, and money on the pursuit of a "perfect" body that shows how successful you are as an insert-dream-life-purpose-here. You don't have to have a "perfect" body to make a difference in the world.

It's okay to have a belly that is a bit bigger.

It's okay if your jeans don't fit sometimes.

It's okay if your arms jiggle.

It's okay to hate going to the gym.

It's okay to eat a slice of chocolate cake for dinner.

None of these things make me or you less human or worse at our jobs, nor should they stand in the way of our realizing our dreams.

My body lets me experience my life well, whether it's 130 pounds or 230. And, if you let it, your body will do the same for you.

Restriction vs. **Choice**

During a recent event, I shared that my body has become quite vocal, telling me (often) what it wants and doesn't want. After the event, a woman approached me and said that there was no way her body knew what it wanted because either she heard nothing at all or it yelled at her for pizza, beer, and ice cream.

Girl, I feel you!

In my experience, when my body is yelling for pizza, beer, and ice cream, it's usually because I'm on a diet where I feel restricted, malnourished, and controlled.

Your body knows what it needs and when it needs it. Forcing yourself to do something completely different denies your body what it needs to thrive, and that's not healthy.

If we're forcing control on our body, of course it is going to respond negatively. It will either rebel by creating false alarms and clamoring for food we don't actually need, or it will shut down completely, making it impossible for us to hear anything it has to say. If you're in this boat, don't fret. It's never too late to get back in sync with your body and then use its signals as a powerful tool to optimize your health.

If you've been restricting your diet for a long time and creating rules around what you can and cannot have, the practice of listening to your body is at first going to seem a bit...weird. You're probably thinking, *But if I tell myself that I can eat anything, I will eat* everything. *I don't trust my body. I would eat cake every day if it were up to my body.*

I'm here to tell you that that is so not true. Even though you've been conditioned to believe that your body can't be trusted, it actually *can* be.

I know this because your body wants to be healthy and balanced. It wants to thrive.

What if I told you that the very things you're using to "improve yourself" are causing you to binge, feel shame, and experience guilt? It's true—the very rules and restrictions you've embraced in your search for balance, health, and bliss are in fact what are ruining you inside.

How can we possibly get past our restrictive mindsets about food, live healthfully, and reach our goal weight, all at the same time? The answer is surprisingly uncomplicated: we let our bodies do the work. Your body knows what weight it feels best at. It knows what it needs and doesn't need. Your role is simply to nourish your body to the best of your ability to help it get where it wants to be.

So if we can just get out of our own way and listen to our bodies, we'll very likely be able to stick to a keto diet, with a much healthier relationship to food.

It is safe to listen to your body. Eat. Eat until you're full. You don't need to restrict foods. You don't need to count calories. You don't need to go to bed hungry or wish you had a different body.

Read that again, only say it out loud and make it personal: It *is safe to listen to my body. I can eat. I'll eat until I'm full. I don't need to restrict foods. I don't need to count calories. I don't need to go to bed hungry or wish I had a different body.*

What feelings come to the surface for you as you're reading this? Perhaps it's the liberating sensation of a weight being lifted?

I first said these words to myself about six months into my keto experience. At the time, I was riddled with rules, had started bingeing, and was generally a hot mess. The moment I gave myself permission to feel and believe these words, it was as if my body said, "WAH?? I don't have to restrict? All of those foods I've told myself I can't have, I can have?! I can have it all! I can say yes!!!"

It was a light-bulb moment for me. I spent the next two weeks eating all the things I'd been denying myself. I ate more than I'd ever eaten before, things I hadn't had in years—candy, toast with jam, bagels, fatty steaks, chocolate, ice cream, you name it. It felt good to allow myself free rein on anything my heart desired, sugar highs and all. And then, as the days turned into a week, and the week became just shy of a second week, I realized eating all the junk food didn't make me feel good—I was experiencing brain fog, imbalanced mood, low energy. I also realized that over the years, I'd given so much power to these "no" foods for no reason at all. I didn't even actually *like* them, and they sure didn't make me feel good, but whenever I tried to diet I felt compelled to eat them *because* they were off-limits. This was around the time that I gradually—and naturally—began gravitating to food that my body was telling me would actually make me feel good, inside and out.

About two months after this realization, I was eating full-blown keto day in and day out, without an ounce of restriction. I was eating foods that made me feel good because these were the foods I was naturally gravitating toward. I learned that, without a doubt, my body craves keto foods. It craves fats and veggies. And because you're reading this, I suspect yours may, too. Pass the broccoli slathered in coconut oil!

Learning to trust your body is even easier when you're eating enough fat.

By eating enough fat, you're giving your brain the fuel it needs to think clearly and your organs the nourishment they need to function optimally. Both help you see things more clearly, make solid choices for yourself, and trust what your body tells you.

By giving yourself permission to trust your body and allowing it to be your guide, you'll quickly realize just how much better off you are—physically improved, mentally balanced, and spiritually sound.

The choice is yours. You can choose to see food as food, as a means of giving your body what it needs, or you can continue to give it the power to control your life. It's all you!

WHY MEASURING IS RUINING YOUR LIFE

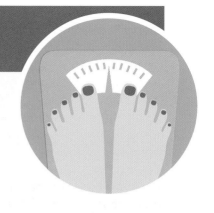

Do you jump on the scale after each meal to see how much weight you've put on? Do you define your worth each day by how much you weigh? Do you obsess and beat yourself up over the daily results?

Let's do a little hypothetical calculation right now, because I know you love calculating. (Cheeky? Yes, you bet!)

 7 min **BREAKFAST** Weighing, measuring food, calculating intake on app

 10 min **LUNCH** Weighing, measuring food, calculating intake on app

 11 min **DINNER** Weighing, measuring food, calculating intake on app

 3 min Double-checking calorie and macro tallies throughout the day

 6 min **STRESSING OUT**

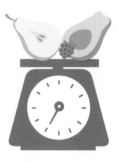

 37 **TOTAL MINUTES PER DAY**

225 HOURS = 9.4 DAYS PER YEAR

How many times have you gotten halfway through your meal and thought, "Wow, I'm not really that hungry anymore, but I have to eat this because I won't stay in ketosis if I don't / it's a long time until my next meal / I've gone to the trouble of making it / I won't be able to build muscle..."?

That little voice inside of you that's telling you you're not hungry is your body's way of trying to reach its happy place.

That's not to say that all tracking is bad, though. There are times where tracking can be helpful, and that's why I've included loads of calculations in chapter 5. Tracking your macros and understanding your intakes are invaluable when you're new to keto, unsure what a carbohydrate is, and totally dumbfounded by just how much fat you need to eat to make all this work. As you learn more about your eating style, you may choose to continue tracking or decide to ditch it. Everything I'm saying here is meant to encourage you to do what's right for you. If that's tracking, have at it. If that's not tracking, that's cool, too. I think so many of us track only because we're told we need to in order to be successful on keto. And this just isn't true.

At the end of the day, if you're pushing and prodding yourself to finish your meal, stopping yourself from eating when you're famished, or struggling to stick to your diet because you get so overwhelmed with tracking that you stop eating keto all together, you are likely ignoring your body's clear signals in the worst possible way. Your body is the food authority. It knows when it's full, when it needs to eat, and even what it needs to eat.

For many of us, tracking sabotages what we're ultimately trying to do—whether that's living a healthier life, losing weight, overcoming an imbalance, or what have you—because we're fighting against what our body is telling us it needs.

On page 234, I'll take you through some exercises you can practice over the course of three days that will hone your instinct and ability to know when you're hungry and what you need to satisfy your hunger, when your body is telling you to stop eating, and how to stop eating at your satiation point.

What's **Holding** You **Back**?

I'm going to let you in on a little secret: no one actually knows what they're doing with their lives, we all get a little lost sometimes, and a *lot* of us know what we need to do to get unstuck but don't do it out of fear, our belief system, our ego, or our lack of connection to ourselves.

For real! Just imagine what life would be like if you didn't have fear. What would you be doing? How would you make money? Who would you surround yourself with? What activities would you enjoy doing? What would you look like? How would you act?

Fear is just one of the many factors that keep us stuck and repeating our experiences over and over and over again, never actually progressing. Let's put an end to that, okay?

Fear and Self-Doubt

I'd love nothing more than to be able to sit here and honestly tell you that I'm this fearless nutritionist-entrepreneur-warrior, but that's just not the truth. (At least, not all the time.) From time to time, we all experience fear. It's doing its job, protecting us from failure—or at least, that's what it thinks it's doing, but in actuality, it may be keeping us from success.

Maybe you want to go back to school but think that you're "too old to do that." You'd like to learn a new language, but you "never follow through with that kind of thing." Or you're thinking about giving this keto thing a go, but you've "tried diets before and they never work." I'm gonna show you how to break down and bust through those fears.

By realizing your fears and busting through them, you'll:

- Appreciate the body you have

- Find it easier to commit to (and stick to) things

- Gain confidence

- Make more money

- And more...

Did you know that I almost didn't start my health and wellness website, Healthful Pursuit, because fear told me that I didn't have anything helpful to share? It's true. I sat on my first YouTube video for a year—that's right, an entire year—before finally moving forward. And even after Healthful Pursuit became a success, I nearly quit writing my first paperback book because fear told me that I had nothing to share—again.

So I know all about the fear game. Sometimes it's about a big thing, like starting a new business, and sometimes it's about a small thing, like your outfit. What's important to keep in mind is that fear thinks it's keeping you safe. "But how is being worried about your outfit keeping you safe?" you ask. That's a great question!

Fear and our fight-flight-or-freeze response are governed by the limbic system, the part of the brain that deals with instinct and basic emotion, not rational thought. It was crucial in keeping our ancestors safe from predators—when you need to run from a saber-toothed tiger, your chances of survival improve if you don't take the time to think through all the possible courses of action first. We wouldn't be around today without it. At the same time, I think we can all lovingly let the limbic system know that it's the twenty-first century, there are no more saber-toothed tigers, and it can stop working against us.

I've found that when it comes to nutrition, fear is usually a process with four stages, each one building upon the other. First, there's the **trigger**: whatever gets the fear ball rolling. This brings up the second stage, thinking about the **norm**: what's socially acceptable, what everyone else is doing, or what everyone else is saying is the right thing to do—what the "safe zone" is. That leads to the third stage, **self-doubt**: the old stories we tell ourselves about who we are and what we're capable of, stories we hold on to even though they're no longer serving us. They're almost always deep down in our subconscious, and we're often not even aware of them. And the result of all this is the fourth stage, **fear**. It could be fear of failing, fear of succeeding, fear of being laughed at or of being alone... Whatever it happens to be, if left unchecked, fear can rule our lives.

On your nutrition journey, some possible triggers could be eating carbs, not tracking your food anymore, not counting macros, starting to eat more fat, scaling back your workouts, emotional eating, or comparing yourself to someone else.

And what does the norm look like? It could be being vegan, eating low-fat, shooting for a certain number on the scale, or taking a doctor's advice even though your body is telling you something different—anything that is informed by other people's advice and opinions.

That leads us to self-doubt, which shows up in those not-so-nice stories that buzz around our brains and often sound like, "I'm not good enough," or "They'll think I'm a joke," or "I don't know enough," "I'm not pretty enough," "I'll never like my body," or "Keto will never work for me, it's all just a waste of time." If it sounds unreasonable and makes you feel terrible, you can bet your bottom dollar that it's self-doubt. But whatever the self-doubt du jour may be, it's less important than what it leads to: fear.

When it comes to fears, hey, we've all got 'em—fear of being disappointed or disappointing someone else, fear of embarrassment, fear of being shamed or called out, maybe even fear of not being noticed at all.

So fear is fueled by and sometimes masks our self-doubt, and sticking to the norm keeps us in the safe zone so we don't have to feel any of this. Ah, feelings... But if we see our fear for what it really is and get underneath the self-doubt to understand what's causing our unhappiness, we can figure out what we want and how to get it.

Here's an example: You may feel like you want more carbs or accidentally eat something that isn't "right" or "according to the plan." That's the trigger. The norm says, "Keto people don't eat carbs." Then the self-doubt pops up with, "See, you knew you wouldn't be able to stick to this," which is followed by the fear of gaining weight.

I get myself out of the fear funk all the time. Here's how.

Take Action! Defeating Fear and Self-Doubt

So you have a big ole case of self-doubt and you don't know how to get over it. These steps can help!

1. **Figure out your self-doubt story.** What are you telling yourself will happen if you do the thing you're presented with? For example, if you doubt your ability to present your ideas in front of your colleagues at tomorrow's general meeting, your self-doubt story could be, "I'll fail and everyone will think I'm a joke."

2. **Come up with the facts.** What experiences from your past do you have that support this fear? What experiences from your past disprove this fear? This one's a doozy because most of us, when we're being honest, can't actually find a past experience that supports the fear!

3. **What are you trying to protect yourself from?** If you're scared that you'll bomb your presentation, could it be that you're afraid of being embarrassed? Or being judged? Maybe you're fearful that you'll lose people's trust?

4. **Best-case and worst-case scenarios.** Ask yourself, "What's the worst that could happen?" Followed by, "Okay, what's the best that could happen?" So you bomb your presentation, so what? You still have a job, a family that loves you, and awesome weekend plans. On the flip side, you could totally crush your presentation, get a bunch of praise from your colleagues, and have the best day ever.

5. **Be kind to the fear.** Now that you know what you're fearful of, you can build a self-affirming statement that shows appreciation for the fear. Maybe it sounds like this: "Thank you for watching out for me. I understand why I am feeling fearful about being embarrassed. I remember how embarrassed I was when I presented my paper in front of the class in ninth grade. I understand that I'm trying to protect myself from reliving this experience. Thank you for wanting to protect me. I am going to present my ideas in tomorrow's meeting and do so confidently."

What we're doing here is respecting what that trusty old limbic system is trying to protect you from. As you run through these five steps, take note of how this particular fear is affecting your life. Maybe you're talking down to people, being critical of others, judging other people's lives and what they have that you don't, or saying no to things you really want to do. When we recognize the negative effects of a fear, it's easier to overcome it.

Finally, and most importantly, do more of the things that make you feel good, whatever that may be—maybe writing a letter to a friend, gardening, or just blasting some fun music—while you make the conscious choice to see love and do it!

Limiting Beliefs

Your core beliefs make up the fabric of your life experience. They act as filters for the world around you, attaching preconceived assumptions to your experiences to help determine your feelings, emotions, and decisions about them. Once these beliefs are formed, they become ingrained through repetition. Often your beliefs are not even objectively "true," but they seem inarguably true to you because somewhere along the way, you decided that they were.

Limiting beliefs are just that—core beliefs that limit our perception and constrain us in some way. Often they originate from personal experience, education, faulty logic, and, the most powerful of all, fear. Once they're ingrained in our belief system, limiting beliefs affect how we relate to others, how we see the world, and how we see our place in it. Addressing our limiting beliefs is essential for overcoming the fear of using intuition to guide our food choices.

Something as seemingly harmless as labeling ourselves based on our roles or occupations can act as a catalyst to trigger a limiting belief. Saying "I am a blogger" can become my story—by omitting the fact that I am also an online marketer and a nutrition educator, I give less importance to those roles, although I am both of those things too.

When we talk about health and wellness, labeling ourselves in any way—whether we say we're keto, Paleo, low-carb, vegan, vegetarian, and so on—strictly defines and narrows our life experiences and sticks us in a box. The longer we stay in that box, the more time we have to reinforce that limiting belief. If we're Paleo, for instance, we tend to think we can't be vegan, too.

All in all, freeing ourselves from limiting beliefs is about being open to seeing ourselves as *more*—the "big picture" or the true form of ourselves. Just rephrasing statements about ourselves can change a limiting belief. For example, we can say, "I intend to eat low-carb, high-fat" instead of "I eat low-carb, high-fat." Say both statements out loud and see which feels more liberating and hopeful. The first? Awesome.

Take Action! Analyzing Limiting Beliefs
Take some time today to explore your limiting beliefs. Some common limiting beliefs are these:

- I am not good enough.

- I do not have enough.

- I have to work harder for my money.

- I do not deserve success or happiness.

What limiting beliefs do you have? Perhaps your feeling of being "not good enough" has limited your relationships. Perhaps when you meet new people, you don't put yourself out there wholeheartedly for fear of rejection, which stems from the belief that you have nothing of value to share. Take a moment to jot down a few of your limiting beliefs below.

My limiting beliefs are:

Once you've created of a list of your limiting beliefs, ask yourself the following questions about each one:

• How has this limiting belief stopped me from experiencing life?

• Can I recall a time that this belief was actually proven to be true? If so, how did it make me feel at that time?

• What upcoming event, experience, or situation can I use to put this limiting belief to the test? (And then actually test it!)

When you got to the second question, you probably realized that there was, maybe, one single time that you felt like this—maybe. But perhaps you discovered that you can't actually recall a single situation where your limiting belief was proven. Yet until now, you believed it to be true with every ounce of your being. Interesting, isn't it?

You're on your way to breaking down the walls!

Losing Sight of Your Why

You are most likely reading this because you want to do right by your body. Awesome, me too! So why are we obsessing about the weight of the kale we had on our plate last night? In the grand scheme of things, it really doesn't matter. Did you want the kale? Yes. Did you enjoy it? Yes. Did you prepare the kale with love? I hope you did. So, moving on.

It can be so very easy to lose sight of what's important and why we are doing all of this, and when we lose sight of that, we can lose our motivation to keep moving forward.

Beyond losing a couple of pounds, why is becoming fat adapted so completely awesome? Here is a list of some of the impressive results, positive words, and uplifting stories people have shared with me over the years:

- *I got my life back.*

- *I can chase after my kids! I run faster than they do.*

- *I was able to have kids.*

- *Sex, lots of sex.*

- *I don't spend my nights alone in my car eating.*

- *My ears have stopped hurting. I was in pain for years!*

- *I get to spend quality time with my partner. I'm present for the first time ever.*

- *I found my confidence, and now I'm singing in front of people, doing what I've always dreamed of.*

- *My brain works! I can think again! I felt like there was a veil over my brain and no amount of medication was helping the problem.*

If you should find yourself obsessing over calories, feeling guilt and shame about your food choices, or building up a wall of rules, come back to this list for inspiration and be reminded of the reasons why you got started on this journey in the first place.

Take Action! Remembering Your Why

Pick five reasons from the list above that most resonate with you, or create your own list of reasons you want to be fat adapted. These reasons should not be tied to how you want to look physically; they should be about how you want your body to function—your emotions, your health, and so on. Place a copy of this list on your fridge, in your car, or in your purse for quick access whenever you feel in danger of losing sight of what's important.

Staying connected to your reasons for wanting to change keeps you focused on the end goal and lowers the risk that you'll become distracted by bright, shiny objects. In the dieting world, these often take the form of the "magic supplement" that promises to get you to your goal weight in record time but fails to deliver or comes with very risky side effects.

In addition to keeping your reasons for going keto on hand, it can pay to dive deeper into your journey so far and your fears and hopes for the future. Answering the following questions will help to keep you focused and probably save you a lot of money and frustration, too.

- Why did *Keto for Women* capture my attention?

- What do I hope will change for me in the future?

- What fears do I have surrounding eating this way, or what challenges have I faced in doing so?

- How do I feel when I think about approaching my nutrition with less rigidity? What feelings come up when I play with the idea of abandoning my plans and just listening to my body?

- Why do I feel like keto will be the solution I've been seeking?

Three Days to
Food Freedom

Beginning your food-freedom journey requires that you connect with your body. No connection translates to no progress. But don't worry, I've got your back. We're in this together.

Connecting with your body makes it possible for you to:

- Tap into your hunger levels

- Understand intuitively exactly which foods your body needs

- Eliminate overeating

- Maintain a healthy weight

Understanding what cues your body is sending you, how they differ from the cues sent by your brain (that is, your reason and emotions), and how to translate them into action will be a dramatic turning point for you. The more you practice getting in touch with your body, the easier it will be to eat what you need, when you need it, and to begin to fill your life with self-gratitude for your awesome abilities to make the right choices.

There are some practical steps you can take to get in touch with your body, and I'll walk you through these in the following pages. I recommend that you practice just one step each day to allow things to marinate, so I've set this up as a process that takes three days. But of course, if you'd like to spend more time or less on any step, it's up to you!

Warning: Uncomfortable feelings may come to the surface as you work through this process. Instead of rejecting them or feeling bad about them, take them as a good sign! Give yourself permission to experience and fully feel all the thoughts and emotions that will no doubt come over you. Feeling is healing. Get comfortable with being uncomfortable (for the time being, at least), and trust that self-love and your desire to discover a better new way of doing things will guide you unerringly down the path you are meant to be on.

Grab your journal, cuddle up in a quiet corner, and scribble. Reflect and let your mind go. Take as little or as much time as you need.

Practice patience.

Trust yourself.

Let it be easy.

And if, after three days, you want to go deeper, I have a twenty-one-day program dedicated to this practice called Whole Keto (healthfulpursuit.com/whole).

Day 1: Setting the Foundation

It's important to get a clear picture of where we are before we try to figure out where we're headed and how we're going to get there. So let's start things off by situating ourselves, shall we?

Close your eyes and think of a few of your past meals (or snacks, lunches, dinners—whatever you can remember). It doesn't matter if you ate them as recently as this morning or as far back as last Christmas.

Got them fixed in your mind? Okay, for each meal, ask yourself some questions.

- What was the tone of the environment, conversations, or events that were going on around me before, during, and after the meal?

- What emotions did I experience before, during, and after the meal?

- What internal dialogue, if any, was running through my mind before, during, and after the meal?

- How did I feel about myself before, during, and after the meal?

- How was my behavior before, during, and after the meal?

- What was my energy level like before, during, and after the meal?

Tip: If relying on your memory to answer these questions is too challenging, set the worksheet down and, for the next day, become a conscious witness to the situations, emotions, dialogue, and feelings you experience around your meals. Then come back to your worksheet—the answers should flow a little easier.

Day 2: Recognizing Your Food-Freedom Drivers

Review your answers from day 1. Note the factors that seem to elicit the strongest responses for you—the ones where you were able to clearly identify feeling crummy, unbalanced, and/or out of control. Do any patterns emerge?

Maybe you eat in the car because you're ashamed to have others see you eating. Perhaps you eat before you get hungry because you're afraid of getting hunger pangs. Maybe you find that you're consistently eating whenever you get anxious or overwhelmed.

Choose the three responses that elicit the most emotion for you and write them down below. Then rate each response on a scale of 1 to 10, with 10 being the strongest, based on the power you believe it has to impede your progress in moving forward with a healthy life.

Its power: 1 2 3 4 5 6 7 8 9 10

Its power: 1 2 3 4 5 6 7 8 9 10

Its power: 1 2 3 4 5 6 7 8 9 10

Keep these situations, feelings, and emotions in mind tomorrow. As you hold them in your mind, remember that these are sensitive issues for you and make a special point of being gentle and kind to yourself around them.

As you become more comfortable with this process, you can practice answering the six "Setting the Foundation" questions from day 1 at the beginning of each meal to keep yourself accountable and focused on your food-freedom goals.

If you're struggling to deal with the emotions that this exercise stirs up, remind yourself that you are creating love in your life, that this action is love, and that you're ready for and deserve a life of love.

Day 3: Acknowledging Your Unkindness

Your thoughts and perceptions create your reality. Your perception of everything around you, everything you're experiencing right now, exists because you yourself have created it. Taking responsibility for your experiences will help you to accept and welcome the true power that you have to create for yourself a new, more loving, and more authentic reality. It's time to get honest with yourself about the reality you've created and flip your negative perceptions and beliefs upside down.

Reflect on the following questions and write down your answers. Be aware that your fears will attempt to sabotage your efforts by making you doubt or criticize your answers, dream up excuses to avoid the questions, and generally poke fun at you. Do not question or judge your answers. Know that love wants to forgive, and that's why we're here—to love ourselves and let go of our ingrained negative beliefs.

- How am I psychologically unkind to myself on a daily basis?

- How am I physically unkind to myself on a daily basis?

- How have I given fear permission and power to control my thoughts and actions?

- What negative statements or stories have I created about myself?

Now, using your answers from above, flip the negative responses and behaviors you've identified into positive affirmations that begin with the words "May I be..."

For example, if you've learned that you tend to be most critical of yourself when you're immersed in a hectic environment, your positive affirmation could be, "May I be calm." If you've identified a pattern of creating negative stories about yourself in response to situations that make you feel something in your life is lacking, your affirmation could be, "May I be abundant."

Compose seven affirmations for yourself, or use the examples provided below. For the next seven days, every day for a full week, pick one affirmation to be your focus. Write it on your palm or a sticky note, record it on your phone or your screensaver—just make sure it is front and center so you'll be able to see it multiple times a day.

May I be loving.

May I be kind.

May I be accepting.

May I be thoughtful.

May I be calm.

May I be abundant.

May I be radiant.

If you see progress and want to go even deeper, head on over to healthfulpursuit.com/whole for twenty-one steps to enriching your relationship with your body.

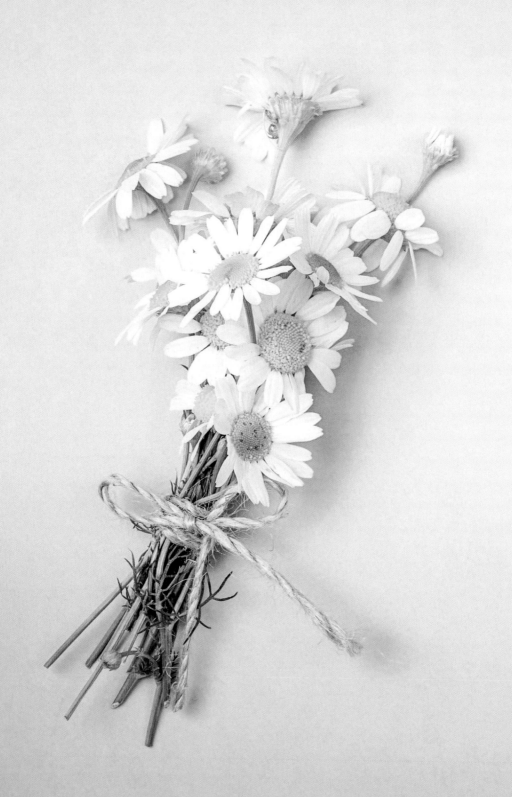

8

OVERCOMING IMBALANCES: SUPPORTING BASIC BODY SYSTEMS

Do you have a thyroid imbalance? What if you haven't gotten your period in a long time? Are you dealing with adrenal dysfunction, chronic pain, or raging PMS? Perhaps you are lacking energy, allergic to eggs, or trying to avoid foods high in FODMAPs. No matter what your personal situation, this chapter is designed to help you reach your goals with actionable step-by-step plans.

Stress as a Common Factor

In the sections in this chapter, the "Test for It" boxes suggest some tests you may find useful if you're concerned about a particular health problem. I do not list "normal" test results because I truly believe that everyone's levels are unique to them. Work with your health-care team to run and interpret the labs, or use a service like Everlywell.com, where you can order your own lab work and collect saliva, urine, and even blood right at home.

I want to start by highlighting something that I'll be bringing up over and over as a contributor to many imbalances we'll be reviewing in this chapter: stress. It can do a lot to a body, forcing us to stay in a hyperaware state and in a constant flood of cortisol, a hormone that, in excess, can make it next to impossible to stay in ketosis, get a good night's rest, maintain balanced hormones, and keep inflammation low.

It's imperative that we work to reduce stress so that we can give power back to the body systems that have been robbed from operating at their best.

In response to an acute stressor, such as a trauma like a car accident, the body responds quickly to keep you alive. Here are the key steps you'll experience in an instant when your brain perceives danger, before you consciously realize what's happening:

1. The hypothalamus in the brain acts as a command center throughout the experience, communicating with the body through the nervous system to prepare for fleeing or fighting.

2. The adrenal glands pump out the hormone epinephrine.

3. Your heart rate increases so that more blood is pushed to the muscles, heart, and vital organs.

4. Your pulse rate, blood pressure, and breath rate all increase to supply as much oxygen as possible to the brain to increase alertness.

5. Your blood sugar rises so more energy is readily available.

6. As the initial surge of epinephrine subsides, the HPA axis—a close linkage between the hypothalamus, pituitary, and adrenals—is activated to stay abreast of the perceived threat. If the brain still perceives something as dangerous, the HPA axis is triggered to release the hormone cortisol.

7. Cortisol continues to be released so that the body stays alert.

8. When the threat passes, cortisol levels fall.

All these reactions are important and necessary, and when they happen during a short period of time, they have no negative long-term effect. When we are chronically stressed, however, the nervous system is *chronically* stimulated, and the end result is chronic immune system suppression, elevated blood sugar, possible high blood pressure, poor circulation, and the suppression of digestion.

Part of the problem is that hormones and the hypothalamus, pituitary, and adrenals play such a large role in a stress response. They all perform many important functions that aren't stress-related—for example, the hypothalamus is in charge of maintaining body temperature, circadian rhythm, hunger, and more—but a stress response takes precedence over these necessary roles. Instead of doing their regular jobs, these hormones and systems are commandeered to respond to stress.

Stress contributes to a vast majority of illnesses. Please don't discount how important it is to lower the amount of stress in your life. While it may feel impossible to do, every little step you take toward reducing stress will make a lasting change to your life. Throughout this chapter, I'll talk about lowering stress as part of addressing specific health concerns, but I really want to drive home how important stress reduction is to your *overall* well-being—not just in relation to a particular problem.

The body is not designed to handle chronic stress, and research shows that chronic stress can be behind such problems as reduced strength, an imbalanced immune system, and increased inflammation.

Autoimmune **Support**

Includes Hashimoto's thyroiditis, rheumatoid arthritis, eczema, psoriasis, asthma, chronic fatigue syndrome, multiple sclerosis, Addison's disease, type 1 diabetes, and lupus

"Autoimmune disease" is the term given to a variety of conditions in which the immune system attacks healthy tissue. By understanding why some people develop autoimmune diseases and connecting the dots behind an autoimmune flare-up, it's possible to go beyond the standard methods of care and live a great life with a dormant autoimmune condition.

Before we get into connecting the dots, let's quickly review how autoimmunity works. All autoimmune diseases are characterized by an overactive immune system. With any autoimmune condition, the immune system loses the ability to differentiate between proteins that belong to the body and proteins that belong to foreign invaders, like bacteria, viruses, or parasites.

This leads to chronic inflammation and tissue destruction. This is true of all autoimmune diseases, but they differ in the type of body tissue that's under attack. For example, rheumatoid arthritis is the result of the immune system attacking the joints, whereas in multiple sclerosis, the immune system attacks the myelin sheath surrounding nerves.

High-sensitivity C-reactive protein (hs-CRP) is a test that measures CRP in the blood to detect inflammation that is associated with autoimmune flare-ups.

Homocysteine levels can indicate whether your body is undergoing a healthy amount of methylation, a process that influences your brain, hormones, immune system, and gut. If homocysteine is imbalanced, it could be a sign of autoimmune or inflammation issues.

25-hydroxy vitamin D looks at levels of vitamin D after the liver has converted it to 25-hydroxy vitamin D (the first of several transformations vitamin D goes through before it can be used by the body). This test is the best way to look at vitamin D levels because it's a good indication of how much vitamin D your body really has.

Vitamin B$_{12}$ level is a good indication of nutrient status and can be low in those with autoimmune conditions.

Heavy metals can be imbalanced in those with autoimmune conditions. A good heavy-metals test will test for arsenic, mercury, cadmium, bromine, selenium, iodine, and urinary creatinine.

While a range of medications are used to treat autoimmune diseases, they generally involve suppressing the immune system and reducing inflammation. And while they can give you relief from a malady, it's important to get to the root of the condition and fix any underlying issues instead of having to rely on medication forever, which could bring about a host of other issues and side effects.

Contributing Factors

Multiple factors can contribute to the development of an autoimmune disease. The specific cause of autoimmunity—what makes one individual get an illness while someone else doesn't—is unknown, but contributors that are often overlooked include whether a family member has a similar autoimmune condition; MTHFR gene mutation; exposure to toxins; infectious agents such as bacteria, viruses, and parasites; chronic or acute stress; chronic gastrointestinal inflammation; food sensitivities; high general inflammation in the body; leaky gut; and hormones.

Hormones

Okay, so you're probably wondering how your hormones can affect the health of your immune system. Hormones can exacerbate autoimmunity or, conversely, keep the immune system in balance. For example, estrogen has been shown to weaken the body's suppressor cells, which keep the immune system in check and prevent it from attacking the body. On the flip side, testosterone can boost the action of suppressor cells.

Excess cortisol can lead to an overworked immune system. Additionally, TSH, the thyroid hormone, has been shown to affect the immune system indirectly by altering the release of T3 and T4 from the thyroid, which in turn affects how the bone marrow and secondary lymphoid tissues (which include your lymph nodes, tonsils, and spleen) produce white blood cells, the foot soldiers of the immune system.

So if you want to support a balanced immune system—and especially if you have an autoimmune condition—you'd be crazy to ignore your hormones.

Simply balancing your hormones might actually improve your autoimmune symptoms dramatically. If you need a refresher on how to address hormonal imbalances, go to page 335. Otherwise, you can rest assured that the actions below will set you on a path to supporting your body.

Leaky Gut

The cells lining your intestines are tightly joined, like a well-constructed brick wall. But with leaky gut, gaps develop between these cells, and tiny particles of food and bacteria escape through the intestinal wall. Outside the digestive tract, your immune system recognizes them as foreign invaders and gets to work to destroy them, just as it should. But when these particles are consistently leaking into the body, the immune system never gets to rest, leading to chronic inflammation, and in some people, the immune system can start overreacting and attack their own tissue.

How do gaps between cells lining the intestines develop? A compound called zonulin is released by the gut wall to moderate its permeability. When too much zonulin is released and those gaps stay open, we have an issue on our hands. If you haven't guessed yet, certain foods trigger larger releases of zonulin than others—for example, gluten is known to increase zonulin. Dysbiosis, an imbalance of the bacteria in the gut, does as well. Leaky gut may also be caused by food sensitivities, bacteria and parasites, and possibly exposure to glyphosate, an herbicide that is often sprayed on crops to kill weeds.

The good news is that you *can* heal leaky gut by changing your diet and lifestyle—the guidelines starting on page 244 will show you how. And once healed, your immune system finally gets to take a break, going back to its normal role of protecting you and not attacking you. From there your tissues are able to heal and your autoimmune symptoms subside.

Understanding Flare-ups

If you have an autoimmune disorder, you already know that sometimes your symptoms subside, maybe even completely, and you're in remission. And then you can suddenly have a flare-up and symptoms ignite overnight.

Flare-ups are a sign that something has aggravated your immune system and more tissue destruction is occurring. It may not always be clear why a flare-up is occurring, but it can be helpful to look at what's going on in your life and identify potential causes, such as:

- Consuming sugar
- Eating inflammatory foods or foods you're sensitive to
- Experiencing high stress
- Being exposed to toxins
- Not moving enough

Diet Adjustments

There's an entire diet dedicated to managing autoimmune conditions. It's called the autoimmune protocol, or AIP.

With my own health journey, I've always felt like it was important for me to know why doing something was better for my health than doing something else. I'll never be one to actively avoid a specific food just because someone's told me that it's bad. I need to completely understand *why*.

So here's why the AIP diet eliminates the foods that it does: these foods have been shown to contribute to leaky gut. When you combine AIP with the high-fat, low-carb approach of keto, inflammation is reduced throughout the body.

Seventy percent of your immune system is in your gut, so if your gut is not healthy, your immune system is not healthy either. A balanced immune system is achieved by restoring a healthy diversity and balance of bacteria to the gut microbiome, healing gaps in the gut lining, providing sufficient amounts of the micronutrients required for the immune system to function normally, and supporting the key hormones that regulate the immune system. The AIP diet, especially when combined with keto, can help with all of this.

The AIP diet is very restrictive and many people find it difficult to follow, but adhering to it for a short period can reset your body so you start feeling better, and then you can start adding eliminated foods back to your diet (more on that on page 246). Because of its restrictiveness, I'd advise against trying out AIP just for kicks. If you don't need to be on an AIP diet, don't do it!

And know that, as helpful as the AIP diet can be, not everyone with autoimmune disease needs to follow it in order to get their symptoms into remission. Some people do quite well by simply following the Fat Fueled Food Pyramid on page 85, which emphasizes whole foods, while others find that addressing lifestyle factors is an essential piece of the puzzle.

AIP

 AVOID THESE!

 GLUTEN & GRAINS*

All foods containing grains or gluten

Amaranth

Barley

Buckwheat

Bulgur

Corn

Millet

Oats

Quinoa

Rice

Rye

Sorghum

Spelt

Wheat

 DAIRY

All sources of dairy, including raw and fermented versions

Butter

Cheese

Cream

Ghee

Milk

Yogurt

 ALL ALCOHOL

 EGGS

 NIGHTSHADES

All peppers
(bell peppers, jalapeños, etc.)

All red spices
(cayenne, paprika, etc.)

Eggplant

Potatoes

Tomatoes

 NUTS & SEEDS

All nuts and seeds and all foods containing nut- or seed-based ingredients, such as nut flour

Almonds

Brazil nuts

Cacao

Canola

Cashew

Chia seeds

Coffee

Flax seeds

Hazelnuts

Hemp seeds

Pecans

Pine nuts

Pistachios

Pumpkin seeds

Safflower seeds

Sesame seeds

Sunflower seeds

Walnuts

 SPICES FROM SEEDS & BERRIES

Allspice

Anise

Black pepper

Caraway seed

Celery seed

Cumin

Dry mustard

Fennel seed

Nutmeg

Poppy seed

 LEGUMES

All legumes in all forms, including cooked, sprouted, and fermented versions

Black beans

Chickpeas

Fava beans

Kidney beans

Lentils

Lima beans

Peanuts

Soybeans

* Gluten and grains should already be avoided on a strict keto diet, but if you're using carb-ups or following another cyclical keto practice, make sure you avoid these.

NSAIDS

Nonsteroidal anti-inflammatory drugs, such as ibuprofen, aspirin, and naproxen, may cause holes to form in the gut and stomach linings, which will worsen autoimmune symptoms (see page 243 on leaky gut).

The Importance of Nutrient-Dense Foods

Your immune system requires an array of vitamins, minerals, antioxidants, essential fatty acids, and amino acids to function normally. Micronutrient deficiencies and imbalances are key players in the development and progression of autoimmune disease—and on the flip side, having a surplus of micronutrients is essential to correct both deficiencies and imbalances and to support the immune system— as well as your hormones, detoxification, and neurotransmitter production. A nutrient-dense diet also provides the building blocks that the body needs to heal damaged tissues.

So, while it's tempting to focus on what you're *not* eating on AIP, it's important to make sure you're also consuming the most nutrient-dense foods available. You can follow the AIP diet perfectly, but if you forget to add in nutrient-dense foods, your ability to heal won't be optimally supported.

For example, liver, fatty fish, and shellfish are rich in vitamins A and D, zinc, choline, and various B vitamins, which are essential for a healthy immune response, energy production in the mitochondria, and healing damaged tissues, especially the gut lining. Liver in particular is crucial on a strict AIP diet because it contains nutrients that would otherwise come from eggs, which are off-limits.

Many people who attempt an AIP diet struggle with consuming some of the more nutrient-dense foods like liver, shellfish, fermented vegetables, and bone broth. But these foods should be considered an integral part of an effective AIP approach, and I strongly encourage those with autoimmune diseases to get comfy with these foods—learn to love 'em.

It's also important to source the best-quality ingredients possible—you really want to avoid toxins and chemicals, such as pesticides, as much as possible—and to eat as much variety as you can. The wider the variety of foods you eat, the wider the variety of micronutrients you consume.

Reintroducing Foods

A lot of people remove all of the non-AIP foods from their diet and think that that's how they'll have to eat for the rest of their lives. Not the case! After you've been following AIP for thirty days, giving your body a chance to heal, you'll want to reintroduce each eliminated food systematically to see if it's something that bothers you or if it can return to being part of your usual lineup.

The benefits of reintroducing non-AIP foods are vast. First, you may actually be able to tolerate nutrient-dense foods like eggs, and the more nutrient-dense foods you can eat, the better. Second, reintroducing foods will give you a better understanding of which foods are more crucial to avoid than others, so you have more freedom in your food choices. And third, a broader diet can significantly improve your ability to enjoy food, both at home and when you're out to eat, which will certainly add to your quality of life.

The reintroduction of foods is likely going to be the most challenging part of personalizing your AIP diet. It can take hours, days, or even weeks for an immune response to kick in to the point that you experience symptoms. While some people get an immediate and strong reaction to a food they've eaten, others have only a minor increase in symptoms that can be hard to recognize.

The good news is that, once they've done some healing, those with an autoimmune disease can frequently tolerate foods like dairy, eggs, nightshades, and nuts and seeds. The effort of determining which foods you can tolerate and which should stay off-limits is absolutely worth it.

Here's what I've found to be the best process for reintroducing foods:

1. Identify the eliminated foods that are most important to you. Maybe you really miss eggs, or tomatoes, or cheese. These are the foods you want to reintroduce first.

2. Reintroduce one food at a time. This doesn't mean a *category* of foods, like dairy as a whole—it means each individual food needs to be reintroduced on its own. So if you're reintroducing nightshades, for example, start with *just* potatoes, then add tomatoes, then eggplant, and so on.

3. Give yourself at least three days before reintroducing another food. During those three days, look for any change in how you're feeling. You may see a return of autoimmune symptoms you've experienced in the past, such as joint pain or skin inflammation, or you may experience a new symptom, like gastrointestinal distress or fatigue.

4. If you've eaten the food consistently for three days and you don't notice any negative side effects, you can generally assume the food is okay for you to eat! But if you do experience symptoms, stop eating the food you reintroduced and see if symptoms abate. If so, you may need to keep avoiding that food for an additional thirty days and then try again using steps 2 and 3 above.

Foods in certain groups need to be reintroduced in a particular order, starting with those that are least likely to cause a reaction. With dairy, for instance, start by reintroducing ghee, which contains the least amount of milk proteins. If you don't have a reaction to ghee, you can continue with other dairy foods, like grass-fed butter and kefir. With eggs, reintroduce the yolk first as egg whites can elicit more of a reaction than the yolks.

Please don't think you'll never be able to eat autoimmune-triggering foods again. With the proper protocol and patience, you should be able to indulge in foods like egg whites, seeds, and chocolate.

Ultra-Healing Foods

THE EXTRAS

- Fresh and dried basil
- Fresh and dried cilantro
- Fresh and dried parsley
- Fresh and dried rosemary (leaves and ground)
- Ground cinnamon
- Ground cumin
- Ground turmeric
- Mushroom elixirs
- Sea vegetables: spirulina and chlorella

STARCHES AND FRUITS

- Bananas
- Beets
- Blueberries
- Butternut squash
- Carrots
- Green plantains
- Sweet potatoes

Keep fructose intake between 10 and 20 grams daily

PROTEIN

- Bone broth
- Collagen
- Fish
- Gelatin
- Grass-fed beef
- Lamb
- Organ meats
- Oysters
- Salmon
- Shellfish

NON-STARCHY VEGETABLES

- Broccoli
- Brussels sprouts
- Cauliflower
- Daikon
- Fermented vegetables, such as
- kimchi and sauerkraut
- Garlic
- Mustard greens
- Spinach
- Swiss chard
- Watercress

HEALTHY FATS

- Avocado oil
- Avocados
- Coconut oil
- Duck fat
- Extra-virgin olive oil
- Lard
- Red palm oil
- Tallow

WATER

Additional Adjustments

Say Yes To

ADDITIONAL GUT SUPPORT & INFLAMMATION SUPPORT

You may progress really well with just the information in this section, or you may find that inflammation or gut health is still an issue for you. If so, follow the protocols in the Gut Support (page 256) and Inflammation Reduction (page 251) sections of this chapter to go even deeper with your healing.

SOFT, WELL-COOKED FOODS

Opt for stews, soups, braised meats, and meals prepared in a slow cooker. These items are easier to digest and may cause less dietary stress on your body.

FILTERED WATER
Water can be a common source of toxins, so filter your water with a reverse osmosis filter.

STRONG SUPPORT SYSTEM
Therapy, a support group, and relationships with kind persons all help to balance the mind, body, and spirit. When left untreated, emotional trauma can lead to physical symptoms and disease; seeking support can be hugely helpful.

DAILY STRESS REDUCTION
If you're not doing some form of regular stress management, you'll sabotage all of your best efforts with diet, exercise, and supplements. Minimizing stress is nonnegotiable for people suffering with autoimmunity. Yoga, meditation, breathing exercises, qigong, and tai chi have all been scientifically proven to reduce stress and inflammation, thus calming the immune system. If none of these feel right to you, find a self-care practice that does—maybe an unhurried walk in nature, or a relaxing bath, or just sitting alone with your headphones on, listening to your favorite music.

ORGANIC PRODUCE
Try for organic as much as possible, especially with crops that are treated with a lot of pesticides and other chemicals. Generally speaking, if you have to choose, foods that don't have a thick peel should be organic, like apples, bell peppers, celery, cherries, cherry tomatoes, cucumbers, grapes, nectarines, peaches, spinach, strawberries, and tomatoes. The Dirty Dozen list on the Environmental Working Group website (www.ewg.org/foodnews/dirty-dozen.php) is updated every year with the produce most likely to be contaminated with pesticides.

MOVING YOUR BODY
Inactivity causes inflammation, and inflammation is a key factor in autoimmune disease. Living a sedentary life causes elevations in inflammatory substances and C-reactive protein (CRP), which is associated with inflammation and negatively impacts every organ in the body, particularly the heart. Also, when we don't move, our lymphatic system cannot drain toxins and waste well. Movement is necessary for health, so exercise daily, get a stand-up desk if you can, park in the back of the lot, and meet a friend for a coffee walk instead of a sitting coffee date.

GOOD SLEEPING PATTERNS
Chronically poor sleep is a source of stress and inflammation. When circadian rhythms get misaligned from weeks or months of inadequate sleep, inflammatory immune cells are produced in excess, leading to an increase in "friendly fire" against the body's own tissues.

VITAMIN D

Vitamin D has been shown to directly influence the activity of the immune system. Vitamin D deficiency has been connected with a higher risk of developing autoimmune disease, and on the flip side, vitamin D supplementation is used to reduce the symptoms of autoimmune disease. The best way to get enough vitamin D is to get out in the sun for twenty to thirty minutes a day—without sunscreen. If regular sun exposure isn't an option for you, you may also benefit from vitamin D supplementation. I recommend fermented cod liver oil, which is best taken in the morning with a fatty meal.

Say No To

TOXINS

A body with an autoimmune condition reacts strongly to toxins by increasing inflammation, which increases autoimmune symptoms. It's important to seek out natural versions of anything that comes in contact with your body, such as body wash, lotions, makeup, shampoo, laundry detergent, and household cleaners. Ingredients to avoid include the following: avobenzone, benzophenone, formaldehyde, fragrance/perfume, homosalate, methoxycinnmate, PABA, parabens, propylene glycol, sodium laureth sulfate, sodium lauryl sulfate, synthetic colors, toluene, and triclosan. Dr. Bronner's is a great brand for castile soap, lotions, and toothpaste. Skindeep.org has recommendations for makeup and shampoo. White vinegar and baking soda are great household cleaners.

OVERTRAINING

Exercise is essential to a healthy life, but it can be overdone. Overtraining can cause depletion in the amino acid glutamine, which is essential for healthy immune response and a healthy gut barrier. Overtraining also causes an increase in inflammatory immune proteins. Athletes who overtrain tend to have high inflammation. If you are training for a competitive sport or like to exercise for over an hour a day, please be mindful that these are possible sources of inflammation.

CIGARETTES, ALCOHOL & CAFFEINE

Consumption of these bad boys decreases the effectiveness of the immune system and can cause increased inflammation, which can exacerbate leaky gut conditions.

FOOD SENSITIVITIES

If you're sensitive or allergic to a food, your immune system goes into overdrive when you consume it, leading to anything from hives to swelling to diarrhea to nausea. And aggravating the immune system can exacerbate symptoms of any autoimmune disease. Figuring out what foods you're sensitive to and avoiding them is an essential step in managing autoimmunity (more on that on page 274).

Supportive Supplements

- Vitamins: A, B_6, E, C, D, methylfolate, methyl B_{12}

- Minerals: zinc, iron, copper, selenium, magnesium

- Herbs and plants: hops, smilax, reishi

- Others: aloe vera juice, L-glutamine, homeopathic remedies recommended by a homeopathic doctor, digestive enzymes, probiotics. If you are dealing with an autoimmune condition that affects your adrenal or digestive system, see the recommended supplements for adrenal support on page 374 and gut support on page 267.

Inflammation **Reduction**

Inflammation has a bad reputation, but it's not all bad. In fact, it's necessary for life. When you bang your knee, or when bacteria or a virus enters your body, inflammation is called to the site thanks to your immune system, bathing the area in fluids, proteins, and blood. This process creates swelling and heat to protect and repair the damage and encourage healing. This is a healthy inflammatory response.

An unhealthy inflammatory response is when inflammation becomes chronic. When that short-term heat and swelling becomes long-term, producing a steady low-grade inflammation, it ultimately contributes to the development of disease. Why does this happen? In part, it's due to an overactive immune system that initiates inflammation even when there is nothing to heal. The body keeps reacting to what it thinks is a problem, never shutting itself off.

Test for It: Inflammation

High-sensitivity C-reactive protein (hs-CRP) is a test that measures CRP in the blood to detect inflammation.

Homocysteine levels can indicate whether your body is undergoing a healthy amount of methylation, a process that influences your brain, hormones, immune system, and gut. If homocysteine is imbalanced, it could be a sign of increased inflammation.

Many of us think of inflammation as a contained reaction or situation, when in reality it affects every part of the body. Inflammation plays a role in autoimmune conditions, cardiovascular disease, cancer, diabetes, and more. It can be triggered by various factors, but the most interesting of all factors is fat cells, which can trigger a steady release of substances that attack healthy nerves, organs, and tissues when there is no actual invader to attack. As we gain weight, more of these substances are released, affecting our bodies' ability to use insulin and sometimes leading to type 2 diabetes.

This same reaction can have an effect on our hormones, possibly leading to amenorrhea or low testosterone, and can cause impaired memory and cognition, depression, suppressed immune function, and pain.

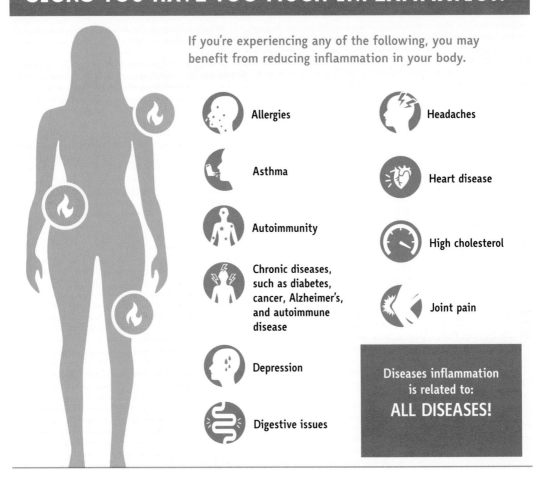

SIGNS YOU HAVE TOO MUCH INFLAMMATION

If you're experiencing any of the following, you may benefit from reducing inflammation in your body.

Allergies

Asthma

Autoimmunity

Chronic diseases, such as diabetes, cancer, Alzheimer's, and autoimmune disease

Depression

Digestive issues

Headaches

Heart disease

High cholesterol

Joint pain

Diseases inflammation is related to:
ALL DISEASES!

Diet Adjustments

Thankfully, the ketogenic diet is in and of itself an anti-inflammatory diet, so following the three steps to Fat Fueled freedom on pages 81 to 213 will do wonders for reducing inflammation. However, if you find inflammation is still lingering after you've become fat adapted, here are some additional dietary adjustments you can make:

- Supplement with exogenous ketones.

- If you don't already follow it, switch to the Classic Keto Fat Fueled Profile (page 199).

- Fast more often, and drink green tea in the morning during your fasts. (See page 138 for more on fasting.)

- Have hot water with lemon and fresh ginger before bed.

- Spend ten to twenty minutes in an infrared sauna two or three times per week.

Ultra-Healing Foods

THE EXTRAS

- Bay leaves
- Fennel
- Fresh dill and dried dill weed
- Fresh and dried basil
- Fresh and dried oregano
- Fresh and dried rosemary
- Fresh and dried sage
- Fresh and dried thyme
- Fresh garlic
- Fresh ginger
- Garlic powder
- Ginger powder
- Ground black pepper
- Ground cinnamon
- Ground coriander
- Ground cumin
- Ground turmeric

STARCHES AND FRUITS

- Blueberries
- Cranberries
- Lemon
- Papaya

PROTEIN

- Chia seeds
- Hemp seeds
- Salmon
- Sardines
- Walnuts

NON-STARCHY VEGETABLES

- Broccoli
- Celery
- Red cabbage

HEALTHY FATS

- Avocados
- Chia seeds
- Flax seeds

WATER

Additional Adjustments

Say Yes To

DISCOVERING FOOD SENSITIVITIES & ALLERGIES

When you eat foods that you're sensitive to, the gut becomes inflamed, which can exacerbate leaky gut issues (see page 243). Follow the elimination protocol on page 277 to determine which foods you might be sensitive to.

HEALING YOUR GUT

Inflammation often goes hand in hand with leaky gut (see page 243), so healing your gut can help reduce inflammation. If you find that your gut needs additional support, follow the advice in the Gut Support section on page 256 in conjunction with this section.

MOVING YOUR BODY

Inactivity causes inflammation. Living a sedentary life causes elevations in inflammatory substances and C-reactive protein (CRP), which is associated with inflammation and negatively impacts every organ in the body, particularly the heart. Also, when we don't move, our lymphatic system cannot drain toxins and waste well. Movement is necessary for health, so exercise daily, get a stand-up desk if you can, park in the back of the lot, and meet a friend for a coffee walk instead of a sitting coffee date.

HIGH-QUALITY FOODS

Poor-quality foods, such as conventionally raised beef, dairy, poultry, and eggs, can increase inflammation due to the imbalance of omega-6 and omega-3 fatty acids. Also avoid highly processed foods, like conventional hot dogs and sausages. And although sugar is already out on strict keto, if you're practicing cyclical ketosis, make sure you choose healthier carbs.

DAILY STRESS REDUCTION

Chronic stress increases systemic inflammation. Yoga, meditation, breathing exercises, qigong, and tai chi have all been scientifically proven to reduce stress and inflammation. If none of these feel right to you, find a self-care practice that does—maybe an unhurried walk in nature, or a relaxing bath, or just sitting alone with your headphones on, listening to your favorite music.

For women, inflammation is more of a problem postmenopausally due to lower levels of protective estrogen.

Say No To

DAIRY

If you're dealing with high levels of inflammation, it's best to avoid all dairy products completely until you've determined whether dairy is safe for your body through the methods described on page 277.

OVERTRAINING

Exercise is essential to a healthy life, but it can be overdone. Overtraining can cause a depletion in the amino acid glutamine, which is essential for a healthy immune response. Overtraining also causes an increase in inflammatory substances. Athletes who overtrain tend to have high inflammation and may experience chronic infections, depression, fatigue, irritability, digestive disturbances, and flu-like symptoms. If you are training for a competitive sport or like to exercise for over an hour a day, please be mindful of these possible outcomes.

SUGAR & REFINED CARBS

If you're practicing carb-ups or another kind of cyclical keto, sugar and refined carbs may cause spikes in insulin and blood sugar, weight gain, and an increase in free radicals—all of which increase inflammation. High blood sugar and high insulin both trigger the release of inflammatory substances. Weight gain, particularly abdominal weight, is associated with inflammation. Abdominal weight is often composed of visceral fat, fat around the internal organs, and that's exceptionally good at stimulating an inflammatory response in the body. Free radicals act like pinballs flying around inside your body and damaging the cells they come in contact with, and the immune system must activate the inflammatory process to heal the damage.

ALCOHOL

Alcohol can trigger chronic inflammation because of its effect on the lining of the gut, which allows bacteria to pass through the gut lining and cause inflammation.

OMEGA-6-RICH FOODS

Conventionally raised beef and dairy have a higher ratio of omega-6 to omega-3, making them more pro-inflammatory. Conventionally raised poultry and eggs, as well as nuts and seeds, also contain high amounts of omega-6 fatty acids. Avoid these foods if you're already dealing with high inflammation!

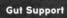

Supportive Supplements

- Vitamins: C, D, E
- Herbs and plants: curcumin, boswellia, willow bark, pycnogenol
- Others: MSM, glucosamine, chondroitin, plant enzymes, omega-3 fatty acids, alpha lipoic acid, grapeseed extract, green tea extract, NAC

Gut **Support**

Includes leaky gut, dysbiosis, mental health, constipation, diarrhea, digestive pain, gas, and bloating

There are many theories about why digestive complaints—from diarrhea and constipation to bloating to stomach pain—have become so common these days. Potential culprits include a decrease in food quality, genetic modification of food, the use of chemicals like pesticides and herbicides in agriculture, and overuse of antibiotics. It's likely that the epidemic of digestive issues is the result of several factors, not just one, but food seems to be one of the biggest contributors to the problem.

Test for It: Gut Health

IgA and IgG are both immunoglobulins, or antibodies, which are created by the immune system to fight bacteria, viruses, and toxins. The five classes of immunoglobulins (IgA, IgG, IgM, IgE, and IgD) combat different things. For the purpose of gut health, IgA and IgG are the most common to test for. When these antibody levels are higher than normal, you can suspect that the gut is affected and inflammation is present.

H. pylori **urea breath test** is used to identify infections of *Helicobacter pylori*, the bacteria that's often behind ulcers.

SIBO breath test can diagnose or rule out small intestine bacterial overgrowth, which may be the cause of chronic diarrhea, bloating, and gas.

For keto women, this is exciting news: it means that we can actively work to prevent and treat digestive disorders by embracing the keto lifestyle and diet. True, everyone is different, so we each need to figure out what works best for us as individuals. But a healthy keto diet is a great place to start because it eliminates so many of the most common food-related causes of digestive complaints. The information in this section will help you go one step further in supporting your gut.

The gut is at the core of our capacity to break down and utilize nutrients from the food we eat. It also produces additional essential vitamins and wards off foreign invaders—in fact, 70 percent of the immune system is found in the gut. In short, it is one of the body's greatest defenders and protectors. When the food we eat cannot be assimilated properly because the gut is damaged or not functioning optimally, we don't get the nourishment we need, and additional imbalances present themselves. So it's crucial to take steps to support and heal the gut.

If you have a strong handle on the issues you're dealing with and are pretty confident in your body's healing powers, everything below should resonate. However, if your symptoms are severe, you might get better results by following the guidelines in the Autoimmune Support section (page 241).

SYMPTOMS OF GUT IMBALANCE

Maybe you got an upset stomach last week. Maybe your bowel movements have been irregular lately. Maybe this week pimples started popping up for the first time since high school. It could be a random occurrence. But it also could be poor gut health.

 Autoimmune disease

 Bloating

 Brain fog

 Constipation

 Diarrhea

 Emotional and mental changes, such as depression, mood changes, or difficulty focusing

 Food sensitivities or allergies

 Inflamed skin and related conditions, including acne, eczema, and psoriasis

 Long-term gastrointestinal symptoms that are really hard to manage despite adherence to a healthy diet and good stress management

 Stomach pain after eating

 Thyroid difficulties

Leaky Gut and Dysbiosis

Leaky gut and dysbiosis are at the core of many gut imbalances.

Leaky gut is exactly what it sounds like: a condition in which the intestines are more permeable than they should be, allowing particles of food and bacteria to escape into the body. It's often associated with autoimmune disorders and gluten intolerance, but it can also lead to gastrointestinal problems like bloating, gas, and cramps, along with fatigue, food sensitivities, joint pain, skin rashes, and chronic inflammation. (For more on how leaky gut develops, see page 243.)

Dysbiosis is an imbalance of the microbiome in our digestive tract, the little environment where microorganisms like bacteria and yeast reside—about one trillion of them, to be exact. These 3 pounds of happy, nice little microbes are crucial to the processes of breaking down food, producing essential vitamins, and preventing foreign invaders from harming us.

With dysbiosis, this microbiome is out of whack. Maybe there are too few beneficial bacteria, too many bad bacteria, or too much or too little yeast, or maybe there's another form of imbalance. Dysbiosis can lead to symptoms such as gas, bloating, diarrhea, constipation, acid reflux, and irritable bowel syndrome.

In order to keep the gut healthy, you need to prioritize high-quality foods. This means more fiber, healthy fats, high-quality proteins, and non-starchy vegetables. It also means cutting out sugar, which damages the microbiome by feeding the unfriendly bacteria. When those bacteria overrun the healthy bacteria in your gut, it can cause an overgrowth of candida, a yeast that lives in the intestines, and promote inflammation. Simply put, sugar is not great for your gut.

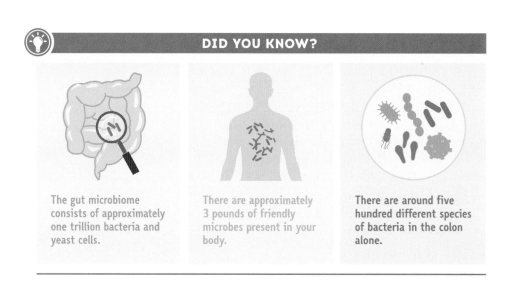

DID YOU KNOW?

The gut microbiome consists of approximately one trillion bacteria and yeast cells.

There are approximately 3 pounds of friendly microbes present in your body.

There are around five hundred different species of bacteria in the colon alone.

THE MICROBIOME PLAYS A KEY ROLE IN:

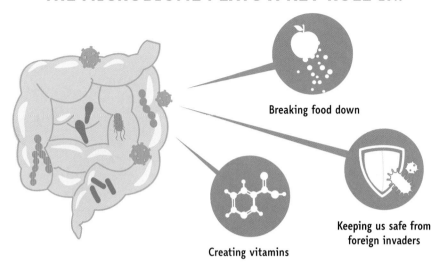

Breaking food down

Creating vitamins

Keeping us safe from foreign invaders

What Your Poop Says About You

I know it is awkward to talk about poop, but surprisingly, bowel movements tell us a lot about the health status of our bodies! In ancient China, imperial physicians would analyze the royals' stool every day—they knew healthy poop was a sign of overall health. I doubt it would go over so well today if we asked our doctors to look at our poop, but we can still help ourselves by paying more attention to our bowel habits.

Normal bowel movements are important for health, and there are so many misconceptions when it comes to what constitutes a normal bowel movement. So often, patients come in and say to me, "I have a bowel movement once every three to four days, but it's been like that my whole life, so that's just my normal." I am here to tell you, that is not normal. Just because you are used to something does not make it balanced or healthy. It means that you've probably had this problem your whole life.

Here are some guidelines on what constitute normal bowel habits:

- Bowel movements should occur one to three times daily, and stool should be a well-formed, long, soft log, light brown in color (with a few exceptions—blueberries, for example, can make your stool darker, and beets can make it red).

- Stool should be fairly easy to pass, and you shouldn't need to bear down hard.

- Food should not be recognizable in the stool (with a few exceptions, such as corn and whole flax seeds).

One Easy Step

There is no quick fix for gut health. But there is one easy step that can help your body get back on the right track: **Every day, drink one cup of bone broth and/or add half a cup of sauerkraut to your meals.** The collagen in the broth helps reduce intestinal inflammation, and the fermented sauerkraut delivers beneficial bacteria to the gut.

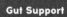

- There should be no blood or mucus in the stool.

- Pelleted stool, like rabbit poop, generally reflects dehydration, yeast overgrowth, lack of good bacteria, food sensitivities, or poor pancreatic function.

- Mushy stool or diarrhea is generally related to parasites, lactose intolerance, food sensitivities, or an imbalanced gut microbiome.

By observing the many signs your body sends to you on a daily basis, even the ever-so-subtle ones, you can get a clear picture of what may be occurring in the gut.

The Gut-Brain Connection

Some signs of poor gut health seem obvious: stomach pain, diarrhea, constipation, and nausea, for instance. It makes sense that a problem in the gut would lead to any of these symptoms. But gut problems can also show up in a much wider array of symptoms—especially in emotional and mental health.

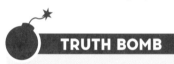

TRUTH BOMB

Ninety percent of serotonin is produced in the gut.

It might seem at first like a stretch that depression could be related to a problem in the gut, but gut imbalance often shows up in our feelings. Poor gut health might end up feeling like unhappiness or a lack of fulfillment, whether mental, emotional, spiritual, or sexual. Mental unfulfillment may show up as mood swings, anger, mental fogginess, or forgetfulness. Spiritual unfulfillment could feel like hopelessness, fatigue, or a general sadness. Sexual unfulfillment could be a libido that's higher or lower than normal.

All this may sound strange, but there are sound scientific reasons that gut problems may result in mental or emotional symptoms. The digestive system actually has its own nervous system, the enteric nervous system, and while its primary function is to deal with local gut issues—moving food along, controlling blood flow to the intestines, producing hormones, managing immune responses, and the like—it also communicates with the brain. This can be seen—or felt—when you are under significant stress or feel anxious and get a stomachache or suffer from some other form of intestinal distress. And this interaction goes both ways, meaning that what you eat and how your gut digests food can send signals to the brain. To use myself as an example, I can get moody when I eat chocolate. This moodiness could be tied to the high amount of oxalates that chocolates contain (more about oxalates on page 299).

In addition, 90 percent of our serotonin, the feel-good neurotransmitter, is made in the gut. When the gut isn't operating optimally, it can't produce as much serotonin, leading to everything from anxiety to depression. Experts have even started connecting gastrointestinal inflammation to inflammation in the brain and a leaky blood-brain barrier, which are factors in the development of neurodegenerative diseases like Alzheimer's and Parkinson's.

And then there is your gut's microbiome. In recent years, it's become more and more clear that there is a link between the presence or absence of certain bacteria and depression, anxiety, ADD, and other emotional and mental conditions.

When we take into account the connection between hormones and mental acuity, the gut takes on even more importance. When gut bacteria is balanced, cortisol is more efficiently regulated, which reduces mental fogginess and focus issues. While traditionally these problems were associated with fatigue and old age, it is becoming ever clearer that digestion can play a big role.

Finally, consider this: proof of the connection between the brain and the gut can be seen in the simple fact that the brain requires energy and the gut provides energy by breaking down food. In fact, in order to function effectively, the brain uses more than 25 percent of the energy that we consume every day. So even if you are eating the right foods, if your gut isn't doing a thorough job of digesting them, your brain won't be getting the energy it needs.

There are a few diets that have been designed to improve neurological disorders. It is noteworthy that these are very similar to the diets designed to improve autoimmune disorders—and to a strict keto diet. By removing all or nearly all sugar, grains, fast food, junk food, dairy, and gluten, most people find their symptoms improve. For those who need a bit more support for mental health concerns, I recommend looking into the Gut and Psychology Syndrome (GAPS) diet.

The Gut-Immune Connection

About 70 percent of your immune system exists in your gut. It's one more reason to prioritize a healthy gut: How can the immune system stay healthy if its host is imbalanced? And when the immune system isn't operating at full capacity or is weakened, it opens up your body to a long list of issues. This is when infections, like colds and flus, flourish. There is also growing evidence that a struggling immune system could contribute to the progression of chronic diseases in the body.

Of course, the development of chronic diseases and a higher risk of catching the flu or a cold are also tied to inflammation, which can be a sign of a problem with the immune system on its own. If you're concerned about inflammation, the information on pages 251 to 256 may be helpful.

The Gut-Weight Connection

Leaky gut and other imbalances of the gut can disrupt estrobolome, the gut bacteria that metabolize estrogens. When estrobolome is imbalanced, it can lead to excess estrogen, otherwise known as estrogen dominance, which can cause weight gain (as well as bloating, breast lumps, mood swings, headaches, hair loss, fatigue, or memory issues).

The gut's role in mental and emotional health also connects it, indirectly, to weight gain. A few pages back, I talked a lot about how the gut plays a major role in keeping us happy and how an unhealthy gut is associated with depression. Depression, in turn, is often accompanied by emotional eating and lack of desire to exercise, both of which contribute to weight gain.

If you experience any of the below, it's best to work alongside a doctor to support your condition and run the appropriate tests.

1. **Candida overgrowth:** Bloating, slight hearing issues, mental fogginess, sinus problems, skin irritations, trouble losing weight. Candida overgrowth is best managed with the steps and strategies outlined in the Candida Support section on page 267.

2. **Small intestinal bacterial overgrowth (SIBO):** Bloating (extremely noticeable, making you look pregnant), constipation, diarrhea, heartburn or acid reflux, excessive burping or flatulence, nausea, abdominal pain. SIBO is a condition characterized by excessive bacteria in the small intestine. It's often the cause of chronic diarrhea, and it can lead to nutritional deficiencies and even osteoporosis. SIBO is usually precipitated by an infection in the gut, such as food poisoning, acute gastroenteritis, or *C. diff*. It's best managed with the strategies in this section and the section on FODMAPs (page 284).

3. **Ulcers:** Sharp pain at the bottom of your sternum, increased or decreased pain with food consumption, a worsening in the sharp pain when stress arises. Ulcers are best managed with the strategies in this section.

4. **Heartburn and acid reflux:** Pain after eating, a chronic cough, pain in your abdomen that worsens when lying down. Heartburn and acid reflux are best managed with the strategies in this section.

Diet Adjustments

Your body has amazing healing powers—you just need the right therapeutic approaches to let them work their magic. Once a gut-healing protocol is in place, many people report other symptoms improving, too, like joint pain, headaches, difficulty sleeping, and so much more—problems that you never would've imagined to be related to the health of your gut!

Keep in mind that optimal gut health doesn't happen overnight. A lot of us have subjected our poor tummies to years of abuse. But know that they *do* want to get better. And with the right actions, they most certainly can.

Ultra-Healing Foods

THE EXTRAS

- Fresh and dried basil
- Fresh and dried cilantro
- Fresh and dried parsley
- Fresh and dried rosemary (leaves or ground)
- Ground cinnamon
- Ground cumin
- Ground turmeric
- Kombucha
- Water kefir

STARCHES AND FRUITS

- Apples, especially the peel
- Berries
- Butternut squash
- Carrots
- Cassava
- Citrus fruits
- Green banana
- Plantains
- Potatoes, cooked and cooled
- Sweet potatoes
- Yacón root

PROTEIN

- Bone broth
- Chicken thighs
- Collagen
- Gelatin
- Grass-fed beef
- Lamb
- Liver
- Oysters
- Salmon
- Shellfish
- Turkey

NON-STARCHY VEGETABLES

- Asparagus
- Bok choy
- Chicory root
- Cucumbers
- Dandelion greens
- Fennel
- Fermented vegetables
- Garlic
- Jerusalem artichokes
- Jicama
- Kale
- Leeks
- Lettuce
- Mushrooms
- Onions
- Spinach
- Zucchini

HEALTHY FATS

- Avocado oil
- Avocados
- Coconut oil
- Duck fat
- Egg yolks
- Lard
- Nondairy yogurt
- Tallow

WATER

Additional Adjustments

Say Yes To

SOFT, WELL-COOKED FOODS

Opt for stews, soups, braised meats, and meals prepared in a slow cooker. These items are easier to digest and may cause less dietary stress on your body.

ZINC-RICH FOODS

Zinc is important for the production of hydrochloric acid, which breaks down food in your stomach. Foods high in zinc include grass-fed beef, oysters, spinach, chicken, and mushrooms. If you have a severe zinc deficiency, you might want to take a supplement.

The easiest way to determine if you're zinc deficient is to do a zinc self-test. To do this, you'll need 1 teaspoon of liquid zinc sulfate heptahydrate. Hold it in your mouth for 15 seconds. The reaction you have will give you a good idea of your zinc status:

Optimal: Immediate unpleasant taste that causes you to grimace
Adequate: A definite but not strongly unpleasant taste that intensifies with time
Deficient: No taste initially, but one develops in 10 to 15 seconds
Extremely deficient: Tastes like water

NUTRIENT-DENSE FOODS

Consume as many nutrient-dense foods as possible, and opting for whole-food sources of fat, such as full-fat grass-fed beef, avocados, and salmon, instead of pure fats and oils. While there's nothing wrong with these healthy fats, like avocado oil, cacao butter, and olive oil, they're less nutrient-dense than their whole-food counterparts. Bone broth and fermented foods are also great choices that will amp up your nutrient load.

QUALITY REST

Every minute you sleep is another minute you're giving your body time to heal. I remind myself of this whenever I have to set my alarm or skip a nap even though my body is begging me for one. Listen to your body and rest when you need to.

DIGESTIVE ENZYMES

Digestive enzymes assist your body to fully digest all of the food that goes into your belly, helping to heal your gut from the inside out.

COCONUT OIL

Coconut oil helps to reduce the overgrowth of bacteria, yeast, and fungus in the small intestine. Once healing is underway, it also helps close the gaps between the cells lining the small intestine. If you like to have a Rocket Fuel Latte (page 144) in the morning, try replacing the MCT oil with coconut oil for more gut love.

L-GLUTAMINE & ALPHA LIPOIC ACID

When your gut is compromised, it reduces your level of glutathione, a powerful antioxidant that attracts toxins and eliminates them from your body.

With lower levels of glutathione, toxins build up, and this stops what's left of glutathione from being recycled in the body. I see this circumstance time and time again—leaky gut with a toxicity problem in need of mega gut healing. Supplementing with L-glutamine and alpha lipoic acid encourages the recycling while also healing the gut (in the case of L-glutamine) and regulating blood sugar (in the case of alpha lipoic acid). L-glutamine is best taken before bed and alpha lipoic acid in the morning.

VITAMIN D

Vitamin D is important for preventing gallstones and helps us digest fat properly. Low levels of vitamin D may play a role in poor stomach emptying, bloating, constipation, and irritable bowel syndrome. The best way to get enough vitamin D is to get out in the sun for twenty to thirty minutes a day—without sunscreen. If regular sun exposure isn't an option, you may find it beneficial to take a supplement. I recommend fermented cod liver oil, which is best taken in the morning with a fatty meal.

FIBER-RICH FOODS

In general, eating lots of fiber-rich foods is good for your gut. But if a whole foods–based diet is a whole new world for you, make sure to increase your vegetable intake slowly—give yourself a chance to adjust before you start throwing back entire heads of cabbage. Also, eating more fiber is not a digestive cure-all. Fiber provides food for the gut flora, but certain imbalances of the gut microbiome can cause fiber intolerance. So if you have a gut reaction every time you eat plants, it could be that fiber is working against you.

PREBIOTIC FOODS

Think of prebiotics as a gut fertilizer: they nourish probiotics, the beneficial bacteria in your colon that help you digest food and absorb nutrients, act as your defense system against harmful bacteria, and prevent digestive disorders. These friendly bacteria simply wouldn't exist if it weren't for prebiotics.

Prebiotics are a type of fiber that's found in certain plant foods and can't be digested in the small intestine, so they enter your colon undigested. This is where they feed probiotics, your friendly gut bacteria. To keep those bacteria happy and doing their very important jobs, eat more prebiotics! Prebiotic foods include garlic, onions, asparagus, bananas, Jerusalem artichoke, dandelion greens, chicory root, yams, tomatoes, coconut meat, radishes, and carrots.

FERMENTED FOODS

Think of fermented foods as a bacterial transplant. They're loaded with probiotics, those beneficial bacteria that prebiotics nourish. Because they contain live organisms, fermented foods can either be an effective health hack or add a damaging bacterial load to an already-burdened system. If you don't have bacterial overgrowth problems, eating probiotic-rich foods is one of the best ways to maintain gut health. But if you *do* have bacterial overgrowth, such as SIBO, be advised that you may react to probiotic-rich items, including certain supplements.

DISCOVERING FOOD SENSITIVITIES & ALLERGIES

When you eat foods that you're sensitive to, the gut becomes inflamed, which can exacerbate leaky gut issues (see page 243). Rule out food sensitivities by following the allergy elimination diet on page 277 to determine which foods you might be sensitive to.

Say No To

CIGARETTES & ALCOHOL

Both cause inflammation of the gut, irritate the intestinal lining, and can further exacerbate an imbalance of healthy bacteria in the gut. However, hard alcohol will increase harmful bacteria, whereas wine may *slightly* increase healthful bacteria due to its polyphenol content. So if you must drink, red wine is best.

PROCESSED OILS

Reducing gut inflammation is yet another reason why you'll want to consume only minimally processed oils. Avoid all vegetable oils like grapeseed and sesame, and highly unstable polyunsaturated fats like hemp and flaxseed oil.

GUT IRRITANTS

Foods known to cause gut irritation include grains, gluten, all forms of dairy (including ghee and butter), eggs, nuts, legumes, seeds, nightshades, and foods high in insoluble fiber, such as strawberries and leafy greens. If you're consuming a good amount of any of these items, you may want to try scaling back or slowly eliminating them from your diet to see if your symptoms improve.

CONSTIPATION

If you're not having a bowel movement two to three times per day, try supplementing with magnesium oxide first thing in the morning on an empty stomach, or have a shot of apple cider vinegar before larger meals.

RUSHED EATING

Chew every mouthful of food at least twenty times before swallowing, and whenever possible, enjoy eating in a quiet space away from distractions.

FODMAP and NIGHTSHADE FOODS

Foods high in FODMAP and nightshade foods may be irritating your condition. Read more about them on page 284 and page 290. Perhaps remove them for a period of time to see if things improve.

Low stomach acid can lead to poor digestion and frustrating symptoms like gas, constipation, indigestion, burping after meals, osteoporosis, diarrhea, and deficiencies in important vitamins and minerals like vitamin B_{12}. Low stomach acid is most commonly caused by overuse of antibiotics, chronic stress, poor diet, eating too quickly, and overuse of NSAIDs. It's also more common as we age and can be influenced by food sensitivities. The primary sign that stomach acid might be low is the feeling that protein-rich foods sit like a rock in your stomach. If you feel like this, then start taking a full-spectrum digestive enzyme with HCl in it.

Supportive Supplements

- Vitamins: A, C, B (including niacin), E, D
- Minerals: zinc, magnesium
- Herbs and plants: milk thistle, peppermint
- Others: L-glutamine, alpha lipoic acid

Candida **Support**

Candida is a benign yeast that lives in all of us, particularly in or on our mucous membranes. In a healthy person, candida is kept in check by all the other microorganisms in the digestive tract, such as bacteria. As part of a balanced internal ecosystem, candida does serve some positive functions. But the boundary between useful and harmful is fairly narrow, and if the body's balance is upset by antibiotics, over-the-counter drugs, birth control pills, or other factors, candida can grow too rapidly, quickly surpassing its useful numbers and bringing on a host of yeast-related symptoms, including vaginal yeast infections, oral thrush, rashes, foggy thinking, or even allergies and arthritis-like symptoms.

The medical community typically only acknowledges that candida overgrowth can occur on the skin, tongue, or reproductive organs, ignoring the digestive tract, one of the most common sites of candida overgrowth.

The problem with candida is that it can cause many random symptoms, making it hard to pinpoint. If you experience three or more of the following symptoms, it may be worth getting the tests listed in the sidebar to determine if you need some candida support:

- acne
- anger
- bloating
- body odor
- brain fog
- constant tiredness
- constipation
- cravings
- depression
- diarrhea
- eczema
- fungal infections
- gas
- headaches
- hormonal imbalances
- increased belly fat
- insomnia
- low energy
- mood swings
- nasal drip
- PMS
- stomach pains
- thrush

If you've been diagnosed with candida overgrowth, the following pages will help you eradicate the excess (we can never remove it all—some candida is necessary for a healthy body) so that your immune system can restore balance and be able to keep it in check once again.

Once you're better, maintain healthy eating habits. Even after the candida is under control, it's best to eat a whole-foods keto diet focused on organic, whole foods with a hefty raw component.

It's important to note that ketones, just as much as sugar, help candida thrive. So it's important not to go too high-carb *or* too high-fat. Be sure your meals are balanced and provide sufficient fat, fiber, and protein. Stick with moderate carbohydrate, neither too much nor too little.

Test for It: Candida

Candida is a bit of a challenge to nail down. Below are some tests that may be helpful, but it's generally a combination of symptoms and a test or two that provides a diagnosis.

DNA stool analysis detects candida, bacteria, fungi, and parasites, painting a very clear picture of the health of your digestion and immune response as it relates to your gut.

Comprehensive stool analysis tests for fungus and yeast.

Organic acids test examines chemical compounds in the urine (and in the blood in lower concentrations) called organic acids. Some of these acids are yeast and fungal markers and could point to candida being present. These markers include citramalic, 5-hydroxymethyl-2-furoic, 3-oxoglutaric, furan-2,5-dicarboxylic, furancarbonylglycine, tartaric, arabinose, carboxycitric, and tricarballylic acids.

A big part of dealing with candida is avoiding sugar, which it feeds on. But candida can feed on ketones, too! So it's super important that, if you determine you have candida, you prioritize the protocol outlined here over ketone generation. If you experience die-off symptoms that don't improve if you stop taking anti-candida supplements, look to your ketones. Generally speaking, if they're over 1.5 mmol/L, they may be too high. Regardless of your ketone level, do not supplement with exogenous ketones, and lower your overall fat intake to 40 to 50 percent instead of 60 to 80 percent.

The treatment for candida overgrowth is multiphased, and you'll need to have patience—it can't be corrected overnight. The anti-candida protocol I recommend is a two-pronged approach:

1. Diet adjustments (outlined below) during month 1

2. Supplement support (see page 271) during months 1, 2, and 3

Diet Adjustments

The anti-candida diet is fairly restricted, so plan to do it during a month when you have minimal events.

Foods to Eat and Foods to Avoid

To treat an overgrowth of candida, you'll need to modify the usual keto diet a bit. Just as on a keto diet, it's important to avoid grains and sugar, but some of the other details need to be adjusted.

One important note: During the month that you're eating an anti-candida diet, you'll need to avoid carb-ups and any other cyclical ketogenic practices that use carbs.

General Guidelines

- Avoid all sources of alcohol.

- Avoid most fermented products including soy sauce. Small amounts of fermented vegetables are fine, as long as they're made without vinegar.

- Avoid all foods containing vinegar, including apple cider vinegar. Common sources are salad dressings, sauces, and pickles.

- Avoid all sources of yeast, including bread, baked goods, and anything containing nutritional yeast.

Vegetables

Many keto-friendly, non-starchy veggies are great, including asparagus, avocados, broccoli, Brussels sprouts, cabbage, cauliflower, celery, cucumbers, eggplant, green bell peppers, leafy greens, onions, parsley, parsnips, peas, radishes, tomatoes, and zucchini.

General rules for vegetables:

- Try to eat six to nine servings (3 to 4½ cups) of veggies daily.

- Eat veggies raw, steamed, or stir-fried.

- Avoid canned, boiled, or microwaved veggies.

- Eat veggies in a wide array of colors. Typically, the darker the color, the more nutrient-dense the veggie.

- Limit all high-glycemic veggies during your carb-ups, including white potatoes, corn, parsnips, rutabaga, and turnips.

- If you use a dressing on your salad, make sure it does not contain sugar or vinegar.

- No mushrooms!

Fruits

No fruits are allowed for the first two weeks of the diet. After that, you can have a maximum of one piece of fresh fruit a day. However, no melons are allowed throughout the entire month.

Animal Protein

Most animal protein is fine: beef, chicken, turkey, lamb, bison, veal, egg, fish, salmon, rabbit, elk, moose, deer, duck, goose, wild birds, pork... They're all good to eat.

General rules for protein:

- Quality is really important. Opt for humanely raised, grass-fed *and* grass-finished animal protein, preferably from a local.

- Eggs should be free-range and organic.

- Limit predatory fish such as tuna, mackerel, sturgeon, swordfish, and shark, as well as orange roughy and snapper—they have higher toxicity levels than other options. Most farmed fish are treated with chemicals and antibiotics, and fed a horrible diet, so look for wild-caught. Atlantic salmon is always farmed and should be avoided. For now, it seems the best fish to eat are small cold-water fish, such as sardines and anchovies, as well as wild Pacific salmon, halibut, cod, and shellfish.

- Roasting is the best way to prepare meat. Barbecuing is the worst way to prepare meat because it creates polycyclic aromatic hydrocarbons (PAHs), which are known carcinogens.

Dairy

- Avoid all dairy. It contains lactose, a simple sugar that provides fuel for candida.

- To replace cow's milk, try unsweetened alternative milks, such as almond or coconut milk.

Nuts and Seeds

- Most types of nuts are fine, but avoid peanuts, pistachios, and cashews because they have a higher risk of developing mold during storage.

- Tahini makes a wonderful sauce and dressing.

- Pure nut butters are fine, so long as they're not coming from peanuts, pistachios, or cashews.

- Do not buy conventional brands of nut butters unless they include *only* nuts—check the label to be sure. It's especially important to avoid sugar and partially hydrogenated oils.

- Nut butters can be stored in the fridge upside down for ease of use.

Beverages

- Water, mineral water, coffee, and herbal teas are all okay.

Oils

- All keto-friendly (minimally processed) oils are fine. See the list on page 97.

Sweeteners

- Stevia is okay in small quantities, around 2 to 4 drops (1/8 teaspoon) per week.

Supportive Supplements

At the same time you begin the diet adjustments, start taking supplements as instructed below. While the diet adjustments will last just one month, supplements should be taken for three months.

One thing to be aware of is that you may experience a die-off reaction: when a large number of candida species die at once, they release a toxic gas that can cause symptoms. This reaction occurs 25 to 35 percent of the time, and symptoms can include dermatological reactions, such as rashes and hives; GI symptoms, such as diarrhea, bloating, or excess gas; neurological symptoms, such as increased fatigue, brain fog, irritability, and memory concerns; and occasionally immune reactions presenting with a flu-like feeling.

If you experience die-off and it's too much to handle, instead of adjusting your diet, which would only further your candida experience, you could stop taking anti-candida supplements and start vitamin C to improve bowel tolerance. Once symptoms die down, you can slowly shift back to your anti-candida supplements with the addition of one to two days of activated charcoal, which may help relieve symptoms more quickly.

For all three months, take a probiotic. Typically, you'll want to start at 50 billion daily and work up to 100 billion.

For the first month, take caprylic acid, an antifungal supplement. Typically, you'll want to start with 100 to 200 mg three times daily and gradually increase over the course of one to two weeks to 500 to 750 mg three times daily.

During the second and third month, choose two of the antifungal options below:

- Grapefruit seed extract: The typical dose is 250 mg twice daily.

- Berberine: The typical dose is 400 to 500 mg twice daily.

- Allicin/garlic: The typical dose is 500 to 800 mg (0.5% to 1% allicin) daily.

If none of the three supplement options above is available to you, the following could offer relief as well: cinnamon extract, pau d'arco, echinacea, neem oil, oregano oil, or clove essential oil.

Additional Adjustments

Say Yes to
ANTIFUNGALS
For some people, prescription antifungals such as Diflucan (fluconazole) or nystatin are necessary to reduce the amount of candida in the body. For moderate and mild cases, herbal antifungals can be strong enough to restore balance. The supplements recommended above are all antifungals.

PROBIOTICS & FERMENTED FOODS
It's likely that a decrease in probiotics in the gut caused your candida imbalance in the first place. Replace them with probiotic supplements, a must for anyone on an anti-candida diet. Aim for high counts (100 billion or more) in a variety of strains (ideally twelve or more). For the widest variety, switch up brands so that you're ingesting different strains with each bottle. Probiotics are also found naturally in lacto-fermented foods (that need to be refrigerated), including sauerkraut and kimchi—as long as they're made without vinegar—as well as natto, miso, and tempeh. (Kefir and kombucha also contain natural probiotics, but save those for later as they contain sugar, too.)

DAILY STRESS REDUCTION

Stress can forcefully affect candida. Manage stress through whatever works best for you: meditation, yoga, laughter, exercise, the company of family and friends, time with pets, getting enough sleep, or anything else that helps you feel relaxed and centered.

BOOSTING THE IMMUNE SYSTEM

Support the immune system so your body can more effectively combat candida. The guidelines in the Autoimmune Support section (page 241) may be helpful.

COFFEE ENEMAS

Check with your health-care provider to see if this process could resonate with you. It acts as a probiotic flush to kill candida.

RAW FOODS

Raw foods have natural enzymes that can provide additional nutrients to the body and ease the digestive load on the body, which can give it more resources to heal your candida overgrowth.

Say No To

SUGAR & SWEETENERS

Yeast thrives on sugar, so if you haven't already, now is the time to seriously cut out the white stuff, plus all the foods in which it hides: cakes, cookies, candies, chocolate, sweet baked goods, prepared foods, packaged foods, granola bars, bread, rolls, muffins, and so on. (But you already omitted most of these when you went keto, right?) Because sugar hides in almost every prepared or packaged food, this also means making most of your food from scratch.

REFINED & PROCESSED FOODS

Refined flours and grains are also sources of sugar (and also should be cut out on keto).

TOXINS

It's important to reduce your exposure to toxic chemicals in food, air, personal care products, and water. For food, opt for organic produce and pasture-raised meat and dairy when possible. If the air quality in your hometown is less than optimal, get a HEPA filter for the room you spend the most time in (your workplace is fair game!). For personal care products, start becoming mindful of the ingredients they use. Ingredients to avoid include the following: avobenzone, benzophenone, formaldehyde, fragrance/perfume, homosalate, methoxycinnmate, PABA, parabens, propylene glycol, sodium laureth sulfate, sodium lauryl sulfate, synthetic colors, toluene, and triclosan. Opt for essential oils instead of perfume, natural deodorant (my favorite is Primal Pit Paste), and natural body wash (my favorite is Dr. Bronner's Castile Soap).

Food Sensitivity and Allergy **Support**

Many people are unaware that a particular food or environmental factor could affect their body so much that it causes anything from fatigue and headaches to chronic nasal congestion, abdominal pain, joint pain, or eczema. Many of these symptoms don't seem like they could be caused by food or your environment, but they can! And by identifying and removing the problem, many people find relief from their symptoms in as few as thirty days.

Food intolerances, sensitivities, and allergies are all a little different, but it can be a challenge to know which reaction you're having. First, if your immune system isn't involved, it's a food intolerance. We'll cover some of the most common food intolerances and how to adjust your diet to avoid them beginning on page 283.

If your immune system is involved—antibodies are produced in response to a particular substance—it's an allergy or sensitivity. Let's go over the difference:

- With a food **allergy**, there's an immediate reaction, often within minutes of ingesting the food. An antibody called IgE (short for immunoglobulin E) is created to fight the food. Common food allergens are milk, eggs, peanuts, tree nuts, wheat, soy, fish, and crustacean shellfish. Even a very small amount of food can trigger a reaction.

- With a food **sensitivity**, there's a delayed reaction that can occur anywhere from 30 minutes to a couple of days following ingestion. A different antibody is formed than with an allergy—IgG instead of IgE. The severity of the reaction depends on the individual and how much of the food is consumed.

How do you know which you're dealing with? By process of elimination, basically. We start with the most serious, allergies.

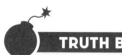

TRUTH BOMB

Intolerances, sensitivities, and allergies stress the body, and stress slows the metabolic rate, interferes with digestion, and leads to a host of health issues.

Allergies

A food allergy generally triggers immediate symptoms and the formation of IgE antibodies, which have an instantaneous and direct impact on our bodies. Despite this, I have encountered many people who have these allergies but are not even aware of it because it's become their "normal." They believe they're fine, even when they're severely reacting to a food.

Symptoms of these allergies generally show up rapidly and can include the following:

- Airway constriction
- Diarrhea
- Dizziness or fainting
- Hives
- Nausea or vomiting

- Rapid heartbeat
- Rashes
- Stomach cramps
- Swelling
- Wheezing

A food allergy is generally something you'll have for life. However, some children grow out of the allergy as they age.

Because allergies can be so serious, it's important to rule out an allergy before investigating whether you have a sensitivity. The following are tests and strategies you can use to determine whether you're dealing with an allergy and, if so, what you're allergic to.

If you test negative for anything below, move on to testing for delayed-onset sensitivities (page 276).

First, **determine if you have an issue:**

- Option 1: Test your level of IgE antibody. If it's over 40 IU/mL, you are likely reacting to something you're eating or something in your environment.

- Option 2: Get an hs-CRP (high-sensitivity C-reactive protein) test to determine if you have inflammation. While this test won't tell you what you're sensitive to, it'll give you an idea of whether inflammation is a concern. If you're not experiencing increased inflammation, you probably don't have a food allergy or sensitivity.

If you do have an issue, **pinpoint what's causing it:**

- Option 1: Run a skin prick test to determine what foods and/or environmental factors you're reacting to. The test involves placing an allergen on your skin, pricking the skin, and waiting for an inflammatory reaction, usually in the form of a rash or hives.

Other Causes?

There are other causes of elevated IgE levels, including parasitic diseases, myeloma, and immunodeficiencies. If your blood tests show elevated IgE and the dots aren't connecting after a skin prick test or IgE panel, I highly recommend connecting with an allergist to help make sense of it all.

- Option 2: Have an IgE panel done, which will measure different IgE antibodies and tell you what they're responding to—different foods, animal dander, pollen, mold, medicine, dust mites, latex, or insect venom.

Next steps: Once you've determined what the culprit is, remove it from your diet for thirty days and then test your IgE or hs-CRP level again. If it's still elevated, you could chat with your doctor about allergy shots and short-term medication to reduce your allergenic load and promote healing. I am wary of advising anyone to turn to medication until they've identified the culprit.

Sensitivities

Sensitivities are different from allergies in two main ways: they involve a different antibody, IgG, and symptoms can sometimes take days to appear, leading to diagnosis frustration and confusion.

To identify sensitivities, here are some things to watch for:

- Acne or bumps on the skin

- Ear pain

- Headaches

- Inflammation

- Irritable bowel syndrome

- Joint pain

The best thing about delayed-onset sensitivities is that you can heal your body and get back on track in a matter of months.

If you test negative for anything below, you are probably not dealing with a sensitivity but perhaps a food intolerance stemming from a gut imbalance. Head to page 283.

First, **determine if you have an issue**. Get an hs-CRP (high-sensitivity C-reactive protein) test to determine if you have inflammation. While this test won't tell you what you're sensitive to, it'll give you an idea of whether inflammation is a concern. If it's not, you probably don't have an allergy or sensitivity.

If you are experiencing increased inflammation, **pinpoint what's causing the issue**:

- Option 1: Have an IgG allergy panel done. This will tell you which foods you are sensitive to, but be aware that the tests can be expensive and aren't always 100 percent reliable—some have a propensity to display false positives, meaning the test will tell you that you're sensitive to a food when you're not. If you consume a food a lot or never consume it, it may get a false positive. Once you have the results, follow the elimination protocol for the foods you know you're sensitive to. In time, you may be able to add them back to your diet.

• Option 2: Determine your sensitivities by following the elimination protocol.

Elimination Protocol

Although it's a tedious process, the elimination protocol will help you determine which foods you're sensitive to and how you react to those foods.

Here's how it works:

1. Remove all potential trigger foods (see the following list) for thirty days.

2. Reincorporate each potential trigger food into your diet, one at a time, for three days and watch for symptoms. (See page 280 for details.)

3. Spotted a problem food? Head to page 282.

Note: If you're practicing cyclical keto (whether that means carb-ups or another method), make sure you test any food you'll be eating during your increased-carb periods when you're reintroducing foods. It may not be part of your regular keto diet, but you'll still need to know whether it can trigger symptoms for you.

Elimination Tips

When you discover more than one sensitivity, think about what food family it belongs to—you could be sensitive to the whole group. If you're sensitive to tomatoes and bell peppers, for instance, you may want to look closely at the whole nightshade family.

And keep in mind that hidden allergens are frequently found in packaged foods. "Flour" usually means wheat; "vegetable oil" may mean corn oil; and "casein" and "whey" are dairy products. Make sure your vitamins are free of wheat, corn, sugar, citrus, yeast, dairy, and artificial colorings. Vary your diet, choosing a wide variety of foods. Do not rely on just a few foods, as you may become allergic to foods you eat every day.

Craving the Foods That Hurt Us

The food you like the *most*—the one you're addicted to and can't live without—is usually the one that you're sensitive to. Generally, the sensitivity came first, but because, ironically, the sensitivity can bring on euphoric feelings, we keep eating the very thing that's harming us. For example, wheat and dairy products contain exorphins, compounds similar to endorphins that are made outside the body. These exorphins bind to the brain's opiate receptors and produce a euphoric, even drug-like haze. This is often why we reach for the ice cream, cheese, bread, or cake to soothe, relax, or calm us.

Elimination Protocol: Foods to Avoid and Foods to Eat

 AVOID

DAIRY

Butter

Casein

Cheese

Cottage cheese

Cream cheese

Ghee

Milk

Sour cream

Whey

Yogurt

Dairy additives found in keto products: sodium caseinate, calcium caseinate

EGGS

Chicken eggs

Duck eggs

Egg protein

Egg whites

Egg yolks

Liquid eggs

Powdered eggs

Egg products found in keto products: silico-albuminate, vitellin, ovomucin, ovotransferrin, livetin, lysozyme, globulin, conalbumin, albumin

NUTS AND SEEDS

Almonds   Sunflower seeds

Brazil nuts   Walnuts

Chia seeds

Flax seeds

Hazelnuts

Hemp seeds

Pecans

CORN PRODUCTS

Baking powder

Cornstarch

Sorbitol

Corn additives found in keto products: food starch, maltodextrin, vegetable gum, vegetable protein, vegetable starch, xanthan gum

CITRUS

Grapefruit

Lemons

Limes

YEAST

Nutritional yeast

Yeast-based ingredients found in keto products: yeast extract, baker's yeast, brewer's yeast

SOY FOODS

Miso

Soy cheese, jerky, milk, nut butter, soy sauce, yogurt

Tempeh

Tofu

Soy-based ingredients found in keto products: soy lecithin, textured vegetable protein

FOOD ADDITIVES

Artificial colors

Artificial flavors

Artificial sweeteners

Preservatives

Texturing agents

NIGHTSHADES

Bell peppers

Cayenne pepper

Chili powder

Chipotle powder

Curry powder

Eggplant

Hot peppers

Hot sauce

Potatoes

Taco seasoning

Tomatoes

SWEETENERS

All sugar alcohols, including erythritol and xylitol, and natural sweeteners like stevia

OTHER

Alcohol

Avocados

Caffeine

Chocolate

Refined vegetable oils

Vinegars (except coconut vinegar and apple cider vinegar)

KNOWN ALLERGENS

Avoid any food you know you are allergic to, even if it is allowed on this diet.

OMITTED ON KETO BUT WORTH MENTIONING (AVOID)

BEVERAGES

Alcohol
Energy drinks
Soft drinks
Sweetened fruit drinks

CORN

Corn chips	Popcorn
Corn oil	Tortillas
Corn sweetener	Vegetable oil from an unspecified source
Corn syrup	
Dextrose	
Glucose	

REFINED SUGARS

Cake
Candy
Cookies
Corn sweetener
Corn syrup
Dextrose
Fructose
Glucose
Levulose
Maltose
Pies
Sucrose
Table sugar

GLUTEN

Baked goods	Most flours
Durum semolina	Oats
Farina	Pasta
Many gravies, sauces, and soups	Rye
Most breads	Spelt

 EAT

THE EXTRAS

Apple cider vinegar
Coconut vinegar
Coconut water
Herbal teas
Herbs and spices

PROTEIN

All animal-based proteins
Bone broth
Collagen
Gelatin

HEALTHY FATS

Avocado oil
Cacao butter
Chicken fat (schmaltz), free-range
Coconut
Coconut butter
Coconut oil
Duck fat, free-range
Goose fat, free-range
Hazelnut oil
Hemp seed oil
Lard, pasture-raised
Macadamia nut oil
MCT oil
Olive oil

NON-STARCHY VEGETABLES (use a wide variety)

Artichoke hearts	Cauliflower	Fennel	Radishes
Arugula	Celery	Garlic	Rhubarb
Asparagus	Chard	Kohlrabi	Shallots
Bok choy	Collards	Lettuce	Spinach
Broccoli	Cucumbers	Mushrooms	Swiss chard
Cabbage	Daikon	Okra	Turnips
Capers	Endive	Olives	Zucchini

Symptoms to Watch For

These symptoms can appear instantly after eating a food you're sensitive or allergic to, or they can be delayed for up to 72 hours.

- Abdominal pain
- Acid reflux
- Anxiety
- Asthma symptoms
- Canker sores
- Constipation
- Depression
- Diarrhea
- Fatigue

- Headaches or migraines
- Heartburn
- Itchy skin, hives, breakouts
- Joint pain
- Nasal congestion or post-nasal drip
- Urinary tract infection
- Autoimmune disease flare-up, such as a bout of eczema or psoriasis

Reintroducing Foods

After thirty days avoiding all potential trigger foods, begin to reintroduce them one at a time. For example, don't choose tomato sauce that contains bell peppers to test tomatoes—bell peppers and tomatoes are *both* on the list of potential triggers, so you need to test them separately. To test tomatoes, eat a raw tomato alongside safe foods, like ground beef and broccoli.

Reintroduce one food every other day. If you experience symptoms after eating it, cross it off your list and wait until the symptoms have gone away completely before reintroducing another food—even if that takes more than forty-eight hours.

Here's how to reintroduce foods:

1. On Day 1, eat a small amount of the specified food during one meal. Do you experience a reaction?

   Yes: You're likely sensitive or allergic to it—cross the food off your list for now.

   You're not sure: Remove it from your diet for now, wait eight days, and then reintroduce it again.

   No: Continue to day 2.

2. On Day 2, eat twice the amount of the food you ate on day 1 during one meal. Do you experience a reaction?

    Yes: You're likely sensitive or allergic to it—cross the food off your list for now.

    You're not sure: Remove it from your diet for now, wait eight days, and then reintroduce it again.

    No: Continue to day 3.

3. On Day 3, eat twice the amount of the food you ate on day 2 during one meal. Do you experience a reaction?

    Yes: You're likely sensitive or allergic to it—cross the food off your list for now.

    You're not sure: Remove it from your diet for now, wait eight days, and then reintroduce it again.

    No: You are probably not sensitive to that food.

Once you are certain a food is safe to eat, you can continue to include that food in your diet as you work through reintroducing the rest of the potential trigger foods. If you already know you are sensitive to a particular food, you do not need to reintroduce or test it.

Here's an example of what the reintroduction process could look like:

1. Start by testing avocado. Have a quarter of an avocado on day 1. If you experience any symptoms, don't eat it again; cross it off your list and wait three days or until the symptoms fully subside before reintroducing another food.

2. Have half an avocado on day 2. If you experience any symptoms, don't eat it again; cross it off your list and wait three days or until the symptoms fully subside before reintroducing another food.

3. Have a whole avocado on day 3. If you experience any symptoms, don't eat it again; cross it off your list and wait three days or until the symptoms fully subside before reintroducing another food.

4. If you don't experience any symptoms on day 3, avocado is a safe food for you. Tomorrow, on day 4, you can reintroduce another food—for example, lemons.

5. On day 4, have 1 tablespoon of lemon juice in water. Then have 2 tablespoons of lemon juice in water on day 5, and 4 tablespoons of lemon juice in water on day 6. Again, if you experience symptoms at any time, stop the test and cross lemons off your list.

6. Continue to add to your safe-foods list using this three-day testing approach.

Note: You don't need to reintroduce every potential trigger food. For example, if you've decided you'd rather live without food coloring, don't test it.

Reintroduction Tips

- You may test foods in any order. Start on a day you feel well—you shouldn't be experiencing symptoms that are unusual for you or feel like you're coming down with something. Recording how you feel each day in a journal or keeping notes on your phone can be helpful.

- When testing dairy, keep in mind that each form of dairy can elicit a different response. That means that you may have a different reaction to cheese than to sour cream, but it also means that you may have a different reaction to cheddar than to Brie. Each form and variety of dairy needs to be tested separately, and it's best to test another food, such as a sweetener or nightshade vegetable, between dairy tests.

- To test food coloring, put ¼ teaspoon of food coloring in a glass of water and drink it. If you want, you can test each color separately.

- When testing eggs, test the yolk and white separately.

- When testing chocolate, use pure unsweetened baking chocolate, unsweetened cocoa powder mixed into a drink, or raw cacao without sugar or added ingredients like soy lecithin. This way, you'll actually test chocolate and not other ingredients found in chocolate products.

- If you've found foods that you're sensitive to, avoid them for at least six months. At that point, you can try reintroducing the food, following the steps starting on page 280. Some people find after six to twelve months, they are able to put a food they were previously sensitive to back in their diet. However, others find they feel better avoiding a particular food for life. Try to rotate your diet, changing the foods you eat on a day-to-day basis, to avoid creating a food sensitivity.

Supportive Supplements

If you're struggling with food sensitivities or allergies, support your immune system by supplementing with any of the following:

- Bromelain (an enzyme) helps to break down foreign proteins, which are responsible for many allergies.

- Catechin is a natural antioxidant that helps minimize the release of histamine during exposure to an allergen.

- Conjugated linoleic acid strengthens the immune system to limit reactions to food allergens.

- Glutathione eradicates free radicals, which can cause allergies. Best taken in the morning.

- MSM helps prevent and treat active allergies. Best taken in the morning.

- Quercetin stabilizes cells, making them less reactive to foreign proteins.

- Vitamin B_6 is a cofactor to the enzyme that breaks down excess histamine production (see page 293).

- Vitamin C reduces the release of histamine.

- Zinc inhibits the release of histamine in the presence of foreign proteins and pauses the inflammation response that occurs during a reaction.

Food **Intolerances**

Unlike food allergies and sensitivities, food intolerances don't involve an immune reaction—but that doesn't mean you don't experience symptoms. With a food intolerance, the body reacts to a food within thirty minutes to forty-eight hours following ingestion. The more of a problematic food you consume, the worse the reaction.

The most common foods that people have trouble with are dairy (see page 99), FODMAPs, lectins, and histamines.

FODMAPs

FODMAP stands for "fermentable oligosaccharides, disaccharides, monosaccharides, and polyols." They're basically types of carbohydrates and sugar alcohols, and in some people, they can trigger gastrointestinal symptoms such as abdominal pain, nausea, diarrhea or constipation, and bloating.

FODMAPs are prebiotics, those foods that nourish the beneficial bacteria in your gut. That's generally a good thing, but if you have an imbalance in your gut bacteria, FODMAPs can tip the imbalance even further, exacerbating the problem.

Studies have shown that a low-FODMAP diet is effective in reducing bloating, abdominal pain, diarrhea, and constipation, and more evidence suggests that a low-FODMAP diet can reduce leaky gut, calm the immune system, and even repair the intestines.

What Causes a FODMAP Intolerance?

There are a few possible reasons that you might develop a FODMAP intolerance.

SIBO: Small intestinal bacteria overgrowth contributes to the development of irritable bowel syndrome and FODMAP intolerance. The overgrowth of bacteria in the small intestine leads to the excessive fermentation of FODMAPs, which increases gas production and allows for further uncontrolled proliferation of gut bacteria.

Lack of enzymes: We need certain enzymes to break down and absorb FODMAPs before they reach the colon. When we don't have enough of these enzymes—due to the quality of our diet, drinking too much water at meals, chronic stress, inflammation, consuming foods we're sensitive to—the fermentation of improperly digested FODMAPs can lead to mega digestive distress.

Emotional and physical stress: Stress makes pretty much any health condition worse. It's known to contribute to the development of irritable bowel syndrome, and it could induce FODMAP intolerance for reasons not yet fully understood—though it may have to do with the fact that stress alters the gut flora significantly.

Managing FODMAP Intolerance

The good news is that a low-FODMAP diet can help you manage your symptoms. Plenty of people have used a low-FODMAP diet to alleviate symptoms associated with various digestive conditions, including irritable bowel syndrome, inflammatory bowel disorders (like Crohn's disease or ulcerative colitis), celiac disease, fructose malabsorption, and SIBO.

- Avoid high-FODMAP foods to allow the damage to your gut lining to heal and the inflammation in your intestines to subside. See the list on page 286.

- Prioritize anti-inflammatory foods (page 253) to reduce overall inflammation, as gut inflammation can irritate the gut and cause intolerances.

- Reduce or eliminate seeds, nuts, and dairy. These aren't high in FODMAPs, but they often irritate the lining of your gut, so avoid them to give yourself time to heal.

- Pack as much nutrition as you can into your low-FODMAP diet. FODMAP intolerance is often associated with nutritional deficiencies, so it's important to give your body all the building blocks it needs for the healing process.

- Find the underlying cause of your digestive issues. If you react to FODMAPs, you most likely have some form of gut dysbiosis, leaky gut, SIBO, or parasites.

- Rebuild healthy gut flora by adding probiotics, those beneficial bacteria that help make your gut a healthier environment. You can get probiotics either from supplements or fermented foods.

If you're taking probiotic supplements, there are a few things to look for:
- The number of strains—generally, the more variety the better

- How much CFU is in each capsule. I personally supplement with two 100 billion capsules each day as I focus on gut healing, but it took time for me to go this high. If you go too high too soon, it could cause major digestive distress.

- Whether the brand you've found is trusted and reputable

- Any other ingredients in the supplement—make sure they don't cause you digestive trouble

- Cost—the more potent and higher-quality the probiotic, the more expensive it's going to be.

Now, for natural probiotics like fermented foods, keep in mind that:
- it's more difficult to control the dose,

- there's a wider variety of strains than found in a supplement,

- they also come with natural *prebiotics*, and

- they're less expensive than supplements, but you have to actually eat them.

Keto Foods to Eat and Avoid

AVOID (HIGH-FODMAP)

THE EXTRAS

Carb powder
Coconut water
Rum
Spices that contain onion or garlic
Xylitol

PROTEIN

Almond meal	Sausages
Cashews	Tahini
Chorizo	Whey protein
Red kidney beans	

STARCHES & LOW-FRUCTOSE FRUITS

Beets
Blackberries

HEALTHY FATS

Most healthy fats are low in FODMAPs!

NON-STARCHY VEGETABLES

Artichokes	Onion
Asparagus	Pickled vegetables
Avocados	Sauerkraut
Cauliflower	Savoy cabbage
Fennel	Scallions (white part)
Garlic	Shallots
Leeks	
Mushrooms	

Note: If dairy is part of your keto protocol, the following dairy items are high in FODMAPs: buttermilk, cow's milk, cream cheese, goat's milk, halloumi cheese, kefir, ricotta cheese, sheep's milk, sour cream, and yogurt (everything but dairy-free, Greek, and goat)

Carb-Up Foods to Eat and Avoid

AVOID (HIGH-FODMAP)

Apples	Honey
Apricots	Mango
Black currants	Nectarines
Cassava	Peaches
Cherries	Pears
Currants	Persimmon
Custard apples	Plums
Dates	Pomegranates
Figs	Prunes
Goji berries	Raisins
Grapefruit	Watermelons

EAT (LOW-FODMAP)

Bananas (unripe only)	Oranges
Beets (canned and pickled only)	Papayas
Bilberries	Parsnips
Cantaloupe	Passion fruit
Clementines	Pineapples (not dried)
Dragon fruit	Plantains
Grapes	Potato chips (plain only)
Guava (ripe only)	Potatoes
Honeydew melon	Rice flour
Kiwis	Sweet potatoes, cooked (limit to ½ cup/100 g)
Mandarins	Tamarinds
Maple syrup	Yams

EAT (LOW-FODMAP)

THE EXTRAS

- Alcohol (limit to 1 glass/1 oz.)
- All spices and herbs free of onion and garlic
- Apple cider vinegar
- Baking powder
- Baking soda
- Balsamic vinegar
- Cacao powder
- Coffee
- Dark chocolate
- Kvass
- Mustard
- Stevia
- Tea (weak only)

STARCHY VEGETABLES & LOW-FRUCTOSE FRUITS

- Blueberries
- Butternut squash (limit to ¼ cup chopped)
- Cranberries (limit to 5 berries)
- Lemons
- Limes
- Pumpkin (limit to ¼ cup/70 g cooked or canned)
- Raspberries
- Rhubarb
- Spaghetti squash
- All forms of squash (limit to 4 oz/115 g fresh)
- Strawberries

PROTEIN

- Egg protein powder
- All fresh seafood and animal protein
- Chia seeds
- Collagen
- Eggs
- Gelatin
- Pumpkin seeds
- Sesame seeds
- Sunflower seeds
- Walnuts

NON-STARCHY VEGETABLES

- Alfalfa
- Bamboo shoots
- Bean sprouts
- Bell peppers
- Bok choy
- Broccoli (limit to ½ cup/50 g)
- Brussels sprouts (limit to 2 sprouts)
- Cabbage (limit to 1 cup/120 g)
- Carrots
- Celeriac
- Celery (limit to 2 inches)
- Chard
- Chicory leaves
- Chives
- Collard greens
- Cucumbers
- Eggplant
- Fennel
- Ginger
- Green beans
- Kale
- Lettuce
- Okra
- Olives
- Pickled gherkins
- Pickled onions
- Radishes
- Scallions (green part)
- Seaweed / nori
- Snow peas (limit to 5)
- Spinach
- Swiss chard
- Tomatoes
- Turnips
- Water chestnuts
- Zucchini

HEALTHY FATS

- All fats in the Fat Fueled Food Pyramid in addition to:
- Avocados (limit to 1/8 avocado)
- Coconut butter
- Coconut cream, inulin-free (limit to ½ cup/125 ml)
- Coconut meat (shredded, fresh, pulverized) (1/4 cup/25 g)
- Coconut milk, inulin-free (limit to ½ cup/125 ml)
- Garlic-infused oil
- Onion-infused oil

WATER

Note: If dairy is part of your keto protocol, the following dairy items are low in FODMAPs: butter, cheese (except those listed in avoid list), cream (limit to ½ cup/120 ml), ghee, yogurt (limit to dairy-free, Greek, goat).

Looking at the Long Term

As effective as a low-FODMAP diet is, you may need to go a step further to heal your gut—that is, unless you want to eat low-FODMAP for the rest of your life and deprive yourself of many delicious and healthy high-FODMAP foods, such as onions, garlic, avocados, cauliflower, broccoli, cabbage, mushrooms, asparagus, and almonds.

As prebiotics, FODMAPs play a crucial role in keeping your gut flora balanced and healthy. In a recent study, twenty-six people with IBS and six healthy people followed two diets, each diet for twenty-one days. One of the diets was low-FODMAP and the other was high-FODMAP. At the end of the twenty-one days, the low-FODMAP diet had caused a dramatic shift in the gut flora by decreasing total bacteria, on average, a whopping 47 percent. On the other hand, eating a high-FODMAP Paleo-like diet seemed to stimulate the growth of beneficial gut bacteria. So, with more and more studies linking the health of your gut flora to your digestion, immune health, weight regulation, hormonal balance, and mental health, it stands to reason that eliminating FODMAPs from your diet for good is not the way to go.

Yes, a low-FODMAP diet can help you feel better in the short term. Sometimes you have to avoid the foods that are causing symptoms to in order to give your body the space to heal. But removing FODMAPs isn't a long-term solution. To really heal your gut, you need to find out what's causing your FODMAP intolerance and address it.

Managing your gut symptoms isn't the same as healing your gut.

I firmly believe that an intolerance to FODMAPs is unlike any other type of food sensitivity stemming from say, a leaky gut, inflammation, or damage to the gut. In my personal and professional experience, it's more likely to be caused by an imbalance in gut flora, whether that stems from SIBO, a lack of digestive enzymes, or another cause. Whatever the source of the dysbiosis, the steps in the Gut Support section (page 256) can help you heal.

I've also seen that FODMAP intolerance doesn't have to be a permanent thing. You should be able to tolerate FODMAPs again once the root cause of your intolerance is healed.

Lectins

Lectins are substances found in plants and seeds that act as the plant's self-defense mechanism: they irritate the gut lining and cause any creature that eats the plant or seed to think twice about doing so again.

Of course, humans have been eating plants and seeds that contain lectins for quite a while. And as a result, we've developed a natural protection against lectins—the mucus layer throughout the gut acts as a protective barrier, neutralizing lectins before they can cause problems.

But if your gut is off balance or you consume high concentrations of lectins, they can get through that protection and damage the intestinal lining. Since the purpose of that lining is to let the good stuff pass into the body and keep the bad stuff contained, it's crucial that it stay healthy and intact.

The immune system is affected by lectins, too. Because we don't digest lectins, we often produce antibodies to them, which unnecessarily amps up the immune system. Plus, if the gut is already injured as the result of another condition, the presence of lectins can stimulate a further unnecessary immune response.

Overconsumption of lectins can also lead to problems such as

- weight gain

- leaky gut

- nutrient deficiencies

- an imbalanced gut microbiome

- increased blood viscosity, meaning the heart has to work harder to do its job

- altered gene expression

- disrupted endocrine function

Many people, especially those with autoimmune disorders, tend to be particularly sensitive to lectins found in certain foods.

Unfortunately, because lectins are found in a ton of plant foods, completely removing them from your diet isn't totally practical. And some lectins actually have health benefits. Still, for many people, consuming high amounts isn't sustainable either. The best course of action is somewhere in the middle: removing foods that have epic amount of lectins.

Lectins are most abundant in peanuts, cashews, unfermented soybean products, and corn-fed meat. (Grass-fed/grass-finished meat is much lower in lectins. This is another reason why high-quality protein is so important.) Corn itself is also a high-lectin food, so while you're likely not consuming corn as part of your regular ketogenic diet, make sure to exclude it as much as possible from your carb-ups as well.

There are some foods high-ish in lectins that you should probably keep to special occasions but aren't nearly as doom-and-gloom as corn and soy: beans and legumes (such as kidney beans and black beans), tree nuts (like almonds, pecans, walnuts, cashews, and pistachios), and nightshade vegetables (including tomatoes, potatoes, eggplant, and peppers).

What's a Nightshade?

Nightshades are a family of plants, both edible and inedible plants (like, so inedible they are poisonous). There are a couple of interesting theories about why edible nightshades can still affect some people negatively, including the way our bodies process the vitamin D in them and the alkaloids (a natural bug repellent) contained in this family of foods.

It's very possible that the low-level toxic properties of nightshades may contribute to a variety of health issues over time, causing symptoms that most of us would never think to attribute to the tomato sauce we slather on our (grain-free) noodles every other day.

Nightshade sensitivity usually appears as inflammation of some sort—joint aches, acne, or gut irritation. I can tell I've had too many nightshades when my face breaks out in small pimples.

Nightshade family members include the following:

- Ashwagandha (used in adrenal and hormone support supplements)
- Bush tomatoes
- Cocoa
- Eggplant
- Garden huckleberries (not regular huckleberries)
- Goji berries
- Paprika
- Peppers, both sweet and hot
- Potatoes (but not sweet potatoes)
- Tomatillos
- Tomatoes

Although many of these are foods that you wouldn't necessarily run into every day, many are often used in supplements and herbal remedies.

If you search online for lectin-rich foods, you're bound to see potatoes on that list. But when a potato is cooked, its lectin content is reduced by up to 60 percent! So have those potatoes during a carb-up and don't worry too much about the lectins. Just don't eat a raw potato and you should be okay.

While it's not a guarantee for success, eliminating or reducing lectins just might be the key to making your gut the healthiest it has ever been. Try it for a couple of weeks and see how you feel.

If you have a favorite recipe that you want to make nightshade-free, here are some suggestions for ingredient alternatives:

Bell peppers

For stir-fries: Add a handful of kale at the end of cooking.

For stuffed vegetables: Use hollowed-out zucchini or butternut squash.

Eggplant

Use zucchini. It slices thin, just like eggplant, and holds up similarly in many recipes.

Potatoes

For roasted potatoes: Use radishes.

For mashed potatoes: Steamed and mashed cauliflower works great.

For potato salad: Try cubed and steamed rutabaga.

Spices containing hot peppers (including paprika, chili powder, and curry powder):

For spice mixtures: Replace with cumin, turmeric, or oregano.

For hot sauce in recipes: Use horseradish.

Tomatoes

It's hard to find a good swap for tomatoes, so the best advice I can give is to look for recipes that don't call for them. That way, you're not stuck eating your salsa sans tomatoes and thinking, "Wow, this really sucks." Instead, you're cooking outside of the box and discovering new ingredients! Often I will simply omit tomatoes in sauces and stews and make up for it with more vegetables and bone broth. For curries, I'll use a coconut milk base instead.

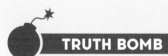

TRUTH BOMB

When a food's ingredients label says simply "spices," it almost always includes paprika.

Lectin Cheat Sheet

High-Lectin Foods

- Corn
- Corn-fed meats
- Casein A1 milk (see page 99)
- Peanuts and cashews
- Unfermented soybean products (if you want to eat soy, make sure it's traditionally fermented)

High-Lectin Foods in Which Lectins Can Be Lowered by Cooking, Soaking, and/or Sprouting

- Legumes, including peas and beans
- Grains, especially whole grains (this is why I recommend white rice for carb-ups instead of brown rice)
- Nightshade fruits and vegetables (see page 290)
- Squash, including pumpkins and zucchini

Low-Lectin Foods

Asparagus	Cauliflower	Olives
Avocados	Celery	Onions
Broccoli	Garlic	Sweet potatoes
Brussels sprouts	Leafy greens	
Cassava	Mushrooms	

Ways to Lower the Lectin Content in Your Food

- Peel fruits and vegetables.
- Remove the skins from nuts and seeds.
- Sprout seeds, grains, and beans (except in the case of alfalfa, in which lectin content increases after sprouting).
- Eat fermented vegetables.
- Pressure-cook your food.
- Opt for white grains over brown during your carb-ups.

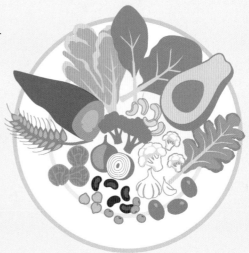

Histamines

Histamine is an extremely important compound in the body. It acts as a neurotransmitter and regulates the production of stomach acid, blood vessel permeability, and contraction of skeletal muscle. It's also a major component of the immune response and thus a key mediator in allergic reactions.

While we all need a certain amount of histamine to function, some people produce excess histamine and/or have a deficiency in the enzyme that breaks down histamine. A few symptoms are dizziness, accelerated heart rate, anxiety, nausea, and difficulty regulating body temperature.

So how does this relate to the gut? Well, many microbes that reside in the gut generate an enzyme called histidine decarboxylase. That enzyme converts an amino acid called histidine, found in certain foods, into histamine. The more of these microbes you have and the more histidine you consume, the higher the amount of histamine produced in your gut. Histamine can then be sent to various sites of the body, exacerbating allergy symptoms.

Histamine intolerance is unlike other food allergies or sensitivities in that the response is cumulative—which can make a histamine intolerance really tricky to recognize. It takes time for the histamine levels to build up. Symptoms may include the following:

- Itching, especially of the skin, eyes, ears, and nose

- Hives

- Tissue swelling

- Reduced blood pressure

- Increased heart rate

- Chest pain

Doctors may identify this as an allergic reaction, but often when standard skin-prick testing is performed, it leads nowhere. This can be a frustrating experience, especially when you don't know that histamine intolerance exists. But hey, now you do!

If you've dealt with any of these symptoms over the years, you may really benefit from a low-histamine diet. This will reduce symptoms so that you can work to repair your gut.

Try avoiding these high-histamine foods and ingredients:

- Alcohol
- Artificial food colors and preservatives
- Chocolate and cocoa
- Citrus
- Eggs
- Fermented foods
- Kefir
- Leftover meats
- Processed, cured, smoked, or fermented meats, such as lunch meat, bacon, sausage, salami, pepperoni

- Most berries and dried fruit
- Seafood
- Spices: cinnamon, chili powder, cloves, anise, nutmeg, curry powder, cayenne
- Spinach
- Tea (herbal and regular)
- Tomatoes
- Vinegar and foods containing vinegar, such as pickles, relishes, ketchup, and prepared mustard
- Yogurt

On top of these tweaks in your diet, you may also want to consider supplementing with quercetin, which is a natural antihistamine, or diamine oxidase, which is the enzyme responsible for the breakdown of histamine. You can also use antihistamine herbs like thyme and holy basil in your cooking.

Over time (how long depends on the severity of your symptoms), your gut will heal and your body will produce less histamine. I've experienced this myself, and now I practice a low-histamine diet on and off—limiting histamine-rich foods when I'm able and not caring too much other times. It hasn't been an issue in years!

Gallbladder **Support**

Includes fat digestion issues, gallbladder imbalances, and gallbladder removal

Some people experience indigestion, nausea, diarrhea, or other gastrointestinal symptoms after they eat fat. These symptoms are often due to a problem with the gallbladder, the organ that stores bile. Bile is essential for digesting fats, and if you have a gallbladder problem—and they're fairly common—bile may not be getting to your digestive tract in sufficient quantities to break down the fat you're eating. And if you've already had your gallbladder removed, you may need to aim for a lower daily fat intake.

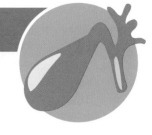

SYMPTOMS OF GALLBLADDER IMBALANCE

If any of these symptoms crop up after you enjoy some fat, or if they're ongoing throughout your ketogenic journey and you can't figure out why, perhaps it's because you're having a hard time digesting fat.

 Oil in the stool

 Pain in the right flank, right below the shoulder blade, at the front or back of the body

 Gas, bloating, and/or nausea that occurs 15 to 30 minutes after a high-fat meal

 A sore or swollen tongue

 Peeling, dryness, and/or blistering of the skin, especially on the palms

Gallbladder symptoms can occur in those who are just beginning a high-fat journey as well as those who have been eating high-fat for many months. Generally, they're due to a plug in the piping and can be relieved by incorporating some of the healing foods listed below. But it's best to book a checkup with your health-care professional to check on the status of your gallbladder and make sure everything is good.

Diet Adjustments

If you do not have a gallbladder, it's very likely that, with patience, you'll be able to get up to 60 percent of your energy coming from fat. But please do not go balls-to-the-wall and eat copious quantities of fat bombs, fatty grass-fed beef, or coconut milk in a single day. Doing so will likely lead to pain, indigestion, nausea, or crazy diarrhea that will make you lose faith in the keto diet quicker than you can say "poo pants." Instead, on a weekly basis, increase your fat consumption by a couple percentage points—as long as you don't experience any symptoms. If you do, back off a little and try again in a couple of days.

Test for It: Gallbladder Health

An abdominal x-ray effectively spots calcium-based gallstones.

A CT scan is effective for spotting gallbladder problems like ruptures and infections, though it's not great at revealing gallstones.

Endoscopic retrograde cholangiopancreatography (ERCP) uses a tube fitted with a small camera and light to help spot gallstones or problems in the bile ducts. It's inserted into the mouth, down through the stomach, and into the small intestine.

An MRI helps to reveal stones in bile ducts and gallbladder cancer, but it doesn't show small stones or infections well.

An ultrasound is helpful in diagnosing gallstones but doesn't reveal inflammation of the gallbladder.

Ultra-Healing Foods

THE EXTRAS

- Cayenne pepper
- Dry mustard
- Fresh and dried cilantro
- Fresh and dried mint
- Fresh and dried parsley
- Fresh ginger
- Ginger powder
- Ground black pepper
- Ground cinnamon
- Ground turmeric

STARCHES AND LOW-FRUCTOSE FRUITS

- Beets
- Carrots

PROTEIN

- Beef
- Chicken
- Salmon
- Turkey

NON-STARCHY VEGETABLES

- Artichokes
- Arugula
- Asparagus
- Beet greens
- Broccoli
- Celery
- Cucumbers
- Fennel
- Kale
- Leeks
- Radishes
- Romaine lettuce
- Spinach
- Fermented vegetables, including sauerkraut, kimchi, and pickled ginger

HEALTHY FATS

- Avocado oil
- Avocados
- Extra-virgin olive oil
- Ghee

WATER

Additional Adjustments

Say Yes To

OX BILE

While you're working on incorporating more fats into your life, it may be helpful for you to include ox bile, a digestive support that aids in the production of bile, with every meal. If you've had your gallbladder removed, this is an essential step, and you will likely need to take ox bile for the rest of your life.

TAKING IT SLOW

If you don't have a gallbladder, slowly increase the amount of fat in your diet over time. Begin by adding 1 tablespoon of fat to each of your meals and increase the amount every couple of days. It should take you about four weeks to get to keto levels of fat, with 60 percent of your daily calories coming from fat. If you experience pain or nausea after a meal, it could be because you ate too much fat. Back off a little and see how you feel. By listening to what your body is trying to tell you, you'll be able to find the amount of fat that works best for you.

BOOSTING DIGESTION

Supplementing with non-flush niacin, B complex vitamins, and a strong digestive enzyme—in addition to ox bile—will help build up your bile and break down fat properly. You could also take a shot of apple cider vinegar or lemon juice before your meals. This helps to signal to the body that a meal is coming and should help to improve overall digestion.

BILE CREATION

There are many things that will help to boost your bile production and encourage proper fat digestion. These include sauerkraut juice (the raw, unpasteurized fermentation liquid of cabbage), fermented liquids, such as kefir or kombucha, and fermented vegetables. Drinking warm water with lemon as soon as you wake may also be helpful.

CHECKING FOR FOOD SENSITIVITIES

Follow the guidelines in the section on allergies and sensitivities (page 274) to identify any foods you may be sensitive to.

ACUPUNCTURE

Acupuncture may aid in bile production and assist with processing the emotions associated with the liver and gallbladder (see below).

SWITCHING TO MCT OIL POWDER

If you love the way you feel on MCT oil but hate what it does to your gut, MCT oil powder may work. My favorite brand is from Perfect Keto. MCT oil powder makes drinks creamy—no dairy needed—and provides your body with all the medium-chain triglycerides, without the digestive issues that can crop up with its oil counterpart.

Say No To

WATER WITH MEALS

To improve overall digestion, avoid drinking too much water with your meals, leaving the bulk of your water intake to in-between meals.

ANGRY FEELINGS

According to Chinese medicine, the liver and gallbladder are areas that hold anger. People who are frustrated and angry, feeling bitter toward other people or situations, have a greater propensity for liver and gallbladder issues. If this describes you, to encourage healing, deal with your anger, frustration, and bitterness by focusing on gratitude and love.

Supportive Supplements

If you have a history of gallstones or gallbladder issues, or suspect that you might have a gallbladder imbalance, it's best to check in with your doctor before trying to boost your ability to digest fats.

- Vitamins: non-flush niacin, B complex

- Minerals: magnesium

- Lipids: phosphatidylcholine, sunflower lecithin

- Herbs and plants: bitters, curcumin, cayenne pepper, black pepper, ginger

- Other: full-spectrum digestive enzyme with ox bile, apple cider vinegar, sauerkraut juice, peppermint tea

Kidney **Support**

It's probably not news to you that the kidneys remove waste products and excess fluid from the body in the form of urine. What you may not know is that the kidneys also regulate the body's salt, potassium, and acid content, remove drugs, produce an active form of vitamin D that promotes bone health, control the production of red blood cells, and even produce hormones.

Test for It: Kidney Health

The albumin-to-creatinine ratio (ACR) tests the protein in your urine. A high amount may mean your kidneys' filtering units have been damaged. The level can be abnormally high due to heavy exercise or a fever, so it's important to test multiple times to get a clear picture.

An organic acids test examines chemical compounds in the urine (and in the blood in lower concentrations) called organic acids. Some of these acids are yeast and fungal markers and could point to candida being present. These markers include citramalic, 5-hydroxymethyl-2-furoic, 3-oxoglutaric, furan-2,5-dicarboxylic, furancarbonylglycine, tartaric, arabinose, carboxycitric, and tricarballylic acids.

So when something goes wrong with your kidneys, it can be very serious. Problem is, imbalanced kidneys are a bit challenging to spot. Things like high blood pressure, fatigue, shortness of breath, nausea, frequent urination, excessive thirst, and puffy eyes are all signs that you could have an imbalance, but they're also signs of other imbalances. If you're experiencing these symptoms, it's best to seek the support of a qualified health professional.

The Trouble with Oxalates

Back in 2017, I dealt with pretty intense pelvic pain. When I met with my doctor, she knew exactly what was wrong: oxalates. A little urine collection for an organic acids test and it was clear that I was reacting to the oxalates in my diet. I didn't know too much about oxalates at the time, only that individuals with kidney stones had to avoid them. I removed foods with moderate and high levels of oxalates from my diet and felt relief almost immediately. Today, I am mindful of my oxalate consumption, but I don't worry about it too much. If I get a touch of pain, I back off for a little while. It's amazing what reducing oxalates for a period did for my overall wellness!

Oxalates are naturally occurring compounds that are found in a wide variety of plant foods. Plants produce this substance for their own protection—oxalates actually damage insects' teeth.

While oxalates aren't going to damage *your* teeth, they may cause other imbalances in your body. Oxalates can build up in the kidneys, leading to a high concentration of oxalates in the urine. If this happens in conjunction with a high concentration of calcium, our kidneys are at risk of forming calcium oxalate kidney stones.

While the number one reason people remove oxalates from their diet is kidney stone–related, those with leaky gut have just as many issues with them. In a healthy gut, oxalates are broken down, which prevents them from traveling to the large intestine and being absorbed by body tissues. But in someone with leaky gut, oxalates escape through those gaps in the intestinal lining and into the bloodstream, damaging body tissues, glands, secretory organs, and the brain. When they're uncontained and running amok, oxalates impair enzymes, oxidize cell membranes, interfere with nutrient absorption, and can even alter the way your DNA is expressed.

Diet Adjustments

If you're fairly healthy and have well-functioning kidneys and a balanced digestive system, you can probably eat a variety of nourishing foods and not worry too much about oxalates. A high-oxalate diet isn't inherently bad. However, it is something to be aware of if you're still struggling with digestive symptoms after transitioning to keto. Additionally, you may want to consider reducing oxalates if you:

- have or have had kidney stones

- have a leaky gut

- have allergies, food sensitivities, or difficulty digesting fat

- have any autoimmune or inflammatory issue, like asthma, arthritis, or fibromyalgia

- have taken antibiotics frequently or for long periods of time

- are on the autism spectrum or have a neurological disorder like ADD, depression, or dyslexia

If any of this applies to you, try omitting foods with high and moderate levels of oxalates, as shown in the following table.

But reducing oxalates doesn't have to be an all-or-nothing thing. You may just need to be mindful of the high-oxalate foods you're currently eating. If your treats are made with nut flour, you could switch to coconut flour. Or you could swap out kale for some romaine here and there. When you do a carb-up, do you eat a bunch of berries? How about enjoying an unripened banana instead? These are areas where you can make an easy change.

If you are reducing your oxalate exposure to prevent kidney stones from forming, limit oxalates to 40 to 50 mg per day. In the table opposite, low-oxalate foods have 0 to 5 mg of oxalates per serving, moderate-oxalate foods have 5 to 10 mg of oxalates, and high-oxalate foods have more than 10 mg of oxalates. If a food is not on the list, it's because it hasn't been tested for oxalates.

Don't feel like you have to go overboard in cutting oxalates, though—in this case, more restriction isn't better, at least initially. If you remove oxalates very quickly, it can actually cause a detox reaction that's not so pleasant. (Believe me, I've experienced it firsthand, and it's no fun.) So instead, be conscious of your choices, but don't stress yourself out over getting to 40 to 50 mg on your first day. Work toward it, and over a couple weeks, you'll get there!

Do you have to avoid these foods forever? Maybe not. Some people benefit from reducing as best they can for thirty days and then setting the intention to go for lower-oxalate foods and allowing it to happen naturally, instead of cutting everything permanently and feeling super-restricted.

And it's entirely possible to consume oxalates again once you heal your underlying imbalance. I think a lot of people get hung up on doing these things and

OXALATE LEVELS

DRINKS

	KETO FOODS		CARB-UP FOODS
LOW	Aloe vera juice Distilled alcohol Lemon juice	Lime juice Mint tea Water	Beer Cider Wine
MEDIUM	Coffee (limit to 8 oz/day) Green tea		
HIGH	Chocolate-containing drinks		

DAIRY*

	KETO FOODS
LOW	All types are fine, but limit to 1 serving per day because of calcium restrictions

MEAT

	KETO FOODS
LOW	All except those listed as medium
MEDIUM	Beef kidney Liver

OTHER PROTEINS

	KETO FOODS		
LOW	Eggs Flax seeds		
MEDIUM	Beans* Lentils* Pumpkin seeds		
HIGH	Almonds Cashews Green beans Hazelnuts Macadamia nuts	Peanuts Pecans Pistachios Sesame seeds Sunflower seeds	Tofu and all soy products Walnuts

FATS

	KETO FOODS
LOW	All types are fine, but limit to 1 serving per day because of calcium restrictions
HIGH	Sesame oil

FRUIT

	KETO FOODS	CARB-UP FOODS	
LOW	Avocados Coconuts	Apples, peeled Cantaloupe Cherries Cranberries, canned Green grapes Honeydew melon	Mangoes Nectarines Papayas Pears, peeled Raisins Watermelon

FRUIT (CONT.)

	KETO FOODS		CARB-UP FOODS	
MEDIUM			Apples with skin Apricots Bananas Black currants Cranberries, dried Grapefruit	Oranges Papayas Peaches Pears, with skin Pineapple Plums Prunes
HIGH	Blackberries Blueberries Lemon peel Lime peel	Olives Raspberries Rhubarb Strawberries	Dates Figs, dried Purple grapes Red currants	Tangerines

VEGETABLES

	KETO FOODS			CARB-UP FOODS
LOW	Alfalfa sprouts Asparagus Bok choy Broccoli tips, cooked Brussels sprouts, boiled	Cabbage, raw Cauliflower Collards, raw Green beans Kohlrabi Onions	Parsley Red peppers Radishes Summer squash Turnips Zucchini	Water chestnuts Winter squash
MEDIUM	Artichokes Broccoli, raw/cooked Brussels sprouts, raw/steamed	Cabbage, steamed Cucumbers, peeled Eggplant Leek Lettuce	Lima beans* Mushrooms Peas, canned Snow peas Tomatoes	Carrots, cooked Plantains Potatoes, red and white
HIGH	Celery Chives Dandelion Escarole Green peppers	Kale Leeks Mustard greens Okra Rutabaga	Spinach Swiss chard Watercress	Beets and beet greens Carrots, raw Parsnips Sweet potatoes Yams

GRAINS

	CARB-UP FOODS
LOW	Corn* White rice

CONDIMENTS & OTHER ITEMS

	KETO FOODS			CARB-UP FOODS
LOW	Apple cider vinegar Baking powder Baking soda	Cream of tartar Dry mustard Gelatin and collagen Ginger	Nutmeg Rosemary Sage Tarragon Thyme Vanilla	Maple syrup
MEDIUM	Basil Sauerkraut			
HIGH	Black pepper Cacao powder Carob	Chocolate Cinnamon Oregano Stevia	Turmeric White pepper	Honey

* These are keto "maybe" foods: not part of the strict protocol, but maybe part of yours.

eliminations *forever*. That's not the goal here. Let's *heal* the body so that you can get back to eating almond flour, and chocolate, and carrots...

And please keep in mind that, while limiting oxalates can be a large part of the solution for those struggling with kidney imbalance, when it comes to kidney disease, it's best to work one on one with your doctor to receive the support you need.

Additional Adjustments

Say Yes To
DRINKING WATER
Keeping a water bottle full and at the ready is always a good idea. Opt for water over coffee, juice, energy drinks, and soda.

MOVING YOUR BODY
Any form of movement is good: walking, biking, hiking, HIIT, anything that makes you feel good. Finding an activity you enjoy doing is best.

REDUCING INFLAMMATION
The guidelines for reducing inflammation on page 251 will be helpful here. Processed oils and carbohydrates should be avoided as much as possible.

DAILY STRESS REDUCTION
Stress can lead to high blood pressure, and high blood pressure can place a strain on the kidneys because they rely on a healthy flow of blood for proper function. Pick up relaxing activities like yoga, walking, and reading—or whatever works for you!

Say No To
SMOKING
Smokers have decreased blood flow, which can lead to issues with kidney function. Like any part of the body, the kidneys can't function well when they don't have adequate blood flow.

OVERTRAINING
While movement is beneficial, If you're working out so hard that everything in your body hurts, is swollen, and is painful to the touch, you've pushed too hard. Overtraining can be very damaging and risky for the kidneys.

Supportive Supplements

Vitamins: D$_3$, A, B complex, C, E

Herbs and spices: turmeric, curcumin, rosemary

Others: green tea, fish oil, GLA, NAC, garlic, ginger

Lymphatic System **Support**

The lymphatic system is a network of vessels, ducts, lymph nodes (like the ones that get swollen when you're sick), organs such as the spleen, and more. Through this system flows lymph, a fluid that travels throughout the body to remove waste from every cell while helping to regulate the immune system. When it passes through lymph nodes, harmful substances are filtered out. The nodes also contain immune cells that fight infection by attacking germs that are carried in the lymph fluid.

Think of the lymphatic system like the plumbing in your home that connects sinks, bathtubs, washers, dishwashers, and the like. When the drains are clogged in your toilet or sink, you can't get rid of waste effectively. The same is true for your body's lymphatic system. Stagnant lymph flow leads to a buildup of waste and toxins, weakening immunity and leading to a wide range of health issues.

Lymph is propelled through the body when you move your muscles and through the movement of breathing. The lymph must flow freely to ensure that waste products and fluids do not build up in the tissues.

These are some signs your lymphatic system isn't draining properly:

- Bloating
- Brain fog
- Breast swelling with each cycle
- Cellulite
- Chronic sinusitis, sore throats, colds, or ear infections
- Cold hands and feet
- Fatigue
- Itchy and dry skin
- Joint pain
- Muscle pain and aches
- Stiffness, especially in the morning
- Stubborn weight gain
- Swelling in lymph nodes (like those in the throat, armpits, and groin)
- Water retention

You need extra lymphatic support if you've experienced any of the following:

- Arthritis
- Cancer
- Chronic fatigue
- Fibromyalgia
- Frequent infections, viruses, or colds
- Tonsillitis

Diet Adjustments

Lymph fluid is about 95 percent water, so when you're dehydrated, it becomes thicker and doesn't flow as easily. In fact, one of the most common causes of lymph congestion is dehydration. Stay well hydrated by sipping warm purified water throughout the day to help keep your lymph flowing well. Avoiding caffeine when dehydrated is best. This includes chocolate, coffee, and caffeinated teas.

Ultra-Healing Foods

THE EXTRAS

- Fresh cilantro
- Fresh garlic
- Fresh ginger
- Fresh parsley
- Garlic powder
- Ginger powder
- Ground turmeric

NON-STARCHY VEGETABLES

- Artichokes
- Bok choy
- Broccoli
- Brussels sprouts
- Cabbage
- Cauliflower
- Dandelion greens
- Kale
- Microgreens
- Sauerkraut
- Spinach
- Watercress

STARCHES AND FRUITS

- Beets
- Berries
- Lemons

HEALTHY FATS

- Chia seeds
- Coconut oil
- Extra-virgin olive oil
- Flax seeds
- Hemp seeds
- Pumpkin seeds

PROTEIN

- Oysters
- Salmon
- Sardines

WATER

Additional Adjustments

Say Yes To

SWEATING TO RELEASE ADDITIONAL TOXINS

Removing as many toxins as possible lowers the burden on the lymph. And the lowest-hanging fruit when it comes to detoxification is sweating! Interestingly, sweat from exercise doesn't help remove toxins: when you're in a state of activity and physical stress, the cells throughout your body aren't open for detoxification. Red light therapy is one good option for sweating in a relaxed state. My favorite red light therapy is Joovv.

REGULAR BOWEL MOVEMENTS

Regular elimination is key to a healthy lymphatic system. Follow the digestion-supporting steps starting on page 256 if you're struggling here.

MOVING YOUR LYMPH

The lymphatic system does not have a built-in pump like the heart, so it relies on the contraction and relaxation of the muscles and joints to keep the lymph moving. Tense and relax all the muscles in your body multiple times a day, laugh deeply, and breathe with your belly to encourage the lymph to move with ease.

Dry brushing and lymphatic massage can also assist with lymphatic movement. For dry brushing, purchase a body brush made for dry brushing and brush your entire body with strokes leading toward the heart. Pay special attention to the head, neck, feet, breasts, and abdomen.

ESSENTIAL OILS

Essential oils can help to stimulate blood and lymph flow. Add 10 to 15 drops of grapefruit oil to 2 tablespoons of coconut oil and rub it all over your body after a dry brushing session, or anytime. Add 10 drops of lemon essential oil to 3 tablespoons of Himalayan salt to make a body scrub for the shower. Add 3 drops of juniper essential oil to 1 tablespoon of avocado oil and rub on swollen glands.

Say No To

EPIC STRESS

Lymph congestion increases with emotional or physical stress. Opt for a meditation practice, get out in nature, or spend quality time with people that adore you. Slow down, pause, take a breath, and allow your lymph to flow freely!

TIGHT CLOTHING AND BRAS

Cutting off circulation can cause lymph to stagnate. This is why I've never understood wearing super-tight workout clothing! Wear loose-fitting clothing when you're able and go braless as much as possible.

INFLAMMATION

Systemic inflammation creates congestion and swelling in the tissues, which impairs lymphatic flow. Follow the guidelines in the Inflammation Reduction section on page 251.

TOXINS

Additional toxins will only burden the system you're trying to support. It's important to reduce your exposure to chemicals in food, air, personal care products, and water. For food, opt for organic produce and pasture-raised meat and dairy when possible. If the air quality in your hometown is less than optimal, get a HEPA filter for the room you spend the most time in (your workplace is fair game!). For personal care products, be mindful of the ingredients they use. Opt for essential oils instead of perfume, natural deodorant (my favorite is Primal Pit Paste), and natural body wash (my favorite is Dr. Bronner's Castile Soap). This is a great start to reducing your toxic load in personal care products and can do wonders for your lymphatic system!

Supportive Supplements

Others: antioxidants, omega-3s, glutathione

Cardiovascular **Support**

Includes heart disease, stroke, and hypertension

Cardiovascular disease is often stereotyped as a man's disease when in reality it's the most common cause of death for women, too.

The ketogenic diet is naturally, at its core, a cardiovascular health diet because of its ability to help balance blood sugar and restore insulin sensitivity. Insulin and blood sugar levels are both directly related to the health of your cardiovascular system. As a general rule, having more body fat increases the risk of insulin resistance, and when there's a high level of insulin in the body, the pathways that shuttle fats through vascular walls are affected, which can lead to atherosclerosis. It also places more stress on the arteries, which can lead to higher blood pressure, and raises inflammation, which causes an increase in LDL and triglycerides, and a drop in HDL—all bad news for cardiovascular health.

You may have heard that saturated fat is the worst fat choice for those affected by heart disease, but this is because saturated fat is a marker for junk food in many studies. If you're eating keto, your saturated fat is coming from grass-fed/ grass-finished steak, coconut oil, and butter, not donuts, potato chips, or cookies. That makes a big difference.

What happens to your cardiac risk factors when you are consuming a healthy high-fat diet?

- The smaller, denser LDL cholesterol particles—the dangerous ones—decrease.

- HDL cholesterol—the good kind—increases.

- Triglycerides—fats associated with heart disease in high concentrations— decrease.

All those are very positive effects, so just by following keto, you're taking a great step to heart health.

If you experience any of the following symptoms, you may want to focus on your cardiovascular health and work with your doctor on coming up with a treatment plan:

- Chest pains or discomfort

- Nausea, indigestion, or stomach pain

- Dizziness and light-headedness with shortness of breath

- Extreme exhaustion or unexplained weakness for days at a time

The triglyceride-to-HDL ratio is the best measure of your cardiovascular health. Anything less than 1.0 means that you are in a great place.

Triglycerides are a type of fat found in the blood. The higher your triglycerides, the greater your risk of heart disease.

HDL, high-density lipoprotein, is referred to as the "good" cholesterol because it carries cholesterol from other parts of your body back to your liver, where it is secreted in bile or converted to bile salts. High HDL is generally good.

LDL, low-density lipoprotein, is referred to as the "bad" cholesterol because high levels can lead to a buildup of cholesterol in your arteries. However, the size of the LDL particles is what's really important. If your test comes back as higher in LDL than the norm, it's important to test next your lipoprotein particle number and size with an NMR test (below).

Lipoprotein(a) and lipoprotein(b) are particles in your blood that carry cholesterol, fats, and proteins. The amounts your body makes are determined by your genes and can increase as estrogen levels decline with menopause. If your health-care professional is concerned that your LDL is high, you could ask them to run this test as part of the NMR test. If your lipoprotein(a) is high and your lipoprotein(b) is low, that's great! On the flip side, if lipoprotein(b) is high, that means more work is needed to support the health of your cardiovascular system.

A nuclear magnetic resonance (NMR) test gives you more detailed information about your cardiovascular markers, including LDL particle size and lipoprotein(a) and (b) levels. In a regular blood test, most doctors only draw for triglycerides, HDL, LDL, and total cholesterol. These are a great first step to understanding the health of your cardiovascular system, but if your results are out of the "normal" range, an NMR test is a good next step to dig deeper into what's going on.

Homocysteine is a product of protein metabolism, and in high concentrations, it's been linked to an increased risk of heart attacks and strokes. Elevated homocysteine levels are thought to contribute to plaque formation by damaging arterial walls.

Fasting insulin tests your level of insulin after at least eight hours of fasting. The more insulin sensitive you are—the lower your insulin level—the lower your risk for cardiovascular disease.

High-sensitivity C-reactive protein (hs-CRP) is a test that measures CRP in the blood to detect inflammation, which is associated with a higher risk of developing cardiovascular disease.

Should You Take Statins?

As discussed on page 60, only half of patients who have heart attacks have high cholesterol, and it's probable that heart disease has more to do with inflammation than cholesterol. But mainstream medicine is still very focused on keeping cholesterol low for heart health. So what if your doctor is recommending that you take a statin?

The big story out there is that statins help lower cholesterol and with that lowered cholesterol, patients experience fewer cardiovascular events. Let's go through a couple of facts to unpack this story so that you can make an educated decision about what's best for your health.

There are eighteen studies funded by Big Pharma that paint the picture that in low-risk individuals, statin use cuts cardiovascular events by 18 percent in a five-year period. Impressive, right? But later, those same studies were reviewed, and it turns out they showed only a 1 percent decrease in events over a five-year period.

So if I were a low-risk individual and wanted to cut down the likelihood of having a cardiovascular event, I wouldn't rely on statins to do it. Fifteen percent of individuals taking statins experience significant side effects, including muscle pain, memory loss, and fatigue. Seems like a lot to go through for a 1 percent chance that you'll decrease your likelihood of a cardiovascular event. Also, some experts believe that cholesterol levels naturally increase as we age to protect our brains and reduce the inflammation caused by aging, in which case lowering cholesterol with a statin would make us more vulnerable to neurological and age-related health problems.

However, if I were a high-risk individual who refused to change my diet and lifestyle, statins could be right for me. Statins are most successful in reducing the absolute risk of a secondary cardiovascular event—if you've already had a cardiovascular event, they'll reduce the risk that you'll have another by 5 to 10 percent. However, research is very clear that reducing your risk for cardiovascular disease using diet and lifestyle will benefit you far more than the drugs currently on the market.

Blood Pressure

Hypertension, aka high blood pressure, is a condition in which blood pressure is consistently above 140/90. High blood pressure is associated with physical inactivity and obesity but can also occur in healthy individuals, likely due to genetics. Recent research has disproved the claim that salt raises blood pressure: it turns out that for most people, salt intake is not significantly correlated with high blood pressure. What is associated with it? A diet dominated by carbs and sugar, too much caffeine, and too little sleep, water, and/or exercise. Chronic stress can also cause high blood pressure.

If your blood pressure is high, the ketogenic diet is a great way to lower blood pressure by managing sugar and carb intake, which leads to weight loss and reduced stress.

Hypotension, aka low blood pressure, is a healthy and natural condition—as long as it's associated with athleticism. The more you exercise, the fitter your heart and the more efficient every heartbeat, so your heart doesn't need to work as hard. In nonathletes, though, low blood pressure can be a sign of low adrenal reserve, malnourishment, or ill health, especially if you experience dizziness going from sitting to standing. If your blood pressure is very low—say, below 90/60—you need to go to a doctor immediately.

If your blood pressure is low but not critically low, check for adrenal dysfunction (see page 378). Also, if you've been eating low-sodium for years, it could be contributing to your low blood pressure. If you are truly salt-deficient, adding some salt to your meals can help improve blood pressure.

Diet Adjustments

If you want to keep your heart and arteries healthy, the most important thing to do is to keep inflammation and oxidative stress low. Just following keto will go a long way—remember to focus on whole foods and healthy fats, and you'll be following the best diet for heart health. But you may also want to review the Inflammation Reduction section on page 251.

Ultra-Healing Foods

THE EXTRAS

- Cayenne pepper
- Curry leaves
- Fenugreek*
- Fresh and dried oregano (ground and leaves)
- Fresh garlic
- Garlic powder
- Ground black pepper
- Ground cinnamon
- Ground and whole cloves
- Ground turmeric

*If you're allergic to peanuts, nuts, or legumes, do not eat this; it is a cross-relative allergy.

STARCHES AND LOW-FRUCTOSE FRUITS

- Blackberries
- Blueberries
- Cassava
- Green plantains
- Parsnips
- Jicama
- Sweet potatoes

PROTEIN

- Mackerel
- Pork
- Salmon
- Trout
- Tuna

NON-STARCHY VEGETABLES

- Alfalfa
- Broccoli
- Garlic
- Horseradish
- Jerusalem artichokes
- Kale
- Lettuce
- Onions
- Spinach
- Tomatoes
- Turnip greens
- Watercress

HEALTHY FATS

- Avocados
- Chia seeds
- Flax seeds

WATER

Additional Adjustments

Say Yes To

DISCOVERING FOOD SENSITIVITIES & ALLERGIES

When you eat a food you're allergic to, a substance called angiotonin is released from the kidneys and causes the arteries to tighten, resulting in higher blood pressure. This allergic reaction, in which blood pressure increases without any other cardiovascular risk factors, is often treated with unnecessary blood pressure medication. Follow the guidelines on page 274 to discover if a food allergy could be behind your elevated blood pressure.

PHYSICAL ACTIVITY

Try to get at least thirty minutes of physical activity each day. Even a walk through your neighborhood counts! Regular exercise can lower triglycerides and boost HDL.

SUPPORTING AN AUTOIMMUNE CONDITION

Women with autoimmune conditions could be at greater risk of heart disease and stroke. Read more about supporting an autoimmune condition on page 241.

DAILY STRESS REDUCTION

A stressful situation sets off a chain of events in which your body releases adrenaline, a hormone that temporarily causes your breathing and heart rate to speed up and your blood pressure to rise. When stress is constant, your body remains in this high gear for days or weeks at a time—which is especially damaging to the cardiovascular system. This chronic state of stress may also cause some people to drink too much alcohol, which can raise blood pressure and damage arterial walls. So reduce your stress by adopting a self-care practice that works for you. Yoga, meditation, breathing exercises, qigong, and tai chi have all been scientifically proven to reduce stress. If none of these feel right to you, find a self-care practice that does—maybe an unhurried walk in nature, or a relaxing bath, or just sitting alone with your headphones on, listening to your favorite music.

Say No To

TOXINS

It's important to reduce your exposure to toxic chemicals in food, air, personal care products, and water because excess exposure to environmental toxins and chemicals is particularly damaging for the liver and kidneys, two organs that work closely with the cardiovascular system. For food, opt for organic produce and pasture-raised meat and dairy when possible. If the air quality in your hometown is less than optimal, get a HEPA filter for the room you spend the most time in (your workplace is fair game also!). For personal care products, start becoming mindful of the ingredients they use. Opt for essential oils instead of perfume, natural deodorant (my favorite is Primal Pit Paste), and natural body wash (my favorite is Dr. Bronner's Castile Soap).

ALCOHOL

Alcohol can increase triglycerides, raise blood pressure, and adds to your overall calorie intake, which could be otherwise be used for more nutrient-dense items like leafy greens.

CALCIUM SUPPLEMENTATION

Calcium is often recommended for postmenopausal women to help prevent bone loss and fractures as estrogen, which previously kept bones in tiptop health, drops. Problem is, it's been shown supplementing with calcium may increase the risk of cardiovascular disease. (Plus, calcium doesn't do a good job at preventing bone loss.)

Supportive Supplements

Vitamins: K, B_3, B_6, E

Minerals: magnesium, zinc

Others: omega-3 oil, CoQ10, garlic, L-carnitine, D-ribose, citrus bergamot, nutritional yeast, apple cider vinegar

Nervous System **Support**

Includes bipolar disorder, depression, mood, dementia, sleep disorders, Alzheimer's, anxiety, ADHD, and autism

Think of the nervous system as the motherboard of electric signaling that keeps the body completely interconnected, from the brain to the lungs to the hands and feet and everything else. There are a lot of health conditions that affect the nervous system, either directly or indirectly. This section will highlight some of the most common dysfunctions, disorders, imbalances, and diseases related to the nervous system.

The ketogenic diet improves neurological health in two main ways: First, because keto switches the body from relying on glucose to relying on fat, the brain has a steady supply of clean fuel that doesn't negatively affect its function, as glucose does over time (as seen in Alzheimer's). Second, when you're fat adapted, your cells are better able to neutralize free radicals, which otherwise would damage them. This includes brain and nerve cells, so they're healthier overall on keto.

Diet-based therapies in the realm of brain disease management go a long way in supporting the brain in forming new connections between brain cells, modifying the connections between nerve cells, and enhancing and normalizing function overall.

It all comes down to choosing the right foods that'll reverse or help us to avoid the chronic diseases that affect the brain and that will lower inflammation as much as possible, because excess inflammation affects the mitochondria, which have a direct impact on our nervous system overall.

The big takeaway here: keto is awesome for the brain!

The Role of Mitochondria in Neurological Imbalances

Mitochondria are the parts of a cell that produce energy, recycle waste products, signals cells to die (which is helpful in avoiding the growth of a tumor), and so much more. Mitochondria produce about 90 percent of the chemical energy a cell needs to survive, so a problem in the mitochondria could result in a serious imbalance for the whole body.

Mitochondria require oxygen in order to perform all of their duties. And just as a fire goes out without oxygen, if mitochondria lack oxygen, they stop working. This is where it gets interesting, because the main ketone, BHB, is more efficient than glucose, requiring less oxygen to create the same amount of energy. That means that there's an abundant amount of oxygen to allow mitochondria to flourish.

Why is this important to understand? Well, when mitochondria aren't able to work as well as they should, your energy wanes, your muscles are weak, and you may experience vision or hearing problems. If left unchecked, mitochondrial dysfunction can lead to neurological disorders such as Alzheimer's disease.

We know that the ketogenic diet and ketone bodies benefit mitochondrial function, so when a metabolism-based neurological imbalance is present, it could make sense to use the ketogenic diet as a form of support for the imbalance.

ADD/ADHD

There's no solid research on whether the ketogenic diet is helpful in the case of ADD/ADHD, but we can use what we do know about keto to form a hypothesis.

We know that ketones are a cleaner fuel for the brain—they don't cause excess neurological damage the way glucose does. We know that ketones increase mitochondrial efficiency, enhance brain cells, and strengthen the metabolism. Last, we know that ketones trigger brain-derived neurotrophic factor (BDNF), a protein that stimulates the growth of neurons. BDNF improves learning, higher thinking, and memory, all areas that those with ADD/ADHD struggle with.

I can speak personally here because I was diagnosed with ADD when I was thirteen years old. I was put on drugs such as Adderall, Dexedrine, and Ritalin, with horrible side effects: insomnia and appetite problems, which further encouraged my eating disorder tendencies. I worked with a family counselor, psychologists, and psychiatrists to try to work through my behavior issues and social skills, and while I managed to get along, I never felt truly okay—almost like a zombie.

FORMS OF ADHD

 Inattentive Type

- Avoids or dislikes tasks that require sustained mental effort
- Does not follow through on instructions; may start tasks and not finish them
- Does not manage time well
- Does not seem to listen when being spoken to
- Forgets to pay bills or do daily tasks
- Has problems staying focused on tasks or activities
- Is easily distracted
- Makes careless mistakes
- Often loses important things
- Struggles with paying attention to detail

 Hyperactive Type

- Always "on the go" or active
- Fidgets and/or squirms constantly when seated
- Has difficulty waiting for things
- Interrupts or intrudes on others without permission
- Not able to stay seated when necessary
- Talks over people
- Unable to play or do leisure activities quietly

When I discovered keto, I was on a high dose of Adderall and had accepted that I'd be on some sort of medication to treat this brain disorder forever. After thirty days of being on keto, the Adderall dosage felt off. I met with my doctor and we agreed to lower it. Another thirty days passed, and I still felt it was too much, so my doctor and I chose a week to go off the medication entirely (it's important to choose a time when you're in a low-stress environment and won't be triggered too much). This was back in 2014, and I haven't gone back on ADD medication since.

When I eat too many carbohydrates, or I eat sugar, or I become highly stressed, I can display a bit of ADD behavior, but a quick diet and lifestyle correction—lowering my carbohydrate intake, taking note of my sugar intake, and meditation—goes a long, long way.

Of course, you should work with your health-care professional if you're thinking about adjusting your medication, but I never thought in a million years that I would be off my meds and be okay for this long.

Current research points to the development of ADHD as multifactorial, meaning it could require a combination of various factors, including genetics, stress in the womb, diet, trauma, and toxin exposure. In my case, I believe it was toxin exposure and diet that led to my symptoms.

Anxiety

I've had women tell me that keto made their anxiety worse, and I've had women tell me that keto has made all the difference in their anxiety. In the end, it really varies according to the individual, and it varies according to the severity of the anxiety, as well as allergens, digestive health, and a slew of other factors. I'm not saying this to overwhelm you or make you feel like there are just too many factors for you to be able to make a difference in your symptoms. What I want you to take from this is that you have the power to change your reality with simple switches here and there.

The keto diet can help alleviate anxiety for many, many reasons, but three in particular come to mind. First, it lowers inflammation in the nervous system, which allows us to better interact with our environment and feel mentally clear, sometimes for the first time in a long time. Second, because we're not using glucose as energy, our body has an abundance of a compound called GABA, which is used in the processing of glucose. GABA increases neuron signaling and reduces brain fog, so having more of it is great for the brain. And lastly, the decrease in sugar intake helps stabilize blood sugar, which leads to better brain functioning. Simple as that!

If you have anxiety, you may have noticed that you found it harder to give up sugar than others did. Perhaps you jumped on social media to explain just how strongly you crave the sweet stuff while on keto only to be told to "try harder." But there's a physiological reason for your sugar cravings. When you experience anxiety, your body looks for a quick shot of serotonin—the neurotransmitter responsible for feelings of well-being and happiness. Sugar can simulate that happy lift. However, sugar will only lead to a crash and can actually worsen anxiety symptoms over time.

This is why I believe carb-ups—which supply the body with longer-lasting carbohydrates, not the sugary stuff that's going to make serotonin spike and then crash—are a fabulous strategy if you have anxiety. It's important, however, to take care with the types of carb-up items you choose. Starchy vegetables are likely going to be better than high-sugar fruits, and if you choose fruits at all, berries and apples will probably be the best choice. Blood sugar regulation is of the utmost importance to you because it's so tightly linked to brain function.

Many women who are diagnosed with an anxiety disorder end up being prescribed a mood stabilizer to reduce intense and sustained mood shifts, to "level out." While this can help, and I'd never ever tell someone not to take medication that their doctor has deemed important, you can also adjust your diet and lifestyle to approach balancing from all angles. Interestingly, being in a state of ketosis changes the brain on a cellular level in ways that all effective mood stabilizers do.

A 2016 study gave rats a ketone supplement along with their high-carb diets. They found that the rats who were given the ketone supplement experienced a reduction in anxious behavior compared to the control group. This led the researchers to believe that nutritional ketosis could alleviate anxiety in humans as well.

Epilepsy

Before anticonvulsant medication came along, fasting was thought to be the magic bullet for preventing epileptic seizures, until researchers discovered that the reason fasting worked to reduce seizures was because it resulted in the production of ketone bodies. It was shortly after that they figured out that a diet high in fat and low in carbohydrates—the ketogenic diet—could replicate this metabolic effect without the need to fast for long periods of time.

It was found that the higher the fat percentage, the better the ketogenic diet could treat epilepsy. So for the diet to be most effective, patients were required to consume at least 90 percent of their calories from fat. Getting this much fat every day is a challenge and raises concerns that such a high fat intake limits the ability to consume enough protein to be healthful, especially for children.

So when anticonvulsant medication came along, the diet became less of a first-response treatment and more of a backup for when the medication does not work as effectively as needed.

A combination of medication and the ketogenic diet may be recommended for those with epilepsy—a balance of both worlds that I've heard is quite beneficial.

As the keto diet becomes more widespread and research into it advances, ketone-promoting approaches will continue to be developed. One such approach is the MCT diet, which focuses on medium-chain triglyceride intake and results in a boost in therapeutic ketones much greater than what long-chain triglycerides can provide. This goes a long way to reducing the overall fat intake required, which allows for a bit more protein in the diet. Also, I would imagine that the accessibility of exogenous ketone products makes adhering to this diet for epilepsy easier, and focusing a bit more on an increase in protein may go a long way, too.

Diet Adjustments

No matter what neurological concern you're dealing with, simply following a keto diet can be nourishing and supportive, especially when you consume very high amounts of fat. Meaning, when you're reading through the healing foods and lifestyle adjustments listed on the following pages, take note of the types of fats suggested and gravitate toward those! The more fats you consume, the better you may feel.

Wanna boost your brain function? Try intermittent fasting a couple of times a week (see page 138 for more).

Ultra-Healing Foods

THE EXTRAS

- Fresh and dried rosemary (leaves and ground)
- Fresh and dried sage
- Ground cinnamon
- Ground cumin
- Ground turmeric

STARCHES AND FRUITS

- Beets
- Blueberries
- Carrots
- Pomegranates
- Pumpkin
- Squash

PROTEIN

- Eggs
- Lamb
- Mackerel
- Organ meats
- Salmon
- Sardines
- Shellfish

NON-STARCHY VEGETABLES

- Asparagus
- Bok choy
- Broccoli
- Cabbage
- Cauliflower
- Collards
- Kale
- Spinach
- Tomatoes

HEALTHY FATS

- Almonds
- Avocados
- Coconut oil
- Flax seeds
- MCT oil
- Pecans
- Pumpkin seeds
- Sunflower seeds
- Walnuts

WATER

Additional Adjustments

Say Yes To

DIGESTIVE SUPPORT

The gut and brain are constantly communicating, and your chronic stress, depression, or anxiety could be tied to the health of your gastrointestinal system. Follow the tips and strategies starting on page 256 for overall gut support. (You can read more about the gut-brain connection on page 260.)

TESTING FOR NUTRIENT DEFICIENCIES

Many neurological issues can be exacerbated by improper nutrition and an imbalance in essential nutrients. Ask your doctor to test your levels of vitamin A, B, and D, calcium, magnesium, potassium, iron, and zinc. You can also request an omega-3 test.

NUTRIENT DENSITY

Choose to consume as many nutrient-dense foods as possible, opting for whole-food sources of fat—such as grass-fed beef, avocados, and salmon—whenever possible.

MOVING YOUR BODY

Any form of movement is great: walking, biking, hiking, HIIT, anything that makes you feel good. You may find that outdoor activities feel better. Alternatively, tai chi, an ancient form of Chinese exercise, is a low-impact activity that improves flexibility, balance, and muscle strength.

DAILY STRESS REDUCTION

Any form of stress, whether it is dietary, emotional, or physical, can aggravate your condition. Yoga, meditation, breathing exercises, qigong, and tai chi have all been scientifically proven to reduce stress and inflammation, thus calming the immune system. If none of these feel right to you, find a self-care practice that does—maybe an unhurried walk in nature, or a relaxing bath, or just sitting alone with your headphones on, listening to your favorite music.

DISCOVERING FOOD SENSITIVITIES & INTOLERANCES

When you eat a substance that you are sensitive to, it can affect your gut health, which in turn can affect your brain. Run through the steps on page 277 for determining which foods you may be sensitive to.

DETOXIFICATION AND COLON HYDROTHERAPY

Talk with your health-care provider about detoxification strategies, specifically to combat heavy metal toxicity, which can interfere with neurotransmitters. To aid in digestion and encourage a slow-moving colon to better remove toxins, look into colon hydrotherapy.

Say No To

ARTIFICIAL INGREDIENTS

Artificial colors, flavors, sweeteners (even if they say "keto"), preservatives such as BHA and BHT (commonly found in packaged and canned food), carrageenan, monosodium or monopotassium glutamate, any hydrolyzed, textured, or modified protein—they all affect brain function and increase the risk of neurological imbalances.

GRAINS & DAIRY

Reducing inflammation is the name of your game, so grains and dairy should always, always be off-limits. Grass-fed ghee and butter are okay.

STARCHY CARBS

Keep carbohydrates to a maximum of 50 grams total carbs a day. If practicing carb-ups is essential for your body, opt for non-starchy carbohydrates from fruit or squash.

REFINED OILS

Keep it clean with minimally processed oils. Avoid all vegetable oils and highly unstable polyunsaturated fats, which contribute to inflammation.

TOXINS

The neurological system reacts strongly to toxins by increasing inflammation and therefore decreasing function. It's important to seek out natural versions of anything that comes in contact with your body, such as body wash, lotions, makeup, shampoo, laundry detergent, and household cleaners. Ingredients to avoid include the following: avobenzone, benzophenone, formaldehyde, fragrance/perfume, homosalate, methoxycinnmate, PABA, parabens, propylene glycol, sodium laureth sulfate, sodium lauryl sulfate, synthetic colors, toluene, and triclosan. Dr. Bronner's is a great brand for castile soap, lotions, and toothpaste. Skindeep.org has recommendations for makeup and shampoo. White vinegar and baking soda are great household cleaners.

SWEETENERS, ALCOHOL, CAFFEINE & CIGARETTES

Any of these can cause further damage to your condition by disrupting sleep patterns, causing blood sugar imbalances, contributing to toxicity, or acting as a stimulant.

Supportive Supplements

- Vitamins: B, C, B$_3$
- Minerals: magnesium
- Essential oils: chamomile, lavender, lemon balm
- Others: exogenous ketones, CoQ10, melatonin, omega-3s

9

OVERCOMING IMBALANCES:
SUPPORTING HORMONES

Think of your hormones as messengers that carry information and instructions among your organs and cells, helping to keep your body balanced and functioning as well as it possibly can. These little messengers are secreted by glands in your endocrine system. Hormones help determine your:

- body temperature
- brain development
- digestion
- energy levels
- heart rate

- mood
- muscle growth
- sleep cycles
- weight

...and so much more.

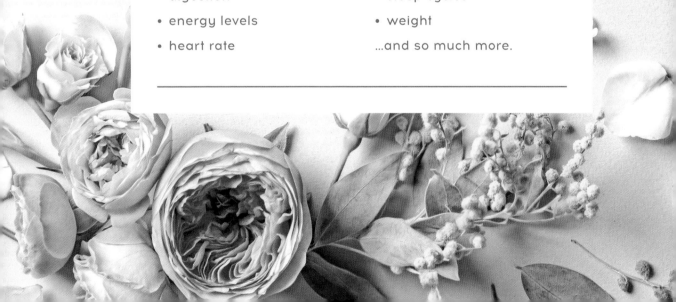

The building blocks that make up hormones are amino acids (read: proteins), fats, and cholesterol. So, no surprise, it's important to consume high-quality fats and proteins. What you eat is used to construct (among other things) hormones, and high-quality building blocks will help your body function optimally. Healthy fats also improve the absorption of vitamin D, a precursor for cholesterol. This is one reason the ketogenic diet is so effective in healing hormonal imbalances: it gives you lots of healthy fats and proteins to create optimally functioning hormones.

But on top of that, keto helps heal the hormonal imbalances that so often accompany a high-carb diet. We talked about this in chapter 3, but here's a quick refresher:

- On a high-carb diet, the adrenal glands secrete higher amounts of norepinephrine, adrenaline, and cortisol—all stress hormones with wide-ranging physiological effects.

- Because keto slows the carb-related excess production of stress hormones, the adrenal glands can focus on creating sex hormones instead, in the case of menopause, and play a more active role in the HPA axis, ending possible imbalances.

- The liver converts excess glucose into triglycerides. Excess triglycerides turn off the gene that produces sex hormone binding globulin, which carries sex hormones into the bloodstream; without it, too much estrogen and testosterone can enter cells. The end result? Dangerously high hormone levels.

- Fat cells produce and store estrogen, so the more body fat you have, the more estrogen you have. On keto, fat is used for energy, which may help balance estrogen levels.

Just following a keto diet is often enough to help us slide back to our hormonal happy place. Now, depending on your physiology, this process could take a couple of weeks, a couple of months, or even a couple of years. But you will get there, and you should be seeing positive changes in your hormones no more than nine months after starting keto.

But if you have specific symptoms or conditions that need addressing, there is more you can do to help support your hormones. That's what we'll look at in this chapter.

Your **Endocrine System**

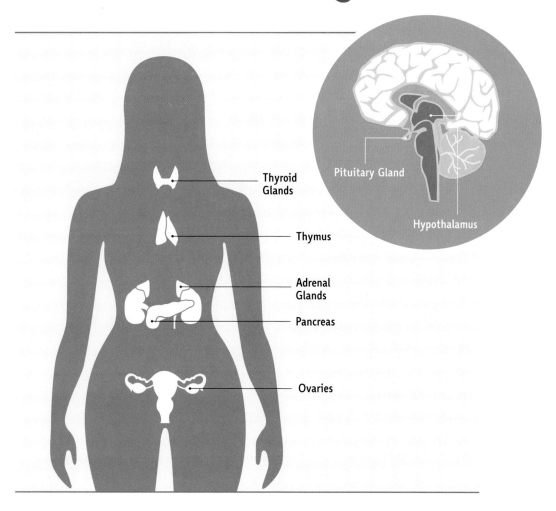

Pituitary Gland

Hypothalamus

Thyroid Glands

Thymus

Adrenal Glands

Pancreas

Ovaries

Before we dive into problems you may be experiencing with your hormones, let's look at an overview of what makes up the endocrine system and the roles hormones play in the body. You don't need to memorize any of this, but reading through this section will help you understand just how truly marvelous your body is, and how important each little hormone is to the big picture.

In Your Brain

Pituitary

This is the master gland of the endocrine system. It controls most of the other hormone-secreting glands.

Involved in:

Adrenal stimulation

Body composition

Menstrual cycle regulation

Metabolism

Milk production

Physical growth

Production of thyroid hormones

Skin and hair color

Things that can go wrong:

Anger

Depression

Difficulty sleeping

Eating disorders

Headaches

Hormone imbalances across the board

Infertility

Lactating when you shouldn't be

Mood swings

Type 2 diabetes

Weight gain

Hypothalamus

The hypothalamus's principal responsibility is to receive information about the internal and external environment—including body temperature, hunger, fullness, and stress—and tell the pituitary gland to start or stop making hormones in response.

Involved in:

Blood pressure maintenance

Memory and selective attention

Milk secretion during breastfeeding

Physical growth

Pituitary gland function

The pleasure response

Regulation of thyroid gland activity

Stress response (appetite suppression and anxiety)

Uterine contractions during childbirth

Water balance throughout the body

Things that can go wrong:

Amenorrhea

Insomnia

Irregular periods

Lack of energy

Thyroid dysregulation

Type 2 diabetes

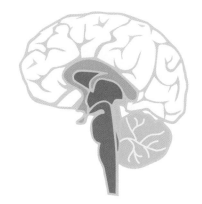

Pineal

The pineal gland is connected to your eyes' retinas, and in response to the amount of light, it signals the sleep center of the brain to regulate the sleep-wake cycle.

Involved in:	*Things that can go wrong:*
Adrenal health	Adrenal dysfunction
Healthy sleep patterns	Drowsiness
Mood regulation	Estrogen/progesterone imbalance
	Insomnia
	Mood swings
	Reduced core body temperature

In Your Neck

Thyroid

This butterfly-shaped organ releases hormones related to metabolism that affect breathing, heart rate, body weight, and more. It creates hormones from the iodine that you consume, so low iodine consumption can cause thyroid problems.

Involved in:

Brain development

Heart function

Maintenance of a balanced mood

Metabolic rate

Muscle control

Proper bone maintenance

Things that can go wrong:

Excess thyroid hormones
(hyperthyroidism):

    Diarrhea

    Racing heartbeat

    Unintentional weight loss

Low thyroid hormones (hypothyroidism):

    Constipation

    Slow heart rate

    Unintentional weight gain

Parathyroid

This is a set of four small glands behind your thyroid. They help control calcium
and phosphorus levels in the body, which are important for bone health.

Involved in:

Calcium regulation and production

Things that can go wrong:

Kidney stones

Muscle cramps and spasms

Osteoporosis

In Your Torso

Thymus

This gland, which is located close to the lungs, shrinks as you age and is slowly
replaced by fat by the time you're a teenager. It plays a pivotal role in protecting
the body against autoimmunity and has strong disease-fighting capabilities.

Involved in:

Immune system development

Things that can go wrong:

Autoimmunity

Cancer

Excess antibody production

Adrenals

The adrenal glands are located at the top of the kidneys. They're best known for their involvement in the stress response: they prepare the body to spring into action in a stressful situation. But there's more to these little glands than you may know—they also release hormones that are essential for survival.

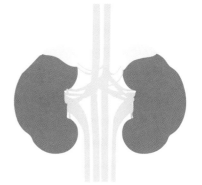

Involved in:

Bodily response to illness

Building muscle and bone

Creation of estrogen

Fight-or-flight response

Libido

Ligament strength

Maintaining balance of water and sodium, which stabilizes blood pressure

Menstrual cycle and fertility

Metabolism

Production of new blood cells

Stimulation of gluconeogenesis

Things that can go wrong:

Abdominal pain

High or low blood pressure

Low estrogen

Low libido

Muscle weakness

Nausea

Salt cravings

Pancreas

The pancreas is part of both the digestive and endocrine systems. On the digestive side, it makes enzymes that break down food. On the endocrine side, it creates hormones that keep blood sugar stable: insulin and glycogen. In people without insulin resistance or diabetes, glucagon is high when insulin is low, and vice versa.

Involved in:

Fat-burning processes

Gluconeogenesis

Glucose storage processes

Glycogen usage processes

Helping muscle cells effectively take up amino acids

Moving glucose from the bloodstream into cells

Things that can go wrong:

Diabetes

Insulin resistance

Hypoglycemia

Ovaries

The ovaries release eggs for fertilization and produce reproductive hormones. These hormones help breasts develop at puberty, regulate the menstrual cycle, and support pregnancy.

Involved in:

Blood clotting

Blood vessel health

Bone formation

Brain function

Inflammation reduction

Libido

Skin and hair health

Triglyceride balance

Things that can go wrong:

Decreased sex drive

Gallbladder problems

Miscarriage

Sex Hormones

From glowing skin to smooth digestion, painless periods, restful sleep, a wild sex life, and everything in between, balanced sex hormones make a world of difference in how you feel in your body. Sex hormones are steroids that are involved in the development and maintenance of your reproductive system, and the main ones are estrogen, progesterone, and testosterone.

While some spiking of estrogen is normal during your cycle, if it stays high, you could be experiencing estrogen dominance, in which estrogen isn't being properly recycled out of the body. It's considered "dominant" relative to progesterone levels—because estrogen and progesterone work closely together, it's imperative that they stay in balance with one another. Symptoms of estrogen dominance include painful menses, headaches, PMS, and irregular cycles. It can be caused by hormonal birth control or hormonal therapy, consuming foods stored in plastic, cycles with no ovulation, weight loss, or chronic stress.

Progesterone works to form the uterine lining and plays an important role in supporting and maintaining a pregnancy, should one occur. The progesterone level increases directly following ovulation to prepare the body for pregnancy and stay elevated until about five days before menstruation, when it begins to steadily decline if no egg has been fertilized.

Testosterone may be known as a male sex hormone, but it plays an important role in women's health: it's needed to maintain a healthy sex drive, energy level, and mood, and it contributes to overall bone health. Levels of testosterone are highest at ovulation and dip back down until a couple of days before menstruation, when it increases slightly.

SYMPTOMS OF SEX HORMONE IMBALANCE

As women, we often discount how important sex hormones are to our overall well-being. It's not normal to experience the following symptoms, and the cause could be imbalanced sex hormones.

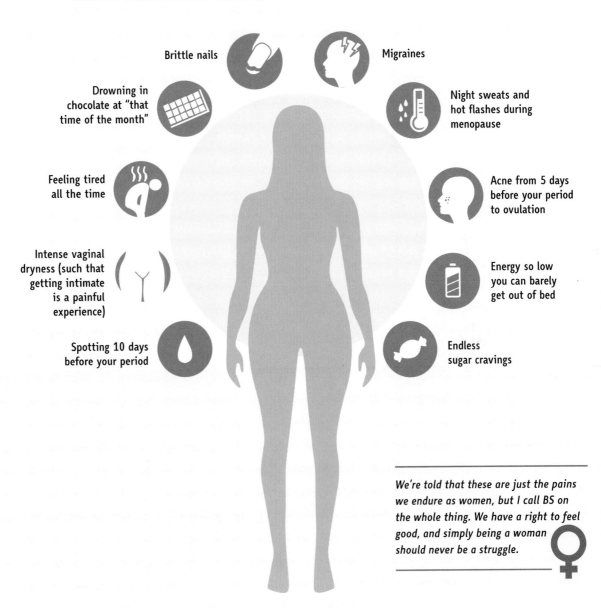

Brittle nails

Migraines

Drowning in chocolate at "that time of the month"

Night sweats and hot flashes during menopause

Feeling tired all the time

Acne from 5 days before your period to ovulation

Intense vaginal dryness (such that getting intimate is a painful experience)

Energy so low you can barely get out of bed

Spotting 10 days before your period

Endless sugar cravings

We're told that these are just the pains we endure as women, but I call BS on the whole thing. We have a right to feel good, and simply being a woman should never be a struggle.

DHEA

While not a sex hormone, DHEA is a hormone produced by the adrenals that influences overall sex hormone balance quite significantly. It's a powerful precursor to estrogen, progesterone, and testosterone, so it plays a key role in hormonal health. In fact, it's the cornerstone of a healthy endocrine system. It's created in the adrenal glands and is the most abundant circulating steroid hormone in the human body!

It is normal for DHEA levels to decline with age, but that's not without symptoms in some women. If your DHEA is low, supplementing with bioidentical DHEA can reduce signs of aging, improve bone density, ease depression, and improve libido. But if you use a supplement, make sure you get frequent DHEA tests so that you don't go overboard. It's all about finding the right level for your body.

THE MENSTRUAL CYCLE

A typical menstrual cycle is between twenty-four and thirty-five days long. The average is twenty-eight days.

Menstruation: Days 1 to 5

Day 1 is the first day of your period. The lining of the uterus, which has thickened in case it's needed to support a fertilized egg, is shed. Estrogen and progesterone both drop.

Follicular Phase: Days 1 to 13

This phase overlaps with menstruation. During this phase, an egg matures in an ovary and the uterine lining again begins to thicken. Estrogen and testosterone both rise.

Luteal Phase: Days 15 to 28

Estrogen and testosterone gradually decline, though estrogen rises again in the second half of this phase. Progesterone rises and the uterine lining continues to thicken.

Ovulation: Day 14

The ovary releases a mature egg. Estrogen and testosterone peak around this time.

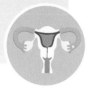

The 8 Most Common Imbalances and Testing Solutions

Of all the hormones active in the endocrine system, these are the top eight that I see women struggle with the most: insulin, leptin, cortisol, DHEA, thyroid, estrogen, progesterone, and testosterone. Further on in the chapter, I'll show you how to balance them using the ketogenic diet, but first you need to understand how to test yourself based on the symptoms you may be experiencing.

	INSULIN		LEPTIN
DESCRIPTION OF IMBALANCE	With insulin resistance, the body produces insulin but is unable to use it properly, so more insulin has to be produced to do the same job. High levels of insulin cause the body to store more fat and makes weight loss a challenge.		Leptin resistance occurs when the body can't use leptin properly. Since leptin triggers fat-burning and tells your brain that you're full, leptin resistance causes a starvation signal to set in and initiates fat storage.
SIGNS OF IMBALANCE	Cravings for sweets that aren't relieved by eating sweets Irritability if meals are missed Dependence on coffee Light-headedness if meals are missed Feeling shaky or jittery, or having tremors Feeling agitated, easily upset, or nervous Poor memory Blurred vision	Fatigue after meals Waist girth that is equal to or larger than hip girth Frequent urination Increased thirst and appetite Difficulty losing weight Weight gain Tiredness after a meal Sleep disturbances Difficulty focusing	Weight gain Difficulty losing weight Constant food cravings Hunger after eating High levels of insulin
TESTS	Serum insulin C-peptide Fasting insulin	Fasting glucose Hemoglobin A1C Triglycerides	Serum leptin
INITIAL SOLUTIONS	Balance your blood sugar Move your body Improve your sleep (page 172) Manage stress (page 165) Check for food sensitivities (page 274) Eliminate alcohol Eliminate refined oils	Supplement with: • Minerals: chromium, magnesium, and zinc • Vitamins: C, B$_6$, E • Herbs: gymnema, cinnamon, berberine • Amino acids: alpha lipoic acid	Eat keto! It will take some time for keto to balance your leptin levels, but be patient, it will happen. If you're practicing carb-ups, stay away from high-sugar foods and opt for starchy vegetables and low-sugar fruits.

	CORTISOL		DHEA	THYROID	
DESCRIPTION OF IMBALANCE	The most common cause of cortisol imbalance is adrenal dysfunction, where cortisol is either too high or too low for certain times of day. This occurs because of a breakdown in communication between the brain and the adrenals and is often caused by stress—it's usually not a physical problem with the adrenal glands themselves.		DHEA is a powerful precursor to estrogen, progesterone, and testosterone. It is normal for DHEA levels to decline with age, but that's not without symptoms in some women.	Every cell in your body requires thyroid hormones to function properly. Some thyroid imbalances don't show up on standard tests, such as problems converting one type of thyroid hormone to another, thyroid resistance (the body doesn't use thyroid hormones properly), or autoimmune attacks against the thyroid gland itself.	
SIGNS OF IMBALANCE	Body aches Difficulty getting started in the morning Salt cravings Sugar cravings Low sex drive Fatigued in the afternoon with a second wind in the evening Low blood pressure Light-headedness Difficulty staying asleep	Body hair loss Dizziness when standing up quickly Afternoon headaches Blood sugar issues Chronic inflammation Weak nails Moodiness Difficulty losing weight	**LOW LEVEL:** Feeling overwhelmed Depression Low levels of estrogen, progesterone, and testosterone Extreme fatigue Decrease in muscle mass Decrease in bone density Aching joints Loss of libido Lowered immunity **HIGH LEVEL:** Acne High levels of testosterone, estrogen, or progesterone PCOS	**LOW LEVEL:** Feeling cold in your hands, feet, or all over Requiring excessive amounts of sleep to function properly Weight gain, even with a low-calorie diet Difficult, infrequent bowel movements Depression or lack of motivation Morning headaches that wear off as the day progresses Outer third of eyebrow is thin Thinning of hair on scalp Dry skin Mental sluggishness Thinning hair or hair loss Difficulty losing weight Constipation Fatigue Dry skin **HIGH LEVEL:** Nervousness Anxiety Mood swings Sensitivity to heat Difficulty sleeping	
TESTS	Serum cortisol Serum DHEA-S Salivary cortisol Salivary DHEA-S		Serum DHEA-S Salivary DHEA-S	TSH Total T4 Free T4 Total T3 Free T3 Reverse T3 T3 uptake Thyroid antibodies	
INITIAL SOLUTIONS	Remove excess stress triggers in your life. This will take time, years even, but every bit of stress you remove from your life will do wonders to your ability to stay healthy. Additionally, follow the steps starting on page 381.		Follow the adrenal support steps on page 381 Find joy in your life. Connect with family and friends, join a class or group of people that share an interest with you. Move your body in a way that feels good and makes you happy. For low DHEA, consider supplementing with bioidentical DHEA to jump-start hormone balance, reduce signs of aging, improve bone density, ease depression, and improve libido.	Follow the thyroid support instructions starting on page 367.	

ESTROGEN	PROGESTERONE	TESTOSTERONE
Estrogen levels rise and fall naturally during our monthly cycles, but during perimenopause, they start to fluctuate and become unpredictable. Eventually, estrogen production falls to a very low level as the ovaries stop producing it and the adrenals take over, making adrenal health of the utmost importance.	The ovaries stop producing progesterone after the final menstrual period and the adrenals take over, producing it in smaller but sufficient quantities. If progesterone is low, estrogen becomes harmful and out of control, a condition referred to as estrogen dominance.	Testosterone may be known as a male sex hormone, but it plays an important role in women's health. If testosterone is high, you may have PCOS (page 357), which may lead to high cholesterol, insulin resistance, or high blood pressure. If testosterone is low, you may experience a reduction in libido, excess fatigue, or bone loss.

ESTROGEN

LOW LEVEL:

Vaginal dryness
Night sweats
Painful sex
Brain fog
Recurrent bladder infections
Feeling lethargic
Depression
Hot flashes

HIGH LEVEL:

Feeling puffy and bloated	Cervical dysplasia (abnormal pap smear)
Rapid weight gain	
Breast tenderness	Insomnia
Mood swings	Brain fog
Heavy menstrual bleeding	Gallbladder problems
Feeling anxious and/or depressed	Feeling weepy and emotional
Migraine headaches	

PROGESTERONE

LOW LEVEL:

PMS
Insomnia
Unhealthy-looking skin
Breast pain
Stubborn weight gain
Cyclical headaches
Anxiety
Infertility

TESTOSTERONE

LOW LEVEL:

Weight gain	Depression
Fatigue	Irritability
Low sex drive	Weight gain
Indecisiveness	Thinning hair
Feelings of low self-worth	

HIGH LEVEL:

Acne	Thinning hair
Polycystic ovary syndrome (PCOS)	Infertility
	Ovarian cysts
Excessive hair on the face and arms	Midcycle pain/cramping
Hypoglycemia and/or unstable blood sugar	

ESTROGEN	PROGESTERONE	TESTOSTERONE
A full blood and salivary female hormone panel, including all estrogen isomers	A full blood and salivary female hormone panel	Blood and saliva testosterone and DHEA panel DHEA-S

ESTROGEN

LOW LEVEL:

Aim for calm movement like yoga or walking.

Increase your body fat: work out less, eat more, and sleep more.

HIGH LEVEL:

Supplement with DIM, which helps upregulate the liver's ability to break down estrogens. Eating broccoli and cauliflower is also helpful.

Support your gut health. More about estrogen and the gut on page 261.

Decrease your body fat by following the steps starting on page 151.

Avoid phytoestrogens, which bind to estrogen receptors. These are found in foods including sesame seeds, greens, licorice root, and alfalfa.

Supplement with vitamin E. You'll want to get a soy-free option with a clear base.

PROGESTERONE

LOW LEVEL:

Seek out vitamin C and vitamin B_6. Loading up on walnuts, red meat, poultry, seafood, spinach, and potatoes during your carb-ups should do the trick.

For increased fertility, seek out zinc. Pumpkin seeds and sunflower seeds are your best bet.

Eat more turmeric. Get a high-quality, organic ground turmeric and add it to sautéed vegetables and grass-fed meats. You can also shave the fresh root over salads and stir-fries, or juice it and add it to smoothies, full-fat coconut milk, or avocado.

HIGH LEVEL:

Move your body.

Support estrogen, which balances progesterone, by following the tips in the column at left.

TESTOSTERONE

LOW LEVEL:

Seek out zinc. Reach for pumpkin seeds and sunflower seeds.

Lift weights. Deadlifts, lunges, step-ups, squats, and Olympic-style lifting are best. Twice a week is generally enough. Sprinting can be beneficial as well.

Light from the sun promotes vitamin D creation, which prevents testosterone from being converted into estrogen. Get bright light in the morning.

Meditation has been shown to increase testosterone levels and lower cortisol levels.

HIGH LEVEL:

Supplement with DIM. Eating broccoli and cauliflower is also helpful.

Drink spearmint tea. Spearmint suppresses testosterone production and acts as an anti-androgen.

Your doctor may be open to running basic labs for your hormone health, but if your results are not in the normal range, you'll likely be prescribed a synthetic hormone medication that could have side effects (more about hormone replacement therapy on page 347). On the flip side, if your results are within the normal range but you know something's wrong, you may be told that your symptoms are part of aging, or you may be told to take an antidepressant or try losing some weight to get things back on track. For the record, I believe there are some other tools you can use to get your life back—we'll talk about them in the rest of this chapter.

Reasons for Hormonal Imbalances

While there are many reasons why hormones can become imbalanced, here are some of the top ones.

Nutritional deficiencies. Nutrients such as magnesium, vitamin C, vitamin A, and B vitamins are important hormone ingredients needed to create a healthy hormone profile. Nutrients also play a critical role in how and when the body excretes hormones, and how the body uses them!

Stress. When we experience stress, cortisol floods our body. If stress becomes chronic, the body has to steal hormones responsible for making progesterone to make more cortisol (a process called "pregnenolone steal"), which renders the body incapable of creating progesterone. Without enough progesterone, estrogen is able to run rampant, which can lead to estrogen dominance. And when the stealing occurs for a long period of time, bones, muscles, strength, energy, libido, and immunity are all seriously affected.

Excess carbohydrates. If we are consuming carbohydrates beyond what our body can process, we can develop insulin resistance—our cells no longer respond easily to insulin's message, and the pancreas has to secrete more and more insulin to keep moving glucose into cells. That leads to weight gain and excess estrogen (to the point of estrogen dominance), and, over time, could lead to an increased risk of cancer and type 2 diabetes.

Xenoestrogens. Many man-made toxins mimic estrogen and accumulate in body fat, wreaking havoc on the balancing mechanisms of the body and raising overall estrogen levels, leading to estrogen dominance.

Lack of high-quality dietary fat and protein. Amino acids, fats, and cholesterol are the building blocks of every hormone. So in order to help your body create the healthiest hormones and efficiently regulate them, you need to eat the best fats and proteins, in sufficient quantities.

Additional contributors to hormone imbalance:

- Chronic inflammation (page 251)

- Conventional dairy products (page 99)

- Dietary stress (page 164)

- Excess alcohol

- Excess caffeine

- Exercising too much (page 162)

- Hormonal birth control (page 339)

- Improper sleep (page 168)

- Lack of physical movement

- Not eating enough (page 34)

- Unfiltered water (page 338)

- Unhealthy digestion (page 256)

- Very low cholesterol levels (page 56)

If you're experiencing symptoms of a hormonal imbalance, you may find that a keto diet alone is enough to balance your system after a month or two. But there are also some adjustments you can make, both to your diet and your lifestyle, to get your hormones on your side once and for all.

How to Support Overall Hormone Health

Say Yes To

FIBER
If you feel constipated, get fiber from nuts, seeds, and non-starchy veggies. On top of that, drink plenty of water to keep things moving.

MAINTAINING ALKALINITY
Remember from chapter 3 that on the alkaline-acid scale, the human body tends to be alkaline, and when it becomes more acidic, it can cause several health problems. Maintaining alkalinity improves your bone density, lowers inflammation, helps with vitamin absorption, and helps you maintain a healthy weight. Test your pH level with a urine-testing kit—it should be between 7.0 and 7.5. If your pH is too acidic, try getting more of these keto-friendly foods:

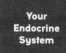
Avocados	Ginger	Mushrooms
Broccoli	Green beans	Oregano
Cabbage	Jicama	Spinach
Celery	Kale	Tomatoes
Cucumber	Lemon juice or apple cider vinegar (mixed in water)	
Garlic		

FERMENTED FOODS

We touched on the importance of gut health in decreasing estrogen on page 260. Well, fermented foods help to rebalance gut bacteria, naturally. My favorites are water kefir and sauerkraut because they're safe to make at home. If you have a severe imbalance, you may also benefit from taking probiotics.

LEGS UP THE WALL

While a regular yoga practice—whether you go to a class or simply stretch at home—can improve numerous aspects of health, there's one particular yoga pose that has a profound ability to balance hormones naturally. It's called "Legs Up the Wall," for good reason: you just lie on your back, lift your legs at the hips, and rest them against a wall. It's suitable for every body type and fitness level.

This pose maximizes lymphatic circulation in the lower body, and lymph moves more progesterone around the body than any other hormone, so making sure that the lymphatic system is flowing well is integral to the health of the endocrine system. By reversing the flow of gravity in your legs with this yoga pose, you help the lymph circulate—and you also encourage the elimination of toxins, which is important for balanced hormones and overall health.

GELATIN

When muscle meat is consumed on its own without the presence of gelatin, the amino acid profile resembles what the body releases in times of extreme stress, when excess cortisol breaks down muscle to provide energy and materials for cell repair. And when this muscle breakdown occurs, tryptophan and excess cysteine flood the body, which suppresses thyroid function. The consumption of a large amount of muscle meat on its own has the same effect.

By helping to balance the tryptophan, gelatin supports healthy thyroid function and adequate thyroid hormones. And our thyroid hormones work synergistically with all other hormones in our body—by supporting our thyroid, we support balanced hormones overall. If you eat a large serving of meat, it's helpful to also have 5 to 10 grams of gelatin at the same time so that the amino acids enter the bloodstream in balance. This can mean enjoying your meat-heavy meals with bone broth, consuming more soups and stews, or simply adding some gelatin powder to a hot liquid such as tea and having it during your meal.

LIVER

Gram for gram, liver is the most nutrient-dense food on the planet, and its unique nutritional profile makes it the ideal superfood for balancing hormones. Most importantly, liver is an excellent source of vitamin A, which improves thyroid function as well as liver health, so we can synthesize and detox hormones optimally.

Contrary to popular belief, we can't get vitamin A from vegetables, and that includes carrots and sweet potatoes. The beta-carotene in veggies must first be converted to vitamin A in the body, and this conversion rate is so poor that it's virtually insignificant—we can eat a ton of beta-carotene and only get a small amount of usable vitamin A. And if you have a hormonal imbalance, it further compromises your ability to convert beta-carotene into vitamin A.

EGG YOLKS

Don't just eat the whites—egg yolks help balance hormones by providing all of the following nutrients:

- **Vitamin A** improves thyroid function and liver health, and you can't get it from vegetables. Egg yolks provide *real* vitamin A!

- **Vitamin D** actually works more like a steroid hormone in the body, so it's vital to get enough of this fat-soluble vitamin.

- **Selenium** is necessary to convert thyroid hormones from the inactive form to the active form, and about 60 percent of an egg's selenium is found in the yolk.

- **Cholesterol** is needed to create sex hormones.

GETTING OUT IN THE SUN

Boosting your intake of vitamin D helps optimize hormones and thousands of other processes in your body. Get ten to thirty minutes in the sunshine without sunblock to increase your level of vitamin D. You may need more or less time required depending on your skin color (the darker your skin, the more time you need in the sun) and location (the closer you are to the equator, the less time needed). Just be careful not to burn!

MAINTAINING A POSITIVE ATTITUDE

If things are bringing you down, try your best to reframe or phase them out of your life. When you're with your friends, dog, significant other, or by yourself, try to have *fun*! Play like you're a kid. Get messy, laugh, get chocolate all over your face—you get the idea.

DAILY STRESS REDUCTION

Try to get seven to nine hours of sleep at night, get moving with moderate exercise, and spend time with people who make you happy. Yoga, meditation, breathing exercises, qigong, and tai chi have all been scientifically proven to reduce stress. If none of these feel right to you, find a self-care practice that does—maybe an unhurried walk in nature, or a relaxing bath, or just sitting alone with your headphones on, listening to your favorite music.

HIGH-QUALITY FOODS

Stick to organic produce where possible to avoid the xenoestrogens present in pesticides. For animal proteins, go for pasture-raised pork, grass-fed beef, and free-range chicken so you know the animal wasn't treated with hormones. If those are inaccessible, opt for the leanest cuts and add your own oils to the proteins.

Say No To

SYNTHETIC ESTROGENS (XENOESTROGENS)

Synthetic estrogens are found in many widely used products and can cause fertility problems and vaginal and breast cancers, not to mention throw your hormones out of whack. Use only glass containers for heating and storing food, avoid using plastic wrap, avoid the consumption of food or drinks from a can, and carry a reusable water bottle and refill it as needed. Below are sources of synthetic estrogens that can contribute to estrogen dominance and throw off the balance between estrogen and progesterone throughout your body:

- Produce that has been sprayed with pesticides, herbicides, and insecticides. Organic is best.

- Bleached paper, including coffee filters, tissue paper, and napkins. Unbleached is best.

- Chlorine-containing bleach. Use disposable gloves and open all the windows— but cleaning with vinegar and water is best.

- Tampons and pads. Menstrual cups, such as those from Peach Life, and unbleached pads are best.

- Nail polish and polish remover

- Unfiltered water. Reverse-osmosis water is best.

- Dryer sheets. Dryer balls work just as well without the estrogen effect!

BLUE LIGHT EXPOSURE

To block stimulating blue light after the sun sets, avoid watching TV, keep your house lights to a minimum, and install an app like f.lux on your computer and cell phone. If, for any reason, you're unable to follow these suggestions, you can always wear blue-light-blocking glasses.

NEGATIVITY

Avoid people who don't make you feel good, situations that weigh you down, and toxic conversations that don't serve your best interests. Instead, surround yourself with uplifting activities, connected conversations, and playfulness.

PROCESSED OILS

Keep it clean with minimally processed oils. Avoid all vegetable oils and highly unstable polyunsaturated fats (more on this on page 98). Vegetable oils are extremely high in omega-6, a pro-inflammation fatty acid. While a little omega-6 in our diet is necessary, too much wreaks havoc on hormones by creating widespread inflammation.

HORMONAL BIRTH CONTROL

Hormonal birth control (including hormonal IUDs, the pill, the Depo-Provera shot, and others) is definitely one area teeming with confusing information. Pharmaceutical companies perpetuate the common misconception that hormonal birth control is not that big of a deal, but that is simply not the truth.

Hormonal birth control works by suppressing your natural hormones so that ovulation cannot occur. But the problem may not be the suppression of your hormones, per se, so much as what is being used to suppress them: synthetic hormones that your body doesn't recognize, as it would bioidentical hormones. These synthetic hormones can create multiple nutrient deficiencies that stand in the way of proper hormone production, including deficiencies in magnesium, zinc, vitamin B_6, vitamin B_{12}, folic acid, and vitamin C.

Personally, I got off hormonal birth control because I wanted a natural period. On hormonal birth control, the uterine lining doesn't thicken, so there's nothing to shed during a period. Instead, the period you get on hormonal birth control is known as withdrawal bleeding, because your body responds to the absence of the artificial hormones it's getting the rest of the month by bleeding somewhat. I wanted to have an actual cycle, to get in touch with my hormones during my cycle, to create my own progesterone, and to ovulate.

But even if that's not a concern for you, hormonal birth control comes with some fairly significant potential side effects. First, there's the increased cancer risk: high-dose, moderate-dose, and triphasic birth control pills, as well as pills containing ethynodiol diacetate, may increase cancer risk. Women with a family history of breast cancer may have a higher risk of breast cancer while on birth control. (On the flip side, while research seems to implicate synthetic birth control for increasing the risk of cervical cancer, there's a decreased risk of ovarian and endometrial cancer. Research on breast cancer overall is mixed and inconclusive.)

The number one side effect of hormonal birth control is headaches and migraines. Other common side effects include nausea, breast tenderness, bloating, mood changes, irregular cycles or no cycles at all, insulin resistance, elevated triglycerides and LDL cholesterol on blood tests, and increased risk for blood clots

- Cycle-tracking apps like Life or MyFlo. When you input your cycle data into apps like these, you will have a 99% efficacy rate in preventing pregnancy. This is the same rate offered by taking a birth control pill! This is the technique I use as our form of birth control.

- Vasectomy or tubal ligation for couples who do not want to conceive in the future

- Condoms and diaphragms are cumbersome but decent options for protection

- Copper IUD, which can be inserted for up to 10 years. It may cause heavier menstrual periods for some women but is a great option for many.

and some autoimmune diseases. Synthetic hormones have also been implicated in the research time and time again as being potential carcinogens.

SOY

Soy milk, soy meat, soy protein, soy-based cereal—all these foods, which are often touted as healthy, wreak havoc on the body. Soy disrupts hormones because it looks like estrogen to the body and therefore causes an imbalance in the estrogen-to-progesterone ratio. Soy also may cause inflammation and leaky gut by inhibiting the protein-digesting enzyme trypsin, and most soy has been genetically modified. The detrimental effects are reduced in fermented soy, such as miso and tempeh, but I believe these should only be eaten in strict moderation. If you're currently trying to balance hormones, I strongly recommend avoiding even fermented soy.

Regulating Your **Cycle** & **Sex Hormones**

If you're experiencing a monthly menstrual cycle, or you're at an age where a monthly cycle is expected, having a regular monthly cycle is key to having balanced hormones. There are ways that you can help regulate your cycle to match its natural rhythms, without hormonal birth control or other artificial means.

If you do not have a period (a condition called amenorrhea—we'll talk more about that on page 349), this information applies to you as well. Your body may still go through the hormonal ebb and flow, but that ebb and flow is not strong enough to produce menstruation. If you're unsure where you are in your cycle, assume that the new moon is day 1 of your cycle and the full moon is day 14 of your cycle.

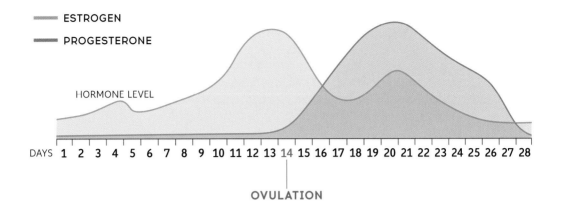

ESTROGEN

PROGESTERONE

HORMONE LEVEL

DAYS 1 2 3 4 5 6 7 8 9 10 11 12 13 14 15 16 17 18 19 20 21 22 23 24 25 26 27 28

OVULATION

Estrogen matures an egg before ovulation. This is why you see an estrogen increase just before ovulation. Additionally, it matures the uterine lining that is shed when a period takes place, which is why the level increases again in the luteal phase.

Signs of excess estrogen: Bloating, decreased sex drive, mood swings, headaches, acne, PMS

Signs of decreased estrogen: Painful intercourse, depression, hot flashes, mood swings, irregular periods, increased instances of UTIs

Progesterone works to balance out the effects of estrogen during the maturation of the uterine lining in the luteal phase. This is why it increases during the estrogen increase.

Signs of excess progesterone: Bloating, decreased sex drive, swelling and tenderness of the breasts in the luteal phase

Signs of decreased progesterone: Low sex drive, thyroid dysfunction (primarily hypothyroidism), weight gain, irregular menstrual cycle

Recognizing Phases of Your Cycle

How do you know what phase of your cycle you're on? You can track your cycle with apps such as MyFlo (Android) or Life (iOS). Your body gives you clues about where you are in your cycle, such as vaginal discharge, body temperature, and cervix position. If you record these factors, you will have a guide to predict when you are ovulating (the days when you can become pregnant) and when you can expect your period.

TRUTH BOMB

Your blood sugar may go up and down during your period. Having unusual blood glucose readings, both highs and lows, is completely normal due to the massive fluctuation in hormones during this time. Don't worry too much about it!

Adjusting Macros

With just a slight tweak to your macro ratio, you can support the healthy, natural ebb and flow of the two main hormones responsible for the menstrual cycle: estrogen and progesterone. A typical menstrual cycle is between twenty-four and thirty-five days long. The following outline assumes that your period lasts for five days, you ovulate on the fourteenth day of your cycle, and your full menstrual cycle is twenty-eight days. If your body is different, you will need to adjust the following to suit your pattern.

Follicular Phase

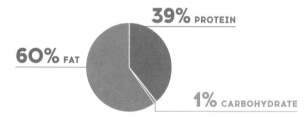

Days 1 to 5
Day 1 is the first day of your period. During your period, your body may respond best to a higher protein intake.

Days 6 to 11
The first day after your period until three days before ovulation. This is when women are most responsive to the ketogenic diet, able to eat very low-carb or no-carb with boundless energy.

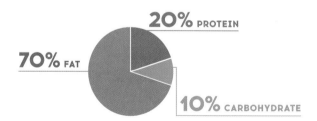

Days 12 to 16*
Two days before ovulation through ovulation to two days after ovulation. Your body is still responding well to eating low-carb during this phase, but you could benefit from a boost in glutathione, an antioxidant, in the evening. Food sources of glutathione include apples, avocados, broccoli, garlic, grapefruit, oranges, parsley, and tomatoes. You could also benefit from increasing your carbohydrate intake after about 5 p.m. Do this each evening during these cycle days, preferably with fruit.

Luteal Phase

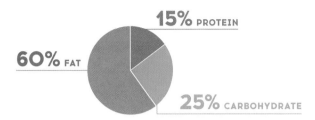

60% FAT

15% PROTEIN

25% CARBOHYDRATE

Days 17 to 28*

The third day following ovulation through the day before you get your period. Your body is likely beginning to crave carbohydrates as you approach the end of your cycle. You could benefit from increasing your carbohydrate intake after about 5 p.m. Do this each evening during these cycle days, preferably with starchy vegetables like cassava, potatoes, sweet potatoes, and plantains.

*Don't worry too much about staying in ketosis. The extra carbohydrates you'll consume are so minimal that you'll be back to burning fat in the morning and feel much better throughout the remaining days of your cycle.

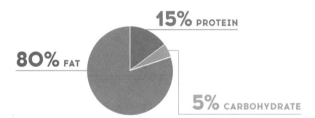

80% FAT

15% PROTEIN

5% CARBOHYDRATE

Menopause

Best for women who are experiencing menopause or have transitioned to postmenopause (for more details, see page 359).

Seed Cycling

Seed cycling is the use of seeds and seed oils to regulate the menstrual cycle. It works because seeds and their oils provide lignans, phytoestrogens, and omega oils, which help balance and support estrogen and progesterone levels.

Start seed cycling on day 1 of your period and continue cycling for at least 3 months. Whenever possible, purchase whole seeds and grind them at home in a coffee grinder, spice grinder, blender, or food processor. Store ground seeds in an airtight container in the fridge. Ground seeds can be added to salads, smoothies, fat bombs, or any other no-bake recipe.

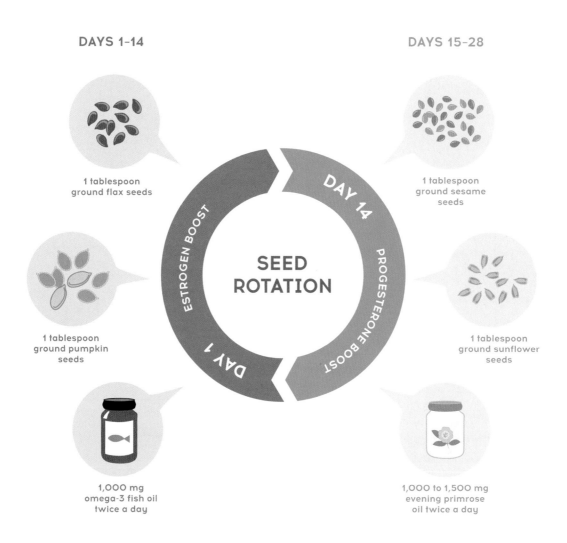

DAYS 1–14

DAYS 15–28

SEED
ROTATION

ESTROGEN BOOST

DAY 14

PROGESTERONE BOOST

DAY 1

1 tablespoon
ground flax seeds

1 tablespoon
ground sesame
seeds

1 tablespoon
ground pumpkin
seeds

1 tablespoon
ground sunflower
seeds

1,000 mg
omega-3 fish oil
twice a day

1,000 to 1,500 mg
evening primrose
oil twice a day

Restoring Your Cycle with Light

When the moon's phases and the menstrual cycle align, it's called "lunaception." Women's menstrual cycles are wired to be in sync with the moon, with ovulation at the full moon and menstruation at the new moon. (This timing is reversed in women who are thought to be more creative—artists and writers, for instance—or are considered healers, like doctors and therapists: they ovulate at the new moon and menstruate at the full moon.)

Just as the ocean is influenced by the moon, so are our bodies. And while science isn't able to pinpoint the cause, when hormones align with the moon's phases, it's a good sign of hormonal balance. But due to hormonal disruption brought on by industrialism (including blue light, processed foods, toxins, and more), this intrinsic hormonal setting is lost to many of us.

The Connection Between Light, Melatonin, and Hormones

We talked earlier in this chapter about the many potential causes of hormonal imbalance. Any of these can alter our cycles so that we're no longer aligned with the moon's cycles—or even have regular cycles of our own.

One factor we haven't discussed in depth, however, is artificial light. It's widely known that blue light (from laptops, phones, TVs, light bulbs, and more) wreaks havoc on our sleep cycles because it has a disastrous effect on melatonin, which helps us fall asleep.

Women's bodies in particular are so sensitive to light patterns that we can manipulate hormones by controlling our nightly light exposure. This is because melatonin also helps control the hormones that regulate our periods. The hypothalamus, which regulates things like blood pressure, emotions, body temperature, and other parts of the endocrine system, is richly supplied with melatonin receptors, and if it doesn't receive sufficient melatonin, its ability to regulate the hormonal system is impaired.

How to Regulate Your Cycles with Light

Achieving lunaception is one of the easiest ways to create regular periods and balance melatonin production, which are two very powerful elements of balanced hormones. Just changing your nighttime lighting the way the moon changes—from complete darkness to a few nights with dim light to darkness again—can help your cycles become more regular. As a result, you'll notice more energy, easier weight management, and fewer PMS symptoms.

If any of the following apply to you, you could benefit from this practice:

- Hormone dysregulation of any kind

- Infertility issues

- Irregular cycles

- Painful menstruation

- Past or current use of hormonal birth control

- PCOS diagnosis

- Skipped periods

The easiest and most natural way to achieve lunaception is to sleep with your curtains open every night to allow your body to sync with the amount of moonlight that enters your bedroom. Now, this approach only works if you live in a place with zero light pollution (read: in the forest).

If you don't have access to moon-only light because of light pollution, where your bedroom is situated, or the shift you are assigned at work, you can use indoor lighting to help align your cycle to the moon (instead of having to live in the woods, four hours away from civilization, or on the ocean, like me).

Here are the steps you can use if simply using moon lighting isn't possible for you:

1. You will need a *very* dark bedroom. Tack down the edges of blackout curtains, put garbage bags over the window, use a towel to cover the crack under your bedroom door—do whatever you need to do to keep all light out. Be sure to test it. If you turn off all the lights at night and aren't able to see your hand in front of your face, move on to step 2.

2. Place a night light with a red light bulb in the hallway if you have frequent bathroom visits at night. The red light—just like firelight—will not trigger early ovulation.

3. If you are not getting a regular period, sleep in complete darkness for one to two months to help reset your body. This is optional, but if your hormones are very imbalanced, it can be an essential step. If your periods are regular and you're quite confident of when you ovulate, sleep in complete darkness until step 4 applies to you.

4. Starting on day 14 of your cycle, the day of ovulation (or, if you're not sure what day you're on in your cycle because you're not getting a consistent period, when the calendar says it's the day before the full moon), sleep with a dim light on in your room for three nights. You can use a night light, leave on a hallway light and keep your door open, or sleep with the blinds open. After three nights, go back to sleeping in complete darkness for the rest of your cycle.

5. Repeat step 4 every month at the same time, forever.

Hormone Replacement Therapy

As a woman who is unable to produce enough DHEA, progesterone, and thyroid hormone to function at her peak performance, I truly appreciate hormone replacement therapy for those who have tried everything to boost their hormones but just can't seem to get them high enough to reap the benefits of healthy hormones. Sometimes the body just needs a little nudge, and when you supplement for a while, the body gets what it needs and can heal itself enough that long-term supplementation isn't necessary.

I've been on both hormone replacement therapy (HRT) and bioidentical hormone replacement therapy (BHRT) in an attempt to rectify my imbalances. And I far prefer BHRT to HRT.

All supplemental hormones are "natural," but not all hormones are bioidentical. Bioidentical hormones are identical to the hormones made by the human body, down to their molecular shape, makeup, and structure. For real, you wouldn't be able to tell the difference between the "real thing" and bioidentical hormones if you stacked them up side by side.

According to medical studies, BHRT has no side effects and can contribute to a reduction in heart attack, stroke, various cancers, diabetes, tooth loss, and cataracts. There's also some evidence that it can help improve skin's thickness, hydration, and elasticity, and even reduce wrinkles. For those with cancer who have undergone treatments that affect estrogen levels, BHRT has been shown to be effective in improving general well-being and quality of life. In one study, people with cancer who underwent BHRT found relief from treatment-related symptoms such as migraines, incontinence, low libido, and insomnia. The study also found their recurrence rate of breast cancer was no higher than average.

If you aren't sure what sort of hormone you've been prescribed, ask your pharmacist for the ingredients. If what you're taking lists esterified estrogens, progestins, or progestogens, the product is not bioidentical.

Bioidentical hormones come in all sorts of delivery systems, from creams and injections to patches, pills, and gels. I prefer creams, vaginal gels, or patches so the hormone can go right into the bloodstream without having to be metabolized by the liver first. This allows for a lower dose of the hormone than pills, where higher doses are prescribed to get the same effect.

Find a doctor familiar with bioidentical preparations who can prescribe a bioidentical prescription based on your lab results and individual needs. They'll likely recommend you to a compounding pharmacy, a pharmacy that specializes in bioidentical hormones and can create a prescription tailored to the individual. While traditional pharmacies may have a small selection of bioidenticals, I've been hard-pressed to find one that can do all of them—DHEA, progesterone, testosterone, thyroid, estrogen, etc.—in one go. The bioidentical hormones used by compounding pharmacies are all FDA approved and are the same hormones that drug companies use in their pills, patches, and vaginal gels.

The easiest way to find a doctor to support you is to search for a compounding pharmacy in your area, and ask them which doctors write prescriptions for bioidenticals that are sent to the pharmacy.

You may be thinking, *Why haven't I heard about BHRT until now? It sounds like magic!* Here's the thing: Hormone replacement drugs became popular after the launch of Premarin in 1942. This medication was derived from the urine of pregnant horses and was used to boost estrogen levels in menopausal women. Women loved it, and it became increasingly popular until the 2002 results of the Women's Health Initiative abruptly altered women's attitudes. The study showed that in menopausal women, taking PremPro (a combination of Premarin and Provera, a synthetic progesterone) led to a greater risk of breast cancer and stroke. After this finding, hormone replacement therapy was lumped all together and labeled dangerous. Bioidentical hormones were tarred with the same brush.

Bioidentical or not, estrogen is a growth hormone and may have adverse effects on uterine and breast tissue, especially if it's not balanced with progesterone. But overall, I've seen BHRT benefit many women, including myself. I would recommend that you try it if you're not having luck with other means of balancing your hormones.

It's always best to chat with your health-care professional before supplementing with hormones; though some are available without a prescription, it can be dangerous to use them if you do not really require the hormone. *Do not* supplement with hormones without testing your levels first, and continue to monitor your levels while on the medication.

Amenorrhea

Amenorrhea is when menstruation is absent for three months or more during reproductive years—either menstruation didn't start during puberty (less common) or periods started but then ceased (more common).

I suffered with amenorrhea from 2007 to 2015 as a result of many factors, including low body fat, excessive training, drug abuse, and immense mental and physical stress. These are among the most common causes of amenorrhea, which also include too few calories, too few carbs, and weight loss.

At first you may think that not having a period sounds a little...freeing. I know I did. I loved it for six out of the eight years I experienced it. But then it became a problem. With a lack of estrogen, progesterone, testosterone, and DHEA flowing through my body, I started to feel severely imbalanced.

Causes of Amenorrhea

Amenorrhea occurs due to the drop in levels of many different hormones, including luteinizing hormone, follicle-stimulating hormone, estrogen, progesterone, and testosterone. These changes can slow some functions in the hypothalamus, the region of the brain responsible for hormone release.

One potential cause of amenorrhea and irregular menstruation is low levels of leptin, a hormone produced by fat cells that helps you feel full. Evidence suggests that women need a certain level of leptin to maintain normal menstrual function. If your carb or calorie consumption is too low, it can suppress your leptin levels and interfere with leptin's role in regulating reproductive hormones. This is particularly true for underweight or lean women on a low-carb diet.

There aren't a lot of studies on the relationship between a low-carb diet and amenorrhea. Studies that report amenorrhea as a side effect of a low-carb diet were usually focusing on women who had been on a low-carb diet for a long period of time and don't comment on the amount of fat consumed or the quality of the food. One study, however, followed twenty teenage girls on a very-low-carb diet for six months—and 45 percent experienced menstrual problems while 6 percent experienced amenorrhea.

This is not to say that a ketogenic diet causes amenorrhea! There are different kinds of low-carb diets, from meat-only to processed-food-only to whole-foods-based. Just as there are thousands of ways to live a glucose-fueled life, there are thousands of ways to live a ketone-fueled life, and some are healthier than others. Really, it boils down to whether your low-carb diet is tailored to your unique

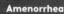

needs, and I think by now you know that that's the name of the game here. Yes, what we're doing is a low-carb diet, but if you add in a high amount of fats, it's a ketogenic diet. And if those fats are *healthy* fats and you focus on whole foods, it's a whole-food or Paleo approach to the ketogenic diet. And if you add in carb-ups, now you're practicing a cyclical approach to a ketogenic diet. See where I'm going with this?

Yes, it's a low-carb diet, but it's a healthy one. Losing your period is rare if you're following a well-formulated ketogenic diet. In fact, keto was a key factor in helping me overcome my amenorrhea, and with patience and the right strategies, you can overcome it too.

Getting Your Period Back

If you've got amenorrhea, know that the holistic keto approach in this book will go a long way toward restoring hormone balance and can also be excellent for fertility. It's the exact protocol that I used to get my period back after eight years of amenorrhea. The changes can be so dramatic that I've even seen menopausal women get their periods again! This is a *good* thing. Of course, the effects vary greatly from woman to woman.

While keto will likely have a dramatically positive effect on your body, failing to address your relationship with stress will hold you back. I've been where you are, so I know how challenging it can be to take stock of your life and simplify things to alleviate stress. But it has to be done, and it has to happen sooner rather than later to get your hormones back on track.

TRUTH BOMB

Once you start ovulating, you're not out of the clear just yet. It's going to take your body a year or two to get to a normal cycle. But you may experience positive results by boosting your carbs three days before ovulation.

In my case, I got my period back with a four-pronged approach: not forcing myself to fast, eating enough, employing carb-ups, and ending my workout obsession. Each action was equally important as the others. If you're struggling with hormonal deficiency, it's likely that these powerful adjustments will play a role in your recovery, too. But I also recommend using the hormone adjustments table from pages 331 to 333 to help to boost hormonal activity, plus the additional adjustments on the following pages.

Additional Adjustments

Remember, these steps are all in addition to the guidelines in "How to Support Overall Hormone Health" on page 335.

Say Yes To
EATING ENOUGH
Abstaining from food puts stress on the body, similar to forcing yourself to fast (which is not the same as fasting naturally, which often happens on keto). Be sure to eat when you're hungry.

CARB-UPS
Carb-ups help boost thyroid function, send signals to your hypothalamus that you're not in starvation mode, and encourage your body to rest as much as possible. If you need a refresher on carb-ups, see page 186. The best carb-up practice for those experiencing amenorrhea is the Daily Fat Burner Fat Fueled Profile (page 201). Or, if you want to get a little wild and create your own plan, eat carbs when it feels right, shooting for at least three carb-up meals a week.

BALANCING INSULIN
Many women who experience amenorrhea also struggle with insulin resistance, so working to become insulin sensitive can bring the body closer to balance. There's no better way to do this than to eat keto! If you need more pointers on insulin-specific support, delve deep into the solutions on page 331.

SUPPORTING YOUR ADRENALS BY REDUCING STRESS
In hypothalamic amenorrhea, the source of the problem is an imbalance with your hypothalamus. The hypothalamus is part of an axis connecting it with the pituitary gland and the adrenals, known as the HPA axis. Think of the axis as a three-legged stool: if one leg has a problem, the whole thing can collapse. Of the three legs, the adrenals are the easiest to support through simple lifestyle changes, and doing so will support the health of your hypothalamus, too.

To support the adrenals, the most important thing is to reduce stress and overexercising. Existing in a constant state of franticness harms your body. Even if you're fully aware that your life is far from stress-free and believe that there isn't much you can do about it, there are small changes that can make stress more manageable and less damaging, Try to get seven to nine hours of sleep at night, get moving with moderate exercise, and spend time with people who make you happy. Yoga, meditation, breathing exercises, qigong, and tai chi have all been scientifically proven to reduce stress. If none of these feel right to you, find a self-care practice that does—maybe an unhurried walk in nature, or a relaxing bath, or just sitting alone with your headphones on, listening to your favorite music.

SUPPORTING YOUR THYROID

The HPT axis is the connection among the hypothalamus, pituitary, and thyroid. As with the HPA axis, any problem with one part of the axis can affect the hypothalamus. The easiest way to support the HPT axis—and therefore support the hypothalamus, which is often associated with amenorrhea—is to support the thyroid. The key for me was finding a doctor who was able to correctly diagnose me with hypothyroidism and prescribe desiccated thyroid to help boost my free T3 and lower my TSH. This gave my body the support it needed to bring my sex hormone production back online. Additionally, by eating keto, I provided my body with all of the precursors needed for hormones, and once my thyroid was being supported, my body was able to put those precursors to work. For more on supporting your thyroid, see page 367.

NUTRIENT DENSITY OVER FATTY COFFEES

While I love fatty coffee drinks, they just don't provide as many nutrients as a plate of kale and grass-fed beef. Fatty coffees are delicious and filling, but greens and meat will go further in helping you heal.

Say No To

FASTING

In women with low hormones, the body can perceive intermittent fasting as a sign of starvation. In response, a signal is sent to the body's various systems that becoming pregnant is not safe because there isn't enough food. As long as this signal is being sent, hormone regulation is next to impossible. Eating three well-formulated keto meals a day floods your body with healing nutrients, turning off the alarm signal so that your hormones can balance out. Although my hormones began to recover as soon as I began eating a Fat Fueled diet, it wasn't until I gave up intermittent fasting that my period returned, about four months later.

PMS

As if I need to explain what PMS is. We've all experienced it at one time or another, whether we're conscious of it or not.

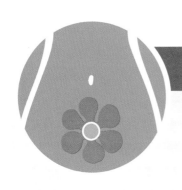

SYMPTOMS OF PMS

Arriving during the latter half of the menstrual cycle (the luteal phase, page 330) and dissipating by the second day of the new menstrual cycle (in the follicular phase, page 330), PMS can bring us ladies:

 Acne

 Changes in vision

 Food cravings

 Aggression

 Constipation

 Forgetfulness

 Back pain

 Cramps

 Bloating

 Increased appetite

 Depression

 Insomnia

 Brain fog

 Fatigue

 Irritability

 Breast tenderness

 Feeling out of control

Mood swings

Basically, PMS comes in a wide range of symptoms, and it can frustrate us and those closest to us if we're not mindful of what's happening.

Just today I freaked out at Kevin, my husband, for leaving his water glass on the kitchen table after dinner. As soon as I realized what I'd done, I yelled out, "PMS, PMS, argh!"

For real, though, a mild case of PMS can be expected, but if PMS is so intense that it gets in the way of your daily life, there's likely an imbalance at play that needs your attention.

Keto can do wonders for PMS symptoms, but it's not magic. Please do not expect PMS to change overnight. In fact, since I used keto to get my period back in 2015, my cycles have kept evolving—even years later, each cycle is a touch better than the last. I started off with painful, even debilitating periods; my flow was heavy, my mind was foggy, and I had a hard time getting through the first five days of each cycle. Now, I barely notice I have my period at all. But this was not an overnight success. Keto will help lessen the symptoms of PMS, but it will take time.

Possible Reasons for PMS

- High levels of estrogen (see page 328)
- Lackluster progesterone levels in the luteal phase (see page 333)
- Breakdown of hormones (particularly estrogen) in the liver is incomplete
- Dysbiosis or imbalance in the microbiome (without proper bacteria balance, estrogen cannot be metabolized properly)
- Imbalanced thyroid (see page 367)
- Imbalanced adrenals (see page 374)

Additional Adjustments

Remember, these steps are all in addition to the guidelines in "How to Support Overall Hormone Health" on page 335.

Say Yes To

CALCIUM-RICH FOODS

Calcium intake can help with any PMS symptoms you're experiencing. Think poppy seeds, sesame seeds, celery, chia seeds, canned sardines or salmon (with bones), almonds, and green veggies, like spinach, kale, broccoli, bok choy, and okra.

BEING OKAY WITH BLOAT

You will probably still have some bloating. It's due to massive surges in estrogen—which can cause quite a bit of extra water to be retained—during the premenstrual part of your cycle, and it's a natural part of the change in hormones during your cycle. So if you tend to bloat or experience puffiness and inflammation during menstruation, this is just how you experience menstruation, and keto probably isn't going to change that. However, if you started out with excessively high estrogen levels, eating keto will help lower estrogen to more normal levels, and in that case, you have full permission to do the happy dance, because your belly is about to get way, way less bloated.

EMBRACING WEIGHT FLUCTUATIONS

It's normal for your weight to fluctuate right before and during menstruation. The best advice I can give you is to stay off the scale for five to seven days before your period, during your period, and for three to four days following your period. There's no reason to make yourself extra miserable by seeing the number on the scale go up during this time. Don't sweat your weight during your period—any added pounds from bloat will go away again once it's over.

IMPROVING SLEEP

PMS is most likely to occur between ovulation and seven days after your period. (Did you do the math on that and think, *Um, so when am I not PMSing?* Fair question.) If you're one of those ladies who experiences sleepless nights or difficulty falling asleep during this time, it's very important to brush up on your sleep skills the week *before* PMS sets in—from day 7 of your cycle to ovulation. The more you practice healthful sleep hygiene then, the easier it will be to continue during your PMS experience.

There's a lot more on good sleep hygiene on pages 171 and 172, but here are the basics: go to bed at the same time every night, wind down a couple of hours before bed, and keep your phone out of your bedroom. Every minute you sleep is another minute you're giving your body to heal. I remind myself of this whenever I have to set my alarm or skip a nap even though my body is begging me for one. Listen to your body and rest when you need to.

MOVEMENT

Physical activity can alleviate the symptoms of PMS by reducing stress, easing cramps, and working to balance progesterone and estrogen. Any form of movement is good here—walking, biking, hiking, HIIT—anything that makes you feel good. You may find that outdoor activities feel better. Tai chi, an ancient form of Chinese exercise, is a low-impact activity that improves flexibility, balance, and muscle strength.

LOWERING ESTROGEN

PMS can be caused by elevated estrogen. Estrogen is produced in fat cells, so the more body fat you have, the higher your estrogen, and that can contribute to hormone imbalance. Whether you need to lose weight or not, adding healthy fats to the diet and reducing carbs and sugar is important for hormone and mood balance. Following the estrogen-lowering tips on page 333 may be helpful, too.

ORGANIC PRODUCE

To avoid the xenoestrogens present in pesticides, try for organic produce as much as possible, especially with crops that are treated with a lot of pesticides and other chemicals. Generally speaking, if you have to choose, foods that don't have a thick peel should be organic, like apples, bell peppers, celery, cherries, cherry tomatoes, cucumbers, grapes, nectarines, peaches, spinach, strawberries, and tomatoes. The Dirty Dozen list on the Environmental Working Group website (www.ewg.org/ foodnews/dirty-dozen.php) is updated every year with the produce most likely to be contaminated with pesticides.

Say No To

EXPERIMENTING WITH DIET BEFORE MENSTRUATION

Don't start a food experiment right before or during your period. There's no reason to make things extra difficult for yourself when you are bleeding. If you're thinking about making a change—for example, giving up dairy or sweeteners—do yourself a favor and wait until your period is over.

TOXINS

Reducing your exposure to chemicals in food, air, personal care products, and water means reducing your exposure to synthetic estrogens. For food, opt for organic produce and pasture-raised meat and dairy when possible. If the air quality in your hometown is less than optimal, get a HEPA filter for the room you spend the most time in (your workplace is fair game!). For personal care products, be mindful of the ingredients they use. Ingredients to avoid include the following: avobenzone, benzophenone, formaldehyde, fragrance/perfume, homosalate, methoxycinnmate, PABA, parabens, propylene glycol, sodium laureth sulfate, sodium lauryl sulfate, synthetic colors, toluene, and triclosan. Opt for essential oils instead of perfume, natural deodorant (my favorite is Primal Pit Paste), and natural body wash (my favorite is Dr. Bronner's Castile Soap).

PCOS

Polycystic ovary syndrome, or PCOS, develops when the ovaries overproduce androgen hormones (one of which is testosterone), and estrogen and progesterone levels drop. Androgen overproduction often begins with the pituitary gland oversecreting luteinizing hormone, which stimulates additional androgen production.

With this hormonal profile, women experience fewer periods than normal. But despite its name, not all women who receive a PCOS diagnosis experience actual cysts. The cysts can develop over time when eggs aren't released.

PCOS is the leading cause of infertility in women. It's closely associated with health concerns that are generally linked to diet: over 50 percent of women who are diagnosed with PCOS are obese or overweight and have symptoms that align with metabolic syndrome (including high blood glucose and insulin resistance).

To be diagnosed with PCOS, you need to have at least two of the following:

- No periods or irregular periods (the time between periods is typically very long)

- Cysts on the ovaries (determined by an ultrasound)

- Increased androgens (determined by blood test)

- Luteinizing hormone and follicle-stimulating hormone irregularities (determined by blood test)

Currently, there's no cure for PCOS, but a ketogenic diet has helped many women overcome it. PCOS is tied to poor glucose metabolism, generally in the form of insulin resistance, and keto is an excellent way to balance blood sugar and improve insulin sensitivity. In several studies, women with PCOS who began following a keto diet showed significant improvements in the levels of both insulin and reproductive hormones. In one study, some women who had been struggling with infertility even became pregnant.

Test for It: PCOS

A pelvic ultrasound can reveal cysts on the ovaries.

Free testosterone is the biologically active form of the hormone and may be elevated in those with PCOS.

Fasting insulin is your level of insulin after at least eight hours of fasting and may be elevated in those with PCOS.

A glucose test measures the amount of glucose in your blood and could be a good indicator if blood sugar imbalance is the cause of your PCOS symptoms.

Hemoglobin A1C is your average level of blood sugar over the past two to three months. It can help pinpoint what's causing your symptoms, if they're related to a blood sugar imbalance, and when they began.

Additional Adjustments

I've seen many women with PCOS benefit just from following a whole foods–based ketogenic diet. But if you want to go a step further, here are some additional adjustments you can make.

Remember, these steps are all in addition to the guidelines in "How to Support Overall Hormone Health" on page 335.

Say Yes To

INCREASED OMEGA-3

Taking fish oil has been shown to decrease testosterone levels in those experiencing PCOS.

MAGNESIUM SUPPLEMENTATION

Women with PCOS often struggle with insulin resistance. Magnesium has been shown to improve insulin sensitivity.

CINNAMON

Ground cinnamon (about 1 teaspoon a day) can help balance blood sugar.

Say No To

CHARRED FOOD

Overcooking food can create advanced glycation end-products, or AGEs—compounds that can accumulate in the body and cause accelerated aging and inflammation. If eaten regularly, they can contribute to intense PCOS symptoms. Avoid roasting, searing, or grilling your foods.

INFLAMMATION

Chronic low-level inflammation may play a role in the development of PCOS, so taking steps to eliminate it can't hurt! Follow the steps starting on page 251.

Symptoms of PCOS

- Acne
- Darkened skin under the arms, at the back of the neck, or in the groin area
- Excess facial or body hair
- Fatigue and low energy
- Headaches
- Infertility
- Insomnia or poor sleep quality
- Insulin resistance
- Irregular periods
- Mood swings, depression, and anxiety
- Pelvic pain during or outside menstruation
- Skin tags
- Thinning scalp hair
- Weight gain or inability to lose weight

Menopause

How many of us are terrified of menopause? I know I was, for a long, long time. The hot flashes, the mood swings... I wanted no part of it. I didn't look forward to the change, and many women don't.

Many of us think that pain and struggle is just part of menopause, brace for impact, and live in agony while we deal with symptom after symptom—for two to ten years. Why do women have it so bad? After the pain of menstruation and childbirth, wouldn't it be grand if entering the last phase of womanhood was a walk in the park? Imagine going through menopause unscathed. Is there such a reality?

Yes! And it starts with the power of hormonal balance in the years leading up to menopause.

Test for It: Menopause

Estradiol measures the level of estrogen in the blood, which can drastically decrease as perimenopause approaches, so it's important to know your levels in order to understand symptoms or avoid them altogether.

Free testosterone is the biologically active form of the hormone and declines as menopause approaches.

Progesterone levels drop as menopause approaches. Lack of progesterone during perimenopause can cause heavier and longer periods.

DHEA-S is the amount of DHEA in your blood and is a good indication of adrenal health. Since the adrenals take up the role of producing hormones during perimenopause and menopause, it's important to test adrenal function.

Sex hormone binding globulin (SHBG) is like Velcro pieces that prevent hormones from doing their job. Too much will cause low hormone function, and not enough will cause high hormone function.

Thyroid-stimulating hormone (TSH) levels can indicate whether the thyroid is being over- or understimulated.

Free T3 is the thyroid hormone T3 unbound in your blood, and free T3 levels are a good indication of what's available for use.

Free T4 is the thyroid hormone T4 unbound in your blood and ready to be converted to free T3.

Cortisol is best tested in the morning, and each test should occur at the same time.

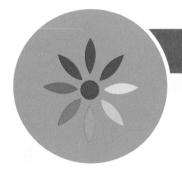

MENOPAUSE SYMPTOMS

 Depression and anxiety

 Difficulty concentrating

 Dry skin, eyes, and mouth

Forgetfulness, from losing your keys to forgetting why you went into a store

 Frequent UTIs

 Hot flashes lasting 1 to 5 minutes, from mild to severe heat

 Increased hair growth on face, chest, back, and neck

Insomnia or difficulty sleeping

Joint pain

 Less breast fullness

 Low sex drive, low arousal, and painful intercourse

 Night sweats

 Reduced muscle mass

 Vaginal dryness

 Weight gain, especially around the waist

So if you're under forty, listen up! If you're as terrified of menopause as I was, now's the time to get over your fear, balance out, and learn to welcome the change when it arrives. Head over to page 335 to read more about how you can balance your hormones now to set yourself up for success later.

For the forty-and-over crowd, don't lose hope. There are countless adjustments you can make to reduce symptoms and feel your best, no matter what you've got going on right now. Whether you're just flirting with the beginning stages of perimenopause or you're well on the other side, things can improve. It doesn't have to be painful, frustrating, or defeating.

First, Perimenopause

During your reproductive years, the follicle-stimulating hormone (FSH) stimulates the release of an egg from one of your ovaries once a month, and when this occurs, it stimulates the ovarian production of estrogen. After ovulation, the follicle that housed the egg produces progesterone. This cycle repeats itself every twenty to thirty-four days or so.

In perimenopause, which begins around four years before menopause, this process becomes a bit sporadic. The body creates less estrogen, progesterone, and testosterone, and in response, the brain's pituitary gland steps up its production of FSH in an attempt to increase estrogen output. During this time, estrogen levels may fluctuate widely, but in the final couple of years before menopause, they steadily decline.

What you'll notice during perimenopause, which generally begins in the mid-to late forties, is that your cycles become more irregular and there's more time between periods. It's also common to experience fatigue, breast tenderness, hot flashes, mood swings, and trouble sleeping. Not everyone experiences perimenopause, however—some women go directly to menopause.

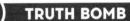

TRUTH BOMB

Proof against the calorie-in-calorie-out mentality: when women reach perimenopause with imbalanced hormones, they put on weight even if they don't eat more than usual. This is due to massive hormonal changes.

STAGES OF MENOPAUSE

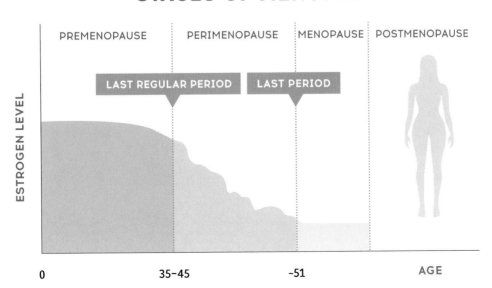

During perimenopause and menopause, the decline in estrogen shifts where weight is stored, from thighs and hips to the abdomen. And body weight overall tends to increase, for the following reasons:

- Lower levels of estrogen promote insulin resistance and higher levels of insulin in the blood, which lead to weight gain. (One of insulin's jobs is to tell the body to store excess glucose.)

- Research suggests that levels of ghrelin, the hunger hormone, increase in the early stages of perimenopause, so women may eat more food than their bodies need.

- Low estrogen levels may impair the production of leptin and neuropeptide Y—hormones that help regulate appetite and weight balance.

- The loss of muscle mass can slow down the metabolism, making it much easier to put on weight and more challenging to lose it.

Then Menopause

Even though we refer to being "in menopause," technically menopause is the final menstrual period. Of course, that's a retrospective diagnosis, as we don't really know it's final until twelve months later. At that point, when there have been no periods for twelve months, someone has "gone through menopause." (To be clear, though, menopause isn't simply not having a period for twelve months. That can happen at any age for a wide variety of reasons, as we explored in the section on amenorrhea earlier in this chapter.) The average age at menopause is fifty-one.

Menopause is one of those double-edged swords. On the one hand, we can finally stop dealing with those pesky monthly periods. But on the other hand, it can cause some pretty nasty symptoms for some women. Not all women—some experience literally no symptoms at all; their periods just stop and life moves on unchanged—but some experience severe dysfunction in mood, weight, sleep, libido, and more.

The good news is, menopause does not have to be a horrific experience! A ketogenic diet is a great way to reduce symptoms like cravings and bloating and help build muscle, which is often lost during menopause. And there are a wide range of things you can do to ease your symptoms.

Overcoming the Issues

BHRT? Head over to page 347 to read more about it.

FOR VAGINAL DRYNESS

- Apply an estrogen gel vaginally.
- Use coconut oil or liquid vitamin E as a lubricant during intercourse.
- Indulge in more foreplay!

FOR HOT FLASHES & NIGHT SWEATS

- Take 2 tablespoons freshly ground flax seeds daily. Purchase the seeds whole and grind them in a coffee grinder or spice grinder. Not appropriate for women with a history of breast cancer.
- Use a natural progesterone cream.
- Try bioidentical estrogen (see page 347). Not appropriate for women with a history of breast cancer.

FOR LOW SEX DRIVE

- Spice things up! Try new things with your partner.
- Check your vitamin D levels. You may need a supplement or to spend more time in the sun.
- Check your DHEA levels. If they're imbalanced, follow the guidelines on page 332.

How Is Menopause Different from Amenorrhea?

Amenorrhea is a medical condition generally brought on by stress, extreme weight loss, or excess exercise. With amenorrhea, you can still release an egg; you just don't have enough endocrine support for menstruation to occur. There's a high chance that by adjusting lifestyle factors, you can get your period back. With true menopause, your ovaries stop releasing an egg every month, and hormone levels decline and transfer from the ovaries to the adrenals. With menopause, menstruation stops and does not return.

- FOR INSOMNIA
- Use a natural progesterone cream.
- Follow the sleep improvement techniques on pages 171 and 172.

FOR JOINT PAIN

- Take 2 tablespoons freshly ground flax seeds daily. Purchase the seeds whole and grind them in a coffee grinder or spice grinder. Not appropriate for women with a history of breast cancer.
- Try bioidentical estrogen (see page 347). Not appropriate for women with a history of breast cancer.

FOR ANXIETY, IRRITABILITY & DEPRESSION

- Use a natural progesterone cream.
- Engage in healthful sleep practices, as outlined on pages 171 and 172.
- Move your body!
- Journaling, goal setting, and finding your passion can be helpful.

Diet Adjustments

In general, keto is great for women transitioning into menopause because it eliminates cravings, increases calcium, reduces bloating, and promotes muscle gain, all quite naturally—you don't have to do much more than eat bacon, loads of coconut oil, kale, and some dark chocolate to stay on point. However, tweaking your keto diet a bit to emphasize healing foods can be helpful.

You may be wondering if carb-ups or another cyclical keto approach is still a good idea during perimenopause and menopause. I find that many women require fewer carb-ups during this time than in their reproductive years.

Ultra-Healing Foods

THE EXTRAS

- Chamomile tea
- Green tea
- Rooibos tea
- Turmeric

STARCHES AND FRUITS

- Butternut squash
- Sweet potatoes

PROTEIN

- Anchovy
- Eggs
- Mackerel
- Organ meats
- Oysters
- Salmon
- Sardines
- Turkey

NON-STARCHY VEGETABLES

- Asparagus
- Broccoli
- Brussels sprouts
- Chinese cabbage
- Collard greens
- Kale
- Okra
- Spinach
- Winter squash

HEALTHY FATS

- Almonds
- Avocados
- Chia seeds
- Coconut oil
- Flax seeds
- Hemp seeds
- Sesame seeds
- Sunflower seeds
- Walnuts

WATER

Additional Adjustments

Remember, these steps are all in addition to the guidelines in "How to Support Overall Hormone Health" on page 335.

Say Yes To

BONE DENSITY

Because estrogen is decreasing, it's important to pay special attention to your bone density. Stand on one leg while washing the dishes, doing the laundry, or standing in line at a store to improve bone density.

MOVEMENT

Staying active is crucial during this time. Studies have shown that in postmenopausal women, regular exercise can help relieve stress, boost metabolism and fat-burning, and prevent loss of muscle mass. In addition, physical activity may relieve hot flashes in some women. Weight-bearing activities like weight training, walking, hiking, jogging, climbing stairs, tennis, and dancing are awesome choices.

YOGA

Yoga is well known for relieving stress, increasing overall well-being, and reducing inflammation.

ACUPUNCTURE

Acupuncture appears to be effective for hot flashes and improving sleep.

BIOIDENTICAL HORMONE REPLACEMENT THERAPY

Exogenous hormones are a true gift for women struggling with menopause. Chat with your health-care provider about options for estrogen, progesterone, DHEA, and other hormones to see if BHRT is right for you. There's more information about BHRT on page 347.

THYROID SUPPORT

There's a cascade effect of hormonal changes that can result in hypothyroidism in menopausal women. When ovulation doesn't occur, it can lead to estrogen dominance. If there's stress in your life, the excess estrogen can be metabolized into stress hormone–like substances that trigger your body to lower its levels of thyroid hormone in order to protect the heart. This may result in hypothyroidism. See page 367 for more on how to support your thyroid.

ADRENAL SUPPORT

As you approach menopause, production of sex hormones starts to move from your ovaries to your adrenal glands. This is why it's so very important to support your adrenals during and after perimenopause and menopause. The stress hormones cortisol and epinephrine, which are produced by the adrenal glands, can wreak havoc on normal hormone metabolism, so what little you do make will be affected by stress hormone levels. Many experts believe that the key to quelling menopausal symptoms lies in getting stress hormone levels under control. See page 374 for more on adrenal support.

Say No To

INFLAMMATION

The decrease in estrogen can cause an increase in joint pain, so staying focused on reducing overall inflammation can be helpful in alleviating symptoms. Follow the steps starting on page 251 to reduce your inflammation.

Thyroid **Health**

The thyroid and metabolism go hand in hand, so it's no wonder the thyroid is the most talked-about endocrine gland when it comes to weight. Blaming the thyroid is an easy explanation for weight gain, but don't be fooled. Studies show that low thyroid function causes an average of 5 to 12 pounds of weight gain, and that's all. If you've experienced extreme weight gain and your thyroid is being blamed, dig a little deeper.

Test for It: Thyroid Health

Anti-TPO (thyroid peroxidase) looks for antibodies in the blood that work against TPO, an enzyme found in the thyroid gland that plays a role in the production of thyroid hormones. When these antibodies are present, it may suggest that you are at risk of developing a thyroid disorder or already have a thyroid-related autoimmune disorder.

Anti-thyroglobulin looks for antibodies against thyroglobulin, a thyroid-created protein. The antibodies affect the function of thyroglobulin, so their presence is a sign you may have a thyroid disorder.

TSH (thyroid-stimulating hormone) tests for the level of TSH in your blood.

Total T4 is mostly metabolically inactive in the body and has to be converted to T3 to be usable. Because of its close relationship with T3, T4 is best measured in conjunction with T3.

Free T4 will tell you the active amount of T4. This will be low in cases of hypothyroidism but can be normal in subclinical, early stages of thyroid dysfunction.

Total T3 is the total amount of active thyroid hormone and will tell you how well your body is converting T4 to T3 to rule out an overactive thyroid.

Free T3 is the more active, usable form of your thyroid hormone and can be helpful if you're supplementing with thyroid hormone, to ensure your body is converting properly.

Reverse T3, an unusable form of the thyroid hormone, can be raised by chronic stress and high cortisol. This test can be helpful to see whether your adrenals are affecting your thyroid health.

T3 uptake is effective at determining whether estrogen and/or testosterone are binding to thyroid hormones.

Tests for adrenal dysfunction (page 375): Adrenal dysfunction can look and feel very similar to hypothyroidism because cortisol binds to thyroid receptors, slowing thyroid production. If you're displaying signs of thyroid imbalance, get tested for adrenal dysfunction as well.

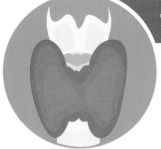

THYROID IMBALANCE SYMPTOMS

Thyroid health is dependent on many variables and doesn't just affect our weight! When the thyroid is out of balance, we can also experience:

 Fertility issues

 Low energy

 Anxiety and irritability

 Growth and development issues

 Mental sluggishness

 Constipation

 Hair loss

 Problems with carbohydrate and fat metabolism

There are two main conditions of thyroid dysfunction: hypothyroidism and hyperthyroidism.

Hypothyroidism occurs when your thyroid hormones are low. In this scenario, your body processes become sluggish and your cells require less energy (aka calories), so any extra is stored as fat. Weight can increase even though the appetite typically decreases. The body produces less heat, so you feel cold, and the sweat glands no longer keep the skin moist, so your skin is dry. Your heart rate slows, your brain wants to sleep all the time, and bowel function slows.

What causes hypothyroidism? There are several possible causes:

- High intake of goitrogens, substances that interfere with the thyroid (see page 370)

- High intake of soy (see page 340)

- Malnourishment from not eating enough, fasting too often, or exercising too hard

- Medication side effects. If you are on meds and have low thyroid, it may be helpful to talk to a pharmacist about possible drug side effects.

- Mineral deficiencies, especially selenium, iodine, and zinc

- Pregnancy

- Stress. High levels of cortisol negatively impacts the conversion of thyroid hormone to the usable form.

Hyperthyroidism is the exact opposite of hypothyroidism: instead of too little thyroid hormone, you have too much. Body processes accelerate and more energy (aka calories) is used, so you can lose weight even if your appetite increases. The body produces more heat and thus perspiration to cool itself down. The heart rate accelerates, bowel activity increases, and cells age at a faster rate. The sleep disruption that occurs makes symptoms worse.

TRUTH BOMB

The adrenals, thyroid, and reproductive system share many of the same pathways. It's rare to see a healthy thyroid in the company of adrenal dysfunction and/or imbalanced sex hormones. Usually when one system fails and isn't tended to, the others fall down with it.

Are Carbs Necessary for Optimal Thyroid Function?

It's true that if you go too low-carb for too long, you could begin to display hypothyroid symptoms. Carbohydrates are needed to convert inactive T4 hormone to active T3 hormone, so if your carb intake is very, very low for a very long time, you could develop hypothyroid symptoms.

The length of time it takes for symptoms to develop is the most reliable indicator of whether your thyroid imbalance was there all along or it was triggered by your switch a low-carb diet. If hypothyroid symptoms develop early on in your keto journey, it's likely that the imbalance was there to begin with and that low-carb eating just brought it to the surface. But if symptoms appear after you've been eating very low-carb for six months, the low-carb diet is probably what spurred the imbalance.

There's an in-depth look at keto and thyroid health on page 367, but basically, if you find that your thyroid doesn't seem happy on keto, adjust your carbohydrate or protein intake by switching your Fat Fueled Profile to one that incorporates carb-ups (see page 200).

Navigating Thyroid Treatments

I lived with hypothyroidism for four years before I found a doctor who would test me for it. I know firsthand how silent this imbalance can be—you don't feel pain, many doctors are reluctant to test for it, and the symptoms read like a hypochondriac's worst nightmare.

Once you receive the proper diagnosis and are placed on the right protocol for you and your body (which may or may not include medication), it's important to understand that thyroid balance is an ongoing affair. Any changes in your life may affect the thyroid and therefore your healing protocol. Once you've found a protocol that works, it's important to get your thyroid levels checked every couple of months to ensure your levels are optimal for your body.

Here are the medication options currently available to those with an imbalanced thyroid:

- Synthetic T4, otherwise known as levothyroxine or Synthroid. It's often beneficial for people with Hashimoto's thyroiditis.

- Desiccated thyroid, otherwise known as naturthyroid. This is a porcine glandular blend of T4 and T3. It provides both inactive hormone and active thyroid hormones.

- Compounded T4 and T3, an alternative to the two options above. It's safe for those with Hashimoto's.

There's no shame in having to supplement with hormones to support your thyroid. Read up more on bioidentical hormones on page 347 and chat with your doctor about options for supporting your thyroid in the best possible way.

Diet Adjustments

You can make a bunch of small adjustments to your eating style that'll have great impact on your thyroid. One of the biggest ones is being conscious of goitrogens—substances found in some foods that can wreak havoc on your thyroid function. Goitrogens interfere with iodine uptake in the thyroid gland, so one way to offset the effects of these foods is to eat foods that are high in iodine. Sea vegetables are your best choice.

If you look at the list of foods high in goitrogens below and think, *What?! I thought that stuff was good for me!* remember: moderation. Rest assured that just because certain foods are high in goitrogens doesn't mean you have to completely

Foods Highest in Goitrogens

Bamboo shoots	Edamame	Rutabagas
Bok choy	Kale	Soy milk
Broccoli	Lima beans	Spinach
Brussels sprouts	Mustard greens	Strawberries
Cabbage	Peaches	Sweet potatoes
Cassava	Peanuts	Tempeh
Cauliflower	Pears	Tofu
Collard greens	Pine nuts	Turnips

avoid them. With the exception of soy, which can interfere with thyroid medication (and doesn't do you any favors for overall hormone health), the benefits of these foods far outweigh the downsides.

Just try not to eat them in their raw form—cooking reduces goitrogen content by up to 30 percent. And keep in mind that eating foods high in goitrogens has a cumulative effect—so, again, eat them in moderation and don't have too many in one day.

If You Have Hashimoto's

These diet adjustments may not work for those with Hashimoto's. For more on autoimmune conditions and support, go to page 241.

Ultra-Healing Foods

THE EXTRAS

- Dried rosemary (leaves and ground)
- Dried sage (leaves and ground)
- Dried thyme (leaves and ground)
- Fresh ginger
- Fresh rosemary
- Fresh sage
- Fresh thyme
- Garlic
- Ground black pepper
- Ground cinnamon
- Ground ginger
- Turmeric

STARCHES AND FRUITS

- Beets
- Cranberries
- Parsnips
- Raisins
- Squash of all kinds
- Strawberries

PROTEIN

- Beef
- Crab
- Eggs
- Lobster
- Organ meats
- Oysters
- Salmon
- Sardines

NON-STARCHY VEGETABLES

- Bell peppers
- Collards
- Daikon
- Fennel
- Fermented vegetables
- Jerusalem artichokes
- Mushrooms
- Sea vegetables, including kelp noodles

HEALTHY FATS

- Almonds
- Avocados
- Brazil nuts
- Ghee
- Pecans
- Pumpkin seeds
- Tahini
- Walnuts

WATER

Additional Adjustments

Remember, these steps are all in addition to the guidelines in "How to Support Overall Hormone Health" on page 335.

Say Yes To

LIMITING FRUCTOSE

Fructose may not raise blood sugar as drastically as other forms of sugar, but because it is metabolized only by the liver, it contributes to an unhealthy fat buildup in the liver. Most of the conversion of T4 to T3 happens in the liver, and a fatty liver does not support adequate conversion.

REDUCING INFLAMMATION

An imbalanced thyroid is likely accompanied by inflammation, so anything that further stimulates inflammation isn't going to help the situation. For this reason, you may want to follow the inflammation reduction guidelines starting on page 251.

IODINE

Iodine deficiency can cause subclinical hypothyroidism—as well as sore breasts, since breast tissue requires 3 mg of iodine per day. If you're eating foods high in goitrogens (see page 370), eating foods rich in iodine at the same time can help overcome the goitrogens' interference with iodine absorption. The safest way to increase your iodine level is to eat kelp tablets, seafood, and two eggs per week.

HIGH-QUALITY SALT

Consume Himalayan pink salt or Celtic sea salt rather than iodized table salt. Sea salt contains more than sixty trace minerals and doesn't pose a risk for overconsumption of iodine, which is a possibility with iodized table salt—it has way more iodine than salt found in nature. Sea salt is also much less processed and tastes better.

EASY MOVEMENT

While physical activity is helpful to maintain the health of your thyroid, imbalance can occur when you're pushing too hard in your workouts, which upsets the hypothalamus-pituitary-thyroid axis and can lead to issues with your thyroid and overall hormone health. If you're obsessed with working out, you could benefit from easing down a little. Keep it light—outdoor walks, gentle swimming, and restorative yoga.

LOVING YOUR ADRENALS

Your adrenals produce hormones that directly affect your metabolic processes: they regulate blood pressure, blood sugar, immune responses, digestion, and electrolyte balance, to name a few. When you perceive stress, your adrenals kick into high gear, producing hormones that will help you deal with the stressor. This process redirects your body's day-to-day functions and deprioritizes anything that's not necessary for survival. And one of the first things to go is thyroid hormone production and distribution.

Normally, stress is a fleeting thing and thyroid hormone function gets back to work in a matter of moments, but if you're experiencing chronic stress, this is not the case. So if you're having issues with your thyroid, it's important to consider whether your adrenals are playing a role in that dysfunction. Support your adrenals by ensuring that you're eating enough, not forcing yourself to fast, maintaining ample nutrient density in your meals, and not sweating the small stuff. Get more adrenal-supporting tips starting on page 381.

TRACKING BODY TEMPERATURE

If you're having symptoms but you're not sure whether your thyroid is the problem, track your body temperature. Things such as stress, illness, and infection can cause fluctuations, but if your average temperature over four days is 97.4°F (36.3°C) or lower, it's probably fair to say that your thyroid may be in need of a little TLC.

To do this, you'll need a thermometer that takes your temperature for ten minutes or more before displaying a reading. When you wake up, before you sit up, get out of bed, or anything, put the thermometer deep in your armpit for ten minutes. Record your temperature readings for four days in a row and calculate the average. If you are menstruating, take your temperature on the second day of menstruation to ensure that your temperature isn't being influenced by ovulation.

Say No To

HALOGENS

Halogens are a group on the periodic table of elements containing molecules such as iodine, bromide, fluoride, and chloride. The thyroid needs iodine in order to produce thyroid hormone, but exposure to high levels of other halogens—such as chlorine from tap water and swimming pools or fluoride from tap water—may impede the thyroid's ability to utilize iodine.

ALCOHOL & SUGAR

Blood sugar fluctuations can aggravate your condition. When practicing carb-ups, consume low-glycemic-index carbohydrates, such as butternut squash, carrots, parsnips, sweet potatoes, oranges, peaches, and pears.

MERCURY TOXICITY

Mercury can attach to thyroid hormone receptors and block thyroid hormone utilization. The best way to limit mercury exposure is to chat with your dentist about removing your amalgam fillings. Many dentists do not support this procedure and argue that mercury-based fillings do not leach mercury into the body.

However, I've met far too many people, my husband included, who have suffered from mercury toxicity, and once their amalgam fillings were safely removed, they were able to clear the mercury from their body quickly and regain their health. If you decide to explore this option, it's best to find a dentist who fully supports removing the fillings and knows how to remove them safely. Additionally, to reduce mercury exposure, avoid high-mercury fish, as outlined on page 93.

SOY
Soy-based foods may inhibit your body's ability to absorb thyroid medication. If you're on medication, it's best to avoid soy wherever possible.

Supportive Supplements

- Vitamins: A, C, B_2, B_3, B_6, B_7, E

- Minerals: selenium, zinc, iodine

- Others: ashwagandha, licorice, kelp, L-tyrosine

Adrenal **Health**

Your adrenal glands sit on top of your kidneys. They're no bigger than walnuts, no heavier than grapes. These little guys are responsible for releasing hormones like cortisol and adrenaline, effectively managing how your body deals with stress and helping you maintain steady blood sugar.

The adrenals are also responsible for creating mineralocorticoids, which are very, very important for sodium-potassium balance and keep fluids at the right levels for proper functioning of the nerves, brain, heart, and many other important organs. The adrenals also produce testosterone, estrogen, and progesterone.

The adrenals, thyroid, and sex hormones are intertwined. If you have imbalanced hormones—especially sex hormones—the first place to look is your thyroid, then your adrenals.

In the case of imbalanced sex hormones, the thyroid is most often to blame. If you haven't read the section about healing the thyroid that begins on page 367, please do. By healing your thyroid, you'll support the healing of your adrenals and sex hormones.

But even when your adrenals are functioning exactly as they're designed to, they can wreak havoc on the body. That's because of the central role they play in one area: responding to stress.

SYMPTOMS OF ADRENAL IMBALANCE

 Afternoon energy lulls

 Irregular menstruation

 Dark under-eye circles

 Low libido

 Difficulty sleeping

 Mental fog

 Fatigue

 Poor digestion

 Feeling overwhelmed

 Puffy, stiff, and sore body

 Frequent colds and infections

 Weight gain

Test for It: Adrenal Health

Serum cortisol tests for the amount of cortisol in your blood. This is the most common test, but there are some drawbacks: if you're having more than one test, it's important to have your blood drawn at the same time of day, and if you tend to get stressed out about needles and the overall blood collection process, this may affect your result.

Saliva cortisol tests for the amount of cortisol in your saliva. It's much more accurate than serum (blood) testing because your saliva contains unbound, bioavailable hormones—meaning a saliva test better represents the level of circulating cortisol.

DHEA-S is the amount of DHEA in your blood and is a good indication of whether the adrenals are producing enough hormones to support your body.

Cortisol, the key stress hormone, stimulates gluconeogenesis and reduces fat-burning. The result? We have more glucose in the blood and less ability to burn fat—plus, excess cortisol and high blood glucose promote fat storage, particularly in the abdomen. Stress also disrupts leptin and other hormones, causing hunger signals to be turned on even when we have just eaten.

Sex hormones can also play a role. The precursor for progesterone, pregnenolone, can also be used to make cortisol, so if we are stressed out or we aren't eating enough and our body needs cortisol, it hijacks that precursor to use for producing cortisol instead of progesterone. If weight loss is your goal, this resulting imbalance can bring it to a halt because excess cortisol affects our ability to burn fat and generate ketones. In addition, when progesterone is lowered, the progesterone-estrogen ratio is imbalanced, which can cause unnecessary weight gain.

So if you have hit a weight-loss plateau or are feeling ravenously hungry all the time, it could be due to high stress. For most people, high stress makes it almost impossible to lose weight despite strict adherence to diet and exercise regimens.

Stress, Cortisol, and Blood Sugar

What happens when your daily life is all about running the kids to soccer, going to the gym, competing for the promotion, and worrying about your diet?

Cortisol increases. It's the primary hormone involved in the response to stress, and it's designed to keep us alive in the face of danger. Everything it does is aimed at that goal—particularly how it affects blood sugar. When we're under stress, cortisol raises blood sugar so that you have the fuel you need to fight or run away from danger. Of course, these days we usually aren't experiencing stress because our lives are in danger, but low-level chronic stress has the same effect on hormones and blood sugar. The greater your stress, the more damaged your metabolism. You aren't processing foods properly, you aren't healing, you aren't managing blood sugar—it becomes a real mess.

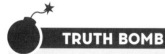

TRUTH BOMB

High cortisol makes it impossible to generate high levels of ketones.

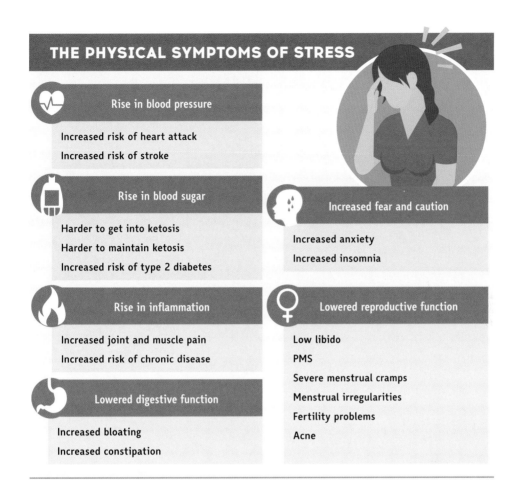

THE PHYSICAL SYMPTOMS OF STRESS

Rise in blood pressure

Increased risk of heart attack

Increased risk of stroke

Rise in blood sugar

Harder to get into ketosis

Harder to maintain ketosis

Increased risk of type 2 diabetes

Rise in inflammation

Increased joint and muscle pain

Increased risk of chronic disease

Lowered digestive function

Increased bloating

Increased constipation

Increased fear and caution

Increased anxiety

Increased insomnia

Lowered reproductive function

Low libido

PMS

Severe menstrual cramps

Menstrual irregularities

Fertility problems

Acne

To make things worse, high blood sugar on its own causes cellular stress, calling on the adrenals to level the playing field. Here's how this cycle works inside a body whose glucose metabolism is impaired:

We eat breakfast, blood sugar rises, cellular stress rises, the rise in stress triggers the adrenals, digestive processes slow down, cortisol is released, insulin is released to move glucose to our cells, some glucose is shuttled into cells, insulin stays high because the body is resistant to insulin, cortisol remains high because blood sugar is still higher, you become hungry, you eat... and the process begins all over again. Only this time, cortisol levels are heightened, your body isn't digesting food properly, and you're likely lethargic, cranky, and a bit on edge.

This constant rise and fall in blood sugar is very hard on the body. The stress you put on your adrenal glands every single day by overeating sugars and starches can't be overcome by breathing techniques, yoga classes, or meditation.

For many, a whole foods–based eating style that's lower in carbohydrates is essential to allow the adrenal glands time to rest and recover, since it doesn't raise blood sugar the way the standard American diet does. However, if constant stress is placed on the adrenals, a condition known as adrenal dysfunction may become your reality.

Adrenal Dysfunction

Adrenal dysfunction is when your adrenals are outputting either too much cortisol or too little. It may be caused by nutrient deficiency, an imbalanced thyroid, a long-term reduction in carbohydrates beyond where your body is most comfortable, overtraining, or copious amounts of dietary, lifestyle, emotional, or psychological stress.

ADRENAL DYSFUNCTION SYMPTOMS

Some symptoms of adrenal dysfunction include:

 Becoming irritable or overwhelmed easily

 Increased energy after 9 p.m.

 Feeling on edge

 Low blood pressure

Sugar and salt cravings

 Feeling "wired but tired"

 Muscle weakness (especially in the legs)

Taking longer than usual to recover after workouts

Adrenal dysfunction is your body trying to tell you that you need more self-care, so if this is your reality right now, try to remember to put the relationship with your body first. Because when you do, you'll be better able to show up in every other aspect of your life.

STAGES OF ADRENAL DYSFUNCTION

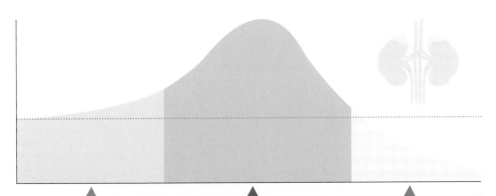

PRE STAGE	HYPER STAGE	HYPO STAGE
Cortisol is on the rise. Usually results from leading a semi-stressful life, not eating enough, eating nutrient-depleted foods, relying on coffee to get going in the morning, and pushing the body to the next level daily.	Cortisol is much higher than it should be, especially at night. When we're exposed to stressful situations, our bodies create more cortisol. This can affect sex hormones and weight, increase depressive tendencies and anxiety, and break down muscle and bone. I highly recommend that anyone at this stage of adrenal dysfunction discontinue working out completely for the time being.	Cortisol has tanked and you've got very little running through you. Your body has been pumping out so much cortisol for so long, and finally it says, "Enough is enough. Screw this." You'll be left with many of the symptoms you experienced in the hyper stage—especially when it comes to your overall hormone health—and on top of that, you will become very, very tired.

Diet Adjustments

Repairing your adrenals can be a bit of an arduous process, but it's always worth the effort. It can take anywhere from six months to several years to heal adrenal dysfunction, depending on the severity of the dysfunction. Needless to say, patience is required.

Ultra-Healing Foods

THE EXTRAS

- Cilantro
- Fresh ginger
- Garlic
- Ginger powder
- Ground cinnamon
- Parsley
- Turmeric

STARCHES AND FRUITS

- Oranges
- Pineapples
- Strawberries
- Sweet potatoes

PROTEIN

- Beef
- Bone broth
- Eggs
- Mackerel
- Organ meats
- Salmon

NON-STARCHY VEGETABLES

- Broccoli
- Brussels sprouts
- Cauliflower
- Dark leafy greens
- Fermented vegetables
- Red bell peppers
- Sea vegetables

HEALTHY FATS

- Avocados
- Chia seeds
- Coconut oil
- Flax seeds
- Olives
- Pumpkin seeds

WATER

Additional Adjustments

Remember, these steps are all in addition to the guidelines in "How to Support Overall Hormone Health" on page 335.

Say Yes To

LESS DIET STRESS

If you tend to track every bite of food, this is a good time to ease up and give yourself a break. The information under "Mindfulness Instead of Tracking" on page 136 may be especially helpful. Sticking to a healthy keto diet is still important, so to make it easier on yourself, try preparing meals ahead of time and keeping keto-friendly snacks on hand. But try to avoid comparing your progress to others', stop justifying yourself to people who challenge your way of eating, and don't stress about how you keto—there are lots of ways to make it work for you. Most of all, be kind to yourself!

BALANCING BLOOD SUGAR

Balancing blood sugar to avoid hypoglycemic or hyperglycemic episodes is important for reducing stress, so keto has your back here yet again. If you incorporate carb-ups, which can be helpful for adrenal healing because of its connection with thyroid healing, opt for items such as sweet potatoes, plantains, cassava, apples, and berries rather than white potatoes, corn, pineapple, or other sweet fruits.

SAYING NO AND REDUCING STRESS

Learning to say no is an important step in stress reduction. Often we think we can do it all, but studies have shown that people who can't say no tend to be less healthy. No one benefits when you overcommit and burn yourself out, so say no every once in a while and use that time for self-care instead. Activities that feed your soul and don't suck your energy are part of a healthy lifestyle: getting into nature, going to a spa, and meeting a friend for coffee offer more than just pleasure; they help reduce stress and keep you healthy.

A REGULAR DAILY ROUTINE

The adrenals like predictability, so eating, sleeping, and working similar hours every day allows them to relax more and heal.

HAPPINESS

Depression contributes to adrenal dysfunction and vice versa, so we must break that cycle. Go dancing, or dance in your living room. Learn to let go and forgive. Love fully and wholeheartedly. Meet up with people face to face (ever-so-challenging in our tech-dominated world). Volunteer. Get good sleep. If you're experiencing more than just a few low days every now and then, see a counselor or talk to your primary care doctor.

SALT INTAKE

Consume ample salt now that you're enjoying a whole foods–based diet. Read more about salt on page 110.

MOVEMENT

Keep it light—outdoor walks, gentle swimming, and restorative yoga. If you really want to work out, here are some guidelines based on the stages of adrenal dysfunction:

- Prestage: One day on, one day off. On your rest day, focus on recovery with a near-infrared sauna, hot/cold therapy, restorative yoga, massage, or yin yoga classes.

- Hyper stage: There is so much cortisol pumping through your veins that working out will only break down the muscle you're trying so hard to build up. Stick to walking, swimming, or restorative yoga.

- Hypo stage: Mega healing needs to happen at this point. You're best off going for short walks, period. But if you're more of an activities person, you can try yoga, yin yoga, yoga nidra, tai chi, or qigong. Sitting out in the sun for a couple of minutes and near-infrared sauna are great for healing, too.

ANTI-INFLAMMATORY FOODS

Chronic stress can cause chronic inflammation. Opt for foods high in anti-inflammatory omega-3 fatty acids, including pecans, walnuts, salmon, mackerel, and flax seeds. Avoid vegetable oils. You may also find that you do better when avoiding nightshade foods (see page 290).

IMPROVING SLEEP

When your adrenals aren't operating optimally, you may find that sleep is hard to come by. Practice proper sleep hygiene: go to bed at the same time every day, wind down a couple of hours before bed, and keep your phone out of your room. Every minute you sleep is another minute you're giving your body to heal. I remind myself of this whenever I have to set my alarm or skip a nap even though my body is begging me for one. Listen to your body and rest when you need to.

ACUPUNCTURE

If meditation isn't your thing and you're looking for a way to receive instant relaxation, calmness, and relief from stress, look into acupuncture treatments.

REAL BREAKFAST

Replace your fatty coffee with a nutrient-packed breakfast, and don't overdo it on the intermittent fasting. Placing too much dietary stress on your body won't help you to overcome adrenal dysfunction.

Say No To

CAFFEINE

People with adrenal dysfunction tend to be negatively impacted by caffeine, and it's a double whammy if you also have the CYP1B1 SNP gene, which is responsible for slowed metabolism of caffeine. These people can literally get insomnia from one cup of coffee they had fifteen hours ago. But for anyone with adrenal dysfunction, it's best to completely remove caffeine from your diet. This includes teas with caffeine, such as green tea, white tea, and black tea, and chocolate.

OVERTRAINING

Intense workouts can cause excessive and unwelcome stress on the body and should be avoided.

NEGATIVE ENVIRONMENTS AND PEOPLE

Avoid people who don't make you feel good, situations that weigh you down, and toxic conversations that don't serve your best interests. Instead, surround yourself with uplifting activities, connected conversations, and playfulness.

Supportive Supplements

Adrenal support comes in an array of varieties and can include the following:

- Vitamins: C, B_5, B_6, B_{12}

- Minerals: magnesium, zinc, chromium

- Herbs: ginseng, rhodiola, eleutherococcus, passion flower, ashwagandha

- Essential oils: lavender, chamomile, orange, lemon balm

- Others: phosphatidylcholine, phosphatidylserine, DHEA (manage with a doctor)

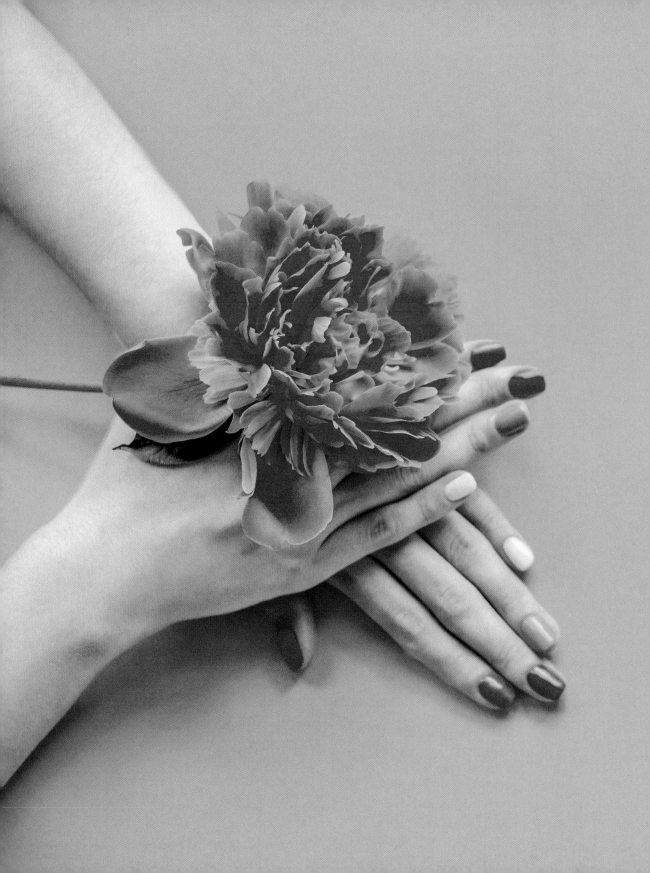

A LITTLE
LOVE LETTER

There's a lot of information on keto out there, so I appreciate your picking up this book. While this is the end of our time together, this is not the end of your keto journey! I appreciate your dedication to your body—in fact, I'm inspired by it. Your desire to make your health your number one priority, even though you may feel a little overwhelmed at times (we all do!), is what fuels me to continue working in this space and providing tools to women like you, based on my experiences. I think it's absolutely rad that you want to put your body first, that you're not discouraged by naysayers, and that you ask yourself the tough questions.

The path to balance isn't easy. You need to build confidence, ask questions, and understand that you are your own best advocate, forever and always. All of the work that leads to good health starts and ends with you. Please never, ever outsource responsibility for your health and wellness to a professional, ever. Challenge them. Try things on for size, and if they don't fit, drop them. If something needs adjusting, do it. You know your body best, and that knowledge is the best tool you can have for getting the life you want. Remember that you have the power to change—and you have the power to *not* change. What you do with that power is up to you.

It's all too easy to stand in our own way. I do it, too: I choose foods that make me feel bad, I don't take care of my body as I know I should, and then I feel like garbage and make even worse choices. But no matter how deep you feel you are in the darkness, remember that there's a way out. There are ebbs and flows to everything in life, including mental and physical wellness. If you're up, enjoy it. If you're down, remind yourself that you'll be up again. Every moment is an opportunity to make a choice that contributes to balance in your life.

Healthfulness isn't about what you eat, where you work out, or how much money you have. It's about your behaviors. Every moment, you have an opportunity to level up your game by choosing a healthy behavior instead of an unhealthy one. It could be choosing to have breakfast instead of running out the door; it could be forcing yourself out for a walk when all you want to do is tell your partner exactly what they did wrong. It could be stepping outside the office when you feel like your emotions have the best of you. All these micro choices and micro behavior shifts make up the balanced woman you are.

You're going to be confronted by people who don't support your way of living. Do not waste your energy and time trying to convince them that the way you've chosen to live is okay. Be selfish in this. Think of your time, energy, and money as the currency of your life and exchange them only for things that light you up, not drag you down. Live happy and your happiness will radiate to people, and those who are truly interested will ask you, with love, what's changed. Then you can share your experiences without having to defend yourself, and you'll find that it's a fair exchange of time and energy and will do wonders in lifting you up.

As you journey toward good health, don't discount how powerful chapter 7 can be to your process. Yes, it's a bit touchy-feely, but being kind to yourself and your body can do wonders to your happiness. Don't believe for a second that you are unworthy of love. *You are worthy.* Being loved is your birthright. You are enough. You are powerful. You have a unique set of gifts to share with the world, gifts that no other human being on this planet has to give. And guess what? None of these gifts has anything to do with how small or large your body is. If you don't believe this down to your core, go back to chapter 7 and dig in.

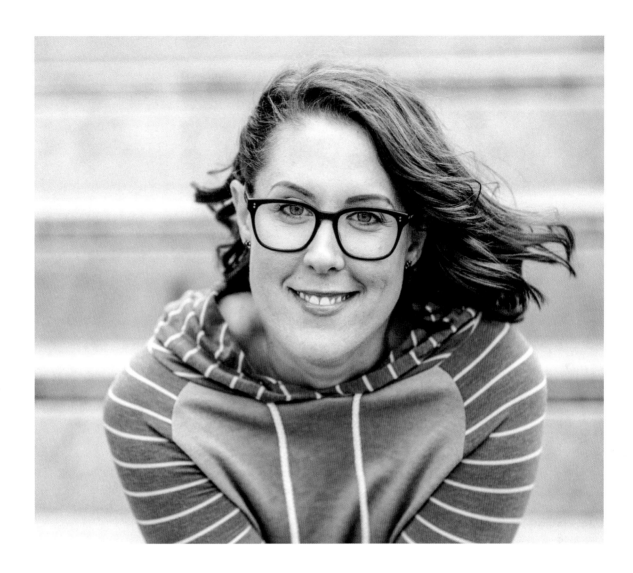

I hope you understand just how inspiring you are and how honored I am to have shared my experiences and knowledge with you. Thank you for giving yourself a chance, for believing in your ability to make a change. I am right here, cheering you on, and I know you have it in you to feel like the powerful, limitless woman that you are.

XO,
Leanne

References

General

Cross, J. H., and E. G. Neal. "The Ketogenic Diet—Update on Recent Clinical Trials." *Epilepsia* 49, Suppl 8 (2008): 6–10. https://doi.org/10.1111/j.1528-1167.2008.01822.x.

Johnstone, A. M., et al. "Effects of High-Protein Ketogenic Diet on Hunger, Appetite, and Weight Loss in Obese Men Feeding Ad Libitum." *American Journal of Clinical Nutrition* 87, no. 1 (2008): 44–55. https://doi.org/10.1093/ajcn/87.1.44.

Kossoff, E. H., and J. L. Dorward. "The Modified Atkins Diet." *Epilepsia* 49, Suppl 8 (2008): 37–41. https://dog.org/10.1111/j.1528-1167.2008.01831.x.

Kossoff, E. H., and J. M. Rho. "Ketogenic Diets: Evidence for Short- and Long-Term Efficacy." *Neurotherapeutics* 6, no. 2 (2009): 406–414. https://doi.org/10.1016/j.nurt.2009.01.005.

Kossoff, E. H., et al. "A Decade of the Modified Atkins Diet (2003–2013): Results, Insights, and Future Directions." *Epilepsy Behavior* 29, no. 3 (2013): 437–442. www.ncbi.nlm.nih.gov/pubmed/24386671.

Mantis, J. G., et al. "Improvement in Motor and Exploratory Behavior in Rett Syndrome Mice with Restricted Ketogenic and Standard Diets." *Epilepsy & Behavior* 15, no. 2 (2009): 133–141. https://doi.org/10.1016/j.yebeh.2009.02.038.

Masino, S. A., and J. M. Rho. "Mechanisms of Ketogenic Diet Action." *Jasper's Basic Mechanisms of the Epilepsies*, 4th edition. Oxford University Press: Bethesda, MD. 2012.

McKay, J. A., and J. C. Mathers. "Diet Induced Epigenetic Changes and Their Implications for Health." *Acta Physiologica* 202, no. 2 (2011): 103–118. https://doi.org/10.1186/1743-7075-3-7.

Noakes, M., et al. "Comparison of Isocaloric Very Low Carbohydrate/High Saturated Fat and High Carbohydrate/Low Saturated Fat Diets on Body Composition and Cardiovascular Risk." *Nutrition & Metabolism* 3, no. 7 (2006). https://doi.org/10.1186/1743-7075-3-7.

Oyabu, C., et al. "Impact of Low-Carbohydrate Diet on Renal Function: A Meta-Analysis of Over 1000 Individuals from Nine Randomised Controlled Trials." *British Journal of Nutrition* 116, no. 4 (2016): 632–638. https://doi.org/10.1017/S0007114516002178.

Ramsey, L., "The 10 Most Popular Prescription Drugs in the US." *Business Insider.* December 28, 2017. www.businessinsider.com/common-popular-prescription-drugs-us-2017-7/#2-synthroid-levoxyl-unithroid-levothyroxine-used-to-treat-hypothyroidism-12-9.

Roth, J., A. L. Szulc., and A. Danoff. "Energy, Evolution, and Human Diseases: An Overview." *American Journal of Clinical Nutrition* 93, no. 4 (2011): 875S–883S. https://doi.org/10.3945/ajcn.110.001909.

Westman, E. C., et al. "Low-Carbohydrate Nutrition and Metabolism." *American Journal of Clinical Nutrition* 86, no. 2 (2007): 276–284. https://doi.org/10.1093/ajcn/86.2.276.

Westman, E. C., J. Mavropoulos, W. S. Yancy, Jr., and J. S. Volek. "A Review of Low-Carbohydrate Ketogenic Diets." *Current Atherosclerosis Reports* 5, no. 6 (2003): 476–483. https://doi.org/10.1007/s11883-003-0038-6.

Wheless, J. W. "History of the Ketogenic Diet." *Epilepsia* 49, Suppl 8 (2008): 3–5. https://doi.org/10.1111/j.1528-1167.2008.01821.x.

Arachidonic Acid

Burgess, J. R., L. Stevens, W. Zhang, and L. Peck. "Long-Chain Polyunsaturated Fatty Acids in Children with Attention-Deficit Hyperactivity Disorder." *American Journal of Clinical Nutrition* 71, no. 1 Suppl (2000): 327S–330S. https://doi.org/10.1093/ajcn/71.1.327S.

Crawford, M. A., et al. "The Potential Role for Arachidonic and Docosahexaenoic Acids in Protection Against Some Central Nervous System Injuries in Preterm Infants." *Lipids* 38, no. 4 (2003): 303–315.

De Souza, E. O., et al. "Effects of Arachidonic Acid Supplementation on Acute Anabolic Signaling and Chronic Functional Performance and Body Composition Adaptations." *PloS one*, 11, no. 5 (2016): e0155153. https//doi.org/10.1371/journal.pone.0155153.

Higgins, A. J., and P. Lees. "The Acute Inflammatory Process, Arachidonic Acid Metabolism and the Mode of Action of Anti-inflammatory Drugs." *Equine Veterinary Journal* 16, no. 3 (1984): 163–175. https://doi.org/10.1111/j.2042-3306.1984.tb01893.x.

Moodley, T., et al. "Arachidonic and Docosahexaenoic Acid Deficits in Preterm Neonatal Mononuclear Cell Membranes. Implications for the Immune Response at Birth." *Nutrition and Health* 20, no. 2 (2009): 167–185. https://doi.org/10.1177/026010600902000206.

Ricciotti, E., and G. A. FitzGerald. "Prostaglandins and Inflammation." *Arteriosclerosis, Thrombosis, and Vascular Biology* 31, no. 5 (2011): 986–1000. https://doi.org/10.1161/ATVBAHA.110.207449.

Richardson, A. J., et al. "Fatty Acid Deficiency Signs Predict the Severity of Reading and Related Difficulties in Dyslexic Children." *Prostaglandins, Leukotriences and Essential Fatty Acids* 63, no. 1–2 (2000): 69–74. https://doi.org/10.1054/plef.2000.0194.

Roberts, M. D., et al. "Effects of Arachidonic Acid Supplementation on Training Adaptations in Resistance-Trained Males." *Journal of the International Society of Sports Nutrition* 4 (2007): 21. https://doi.org/10.1186/1550-2783-4-21.

Seeds, M. C., and D. A. Bass. "Regulation and Metabolism of Arachidonic Acid." *Clinical Reviews in Allergy & Immunology* 17, no. 1–2 (1999): 5–26. https://doi.org/10.1007/BF02737594.

Blood Sugar

González Centeno, A., P. Nahum Hernández, R. Mendoz, and A. R. Ayala. "[Correlation Between Menstruation Disorders and Insulin Resistance] Spanish translation." *Ginecologia y Obstetricia de México* 71 (2003): 312–317. www.ncbi.nlm.nih.gov/pubmed/14515662.

Gordon, E. E., and J. Duga. "Experimental Hyperosmolar Diabetic Syndrome: Ketogenic Response to Medium-Chain Triglycerides." *Diabetes* 24, no. 3 (1975): 301–306. https://doi.org/10.2337/diab.24.3.301.

Kolaczynski, J. W., et al. "Acute and Chronic Effects of Insulin on Leptin Production in Humans: Studies in Vivo and In Vitro." *Diabetes* 45, no. 5 (1996): 699–701. https://doi.org/10.2337/diab.45.5.699.

Muzykewicz, D. A., et al. "Efficacy, Safety, and Tolerability of the Low Glycemic Index Treatment in Pediatric Epilepsy." *Epilepsia* 50, no. 5 (2009): 1118–1126. https://doi.org/10.1111/j.1528-1167.2008.01959.x.

Woodyatt, R. T. "Objects and Method of Diet Adjustment in Diabetics." *Archives of Internal Medicine* 28, no. 2 (1921): 125–141.

Yamada, K. A., N. Rensing, and L. L. Thio. "Ketogenic Diet Reduces Hypoglycemia-Induced Neuronal Death in Young Rats." *Neuroscience Letters* 385, no. 3 (2005): 210–214. https://doi.org/ 10.1016/j.neulet.2005.05.038.

Yancy, Jr., W. S., et al. "A Low-Carbohydrate, Ketogenic Diet to Treat Type 2 Diabetes." *Nutrition & Metabolism* 2, no. 34 (2005). https://doi.org/10.1186/1743-7075-2-34.

Brain Health

Algattas, H., and J. H. Huang. "Traumatic Brain Injury Pathophysiology and Treatments: Early, Intermediate, and Late Phases Post-Injury." *International Journal of Molecular Science* 15, no. 1 (2014): 309–341.

Babikian, T., et al. "Molecular and Physiological Responses to Juvenile Traumatic Brain Injury: Focus on Growth and Metabolism." *Developmental Neuroscience* 32, no. 5–6 (2010): 431–441. https://doi.org/10.1159/000320667.

Costantini, L. C., L. J. Barr, J. L. Vogel, and S. T. Henderson. "Hypometabolism as a Therapeutic Target in Alzheimer's Disease." *BMC Neuroscience* 9 Suppl 2 (2008): S16. doi:10.1186/1471-2202-9-S2-S16.

Davis, L. M., et al. "Fasting Is Neuroprotective Following Traumatic Brain Injury." *Journal of Neuroscience Research* 86, no. 8 (2008): 1812–1822. https://doi.org/10.1002/jnr.21628.

Krikorian, R., et al. "Dietary Ketosis Enhances Memory in Mild Cognitive Impairment." *Neurobiology of Aging* 33, no. 2 (2010): 425.e19–425.e27. https://doi.org/10.1016/j.neurobiolaging.2010.10.006.

Newport, M. T., et al. "A New Way to Produce Hyperketonemia: Use of Ketone Ester in a Case Alzheimer's Disease. " *Alzheimer's & Dementia* 11, no. 1 (2015): 99–103. https://doi.org/10.1016/j.jalz.2014.01.006.

Prins, M. L., L. S. Fujima, and D. A. Hovda. "Age-Dependent Reduction of Cortical Contusion Volume by Ketones After Traumatic Brain Injury." *Journal of Neuroscience Research* 82, no. 3 (2005): 413–420. https://doi.org/ 10.1002/jnr.20633.

Prins, M. L., S. M. Lee, L. S. Fujima, and D. A. Hovda. "Increased Cerebral Uptake and Oxidation of Exogenous BetaHB Improves ATP Following Traumatic Brain Injury in Adult Rats." *Journal Neurochemistry* 90, no. 3 (2004): 666–672. https://doi.org/10.1111/j.1471-4159.2004.02542.x.

Stafstrom, C. E., and J. M. Rho. "The Ketogenic Diet as a Treatment Paradigm for Diverse Neurological Disorders." *Frontiers in Pharmacology* 3 (2012): 59. https://doi.org/10.3389/fphar.2012.00059.

Cancer

Branhouse, D. H., et al. "Staged Treatment of Invasive Carcinoma of Bladder." *Urology* 5, no. 5 (1975): 606–609. https://doi.org/10.1016/0090-4295(75)90109-0.

Cléro, E., et al. "Dietary Patterns, Goitrogenic Food, and Thyroid Cancer: A Case-Control Study in French Polynesia." *Nutrition and Cancer* 64, no. 7 (2012): 929–936. https://doi.org/10.1080/01635581.2012.713538.

Lussier, D. M., et al. "Enhanced Immunity in a Mouse Model of Malignant Glioma Is Mediated by a Therapeutic Ketogenic Diet." *BMC Cancer* 16 (2016): 310. https://doi.org/10.1186/s12885-016-2337-7.

Ohio State University Medical Center. "How Inflammation Can Lead to Cancer." ScienceDaily. April 19, 2011. http://www.sciencedaily.com/releases/2011/04/110419091159.htm.

Paul, B., et al. "Influences of Diet and the Gut Microbiome on Epigenetic Modulation in Cancer and Other Diseases." *Clinical Epigenetics* 7, no. 112 (2015). https://doi.org/10.1186/s13148-015-0144-7.

Seyfried, T. N., and L. M. Shelton. "Cancer as a Metabolic Disease." *Nutrition & Metabolism* (Lond) 7 (2010): 7. https://doi.org/10.1186/1743-7075-7-7.

Seyfried, T. N., et al. "Metabolic Management of Brain Cancer." *Biochima et Biophysica Acta (BBA) Bioenergetics* 1807, no. 6 (2011): 577–594. https://doi.org/10.1016/j.bbabio.2010.08.009.

Seyfried, T. N., et al. "Role of Glucose and Ketone Bodies in the Metabolic Control of Experimental Brain Cancer." *British Journal of Cancer* 89, no. 7 (2003): 1375–1382. https://doi.org/10.1038/sj.bjc.6601269.

Warburg, O. "On the Origin of Cancer Cells." *Science* 123, no. 3191 (1956): 309–314. https://doi.org/10.1126/science.123.3191.309.

Cardiovascular System

Adler, A. J., et al. "Reduced Dietary Salt for the Prevention of Cardiovascular Disease." Cochrane Library. December 18, 2014. www.cochrane.org/CD009217/VASC_reduced-dietary-salt-prevention-cardiovascular-disease.

Campos, H., et al. "Low Density Lipoprotein Particle Size and Coronary Artery Disease." *Arteriosclerosis, Thrombosis, and Vascular Biology* 12, no. 2 (1992): 187–195. https://doi.org/10.1161/01.ATV.12.2.187.

de Lorgeril, M., et al. "Mediterranean Diet, Traditional Risk Factors, and the Rate of Cardiovascular Complications After Myocardial Infarction: Final Report of the Lyon Diet Heart Study." *Circulation* 99, no. 6 (1999): 779–785. https://doi.org/10.1161/01.CIR.99.6.779.

Epping, Janet. "Statins: Benefits Questionable in Low-Risk Patients." Medical News Today. January 20, 2011. www.medicalnewstoday.com/articles/213783.

Ginsberg, H., et al. "Induction of Hypertriglyceridemia by a Low-Fat Diet." *Journal of Clinical Endocrinology & Metabolism* 42, no. 4 (1976): 729–735. https://doi.org/10.1210/jcem-42-4-729.

Halton, T. L., et al. "Low-Carbohydrate-Diet Score and the Risk of Coronary Heart Disease in Women." *New England Journal of Medicine* 355, no. 19 (2006): 1991–2002. https://doi.org/10.1056/NEJMoa055317.

Hu, F. B., et al. "Dietary Saturated Fats and Their Food Sources in Relation to the Risk of Coronary Heart Disease in Women." *American Journal of Clinical Nutrition* 70, no. 6 (1999): 1001–1008. https://doi.org/10.1093/ajcn/70.6.1001.

Kaptein, E. M., et al. "Relationship Between the Changes in Serum Thyroid Hormone Levels and Protein Status During Prolonged Protein Supplemented Caloric Deprivation." *Clinical Endocrinology* 252, no. 1 (1985): 1–15. https://doi.org/10.1111/j.1365-2265.1985.tb01059.x.

Kothawade, K., and C. N. Bairey Merz. "Microvascular Coronary Dysfunction in Women: Pathophysiology, Diagnosis, and Management." *Current Problems in Cardiology* 36, no. 8 (2011): 291–318. http://doi.org/10.1016/j.cpcardiol.2011.05.002.

Mackey, R. H., et al. "Rheumatoid Arthritis, Anti-cyclic Citrullinated Peptide Positivity, and Cardiovascular Disease Risk in the Women's Health Initiative." *Arthritis & Rheumatology* 67, no. 9 (2015): 2311–2322. http://doi.org/10.1002/art.39198.

Majka, D. S., et al. "Association of Rheumatoid Factors with Subclinical and Clinical Atherosclerosis in African American Women: The Multiethnic Study of Atherosclerosis." *Arthritis Care & Research* 69, no. 2 (2017): 166–174. http://doi.org/10.1002/acr.22930.

McBride, P. E. "Triglycerides and Risk for Coronary Heart Disease." *JAMA* 298, no. 3 (2007): 336–338. https://doi.org/10.1001/jama.298.3.336.

Mensink, R. P., and M. B. Katan. "Effect of Dietary Fatty Acids on Serum Lipids and Lipoproteins. A Meta-Analysis of 27 Trials." *Arteriosclerosis, Thrombosis, and Vascular Biology* 12, no. 8 (1992): 911–919. https://doi.org/10.1161/01.ATV.12.8.911.

Novella, Steven. "Statins—The Cochrane Review." *Science-Based Medicine.* January 26, 2011. https://sciencebasedmedicine.org/statins-the-cochrane-review/.

Parks, E. J., et al. "Effects of a Low-Fat, High-Carbohydrate Diet on VLDL-Triglyceride Assembly, Production, and Clearance." *Journal of Clinical Investigation* 104, no. 8 (1999): 1087–1096. https://doi.org/10.1172/JCI6572.

Rosenberg, H. G., and D. Allard. "Evidence for Caution: Women and Statin Use." *Canadian Women's Health Network* 10, no. 1 (2008). www.cwhn.ca/en/node/39417.

Sachdeva, A., et al. "Lipid Levels in Patients Hospitalized with Coronary Artery Disease: An Analysis of 136,905 Hospitalizations in 'Get with the Guidelines.'" *American Heart Journal* 157, no. 1 (2009): 111–117. http://doi.org/10.1016/j.ahj.2008.08.010.

Santos, F. L., et al. "Systematic Review and Meta-Analysis of Clinical Trials of the Effects of Low Carbohydrate Diets on Cardiovascular Risk Factors." *Obesity Reviews* 13, no. 11 (2012): 1048–1066. https://doi.org/10.1111/j.1467-789X.2012.01021.x.

Shepherd, J., et al. "Pravastatin in Elderly Individuals at Risk of Vascular Disease (PROSPER): A Randomised Controlled Trial." *Lancet* 360, no. 9346 (2002): 1623–1630. https://doi.org/10.1016/S0140-6736(02)11600-X.

St-Pierre, A. C., et al. "Low-Density Lipoprotein Subfractions and the Long-Term Risk of Ischemic Heart Disease in Men." *Arteriosclerosis, Thrombosis, and Vascular Biology* 25, no. 3 (2004): 553–559. https://doi.org/10.1161/01.ATV.0000154144.73236.f4.

Taylor, F., et al. "Statins for the Primary Prevention of Cardiovascular Disease." Cochrane Library. January 31, 2013. www.cochrane.org/CD004816/VASC_statins-primary-prevention-cardiovascular-disease.

Yan, M. U., and T. B. van Itallie. "Variability in Body Protein Loss During Protracted, Severe Caloric Restriction: Role of Triiodothyronine and Other Possible Determinants." *American Journal of Clinical Nutrition* 40, no. 3 (1984): 611–622. https://doi.org/10.1093/ajcn/40.3.611.

Cigarettes & Alcohol

Calkins, B. M. "A Meta-Analysis of the Role of Smoking in Inflammatory Bowel Disease." *Digestive Diseases and Sciences* 34, no. 12 (1989): 1841–1854.

CDC Newsroom. "Smoking Is Down, but Almost 38 Million American Adults Still Smoke." Centers for Disease Control and Prevention. January 18, 2018. https://www.cdc.gov/media/releases/2018/p0118-smoking-rates-declining.html.

Mutlu, E. A., et al. "Colonic Microbiome Is Altered in Alcoholism." *American Journal of Physiology. Gastrointestinal and Liver Physiology*, 302, no. 9 (2012): G966–G978. https://doi.org/10.1152/ajpgi.00380.2011.

Nos, P., and E. Domènech. "Management of Crohn's Disease in Smokers: Is an Alternative Approach Necessary?" *World Journal of Gastroenterology* 17, no. 31 (2011): 3567–3574. https://doi.org/10.3748/wjg.v17.i31.3567.

Queipo-Ortuño, M. I., et al. "Influence of Red Wine Polyphenols and Ethanol on the Gut Microbiota Ecology and Biochemical Biomarkers." *American Journal of Clinical Nutrition* 95, no. 6 (2012): 1323–1334. https://doi.org/ 10.3945/ajcn.111.027847.

Wang, H. J., S. Zakhari, and M. K. Jung. "Alcohol, Inflammation, and Gut-Liver-Brain Interactions in Tissue Damage and Disease Development." *World Journal of Gastroenterology* 16, no. 11 (2010): 1304–1313. https//:doi.org/10.3748/wjg.v16.i11.1304.

Dairy

Bartley, J., and S. R. McGlashan. "Does Milk Increase Mucus Production?" *Medical Hypotheses* 74, no. 4 (2010): 732–734. https://doi.org/10.1016/j.mehy.2009.10.044.

Chan, J. M., et al. "Dairy Products, Calcium, and Prostate Cancer Risk in the Physicians' Health Study." *American Journal of Clinical Nutrition* 74, no. 4 (2001): 549–554. htttps://doi.org/10.1093/ajcn/74.4.549.

Mattar, R., D. F. de Campos Mazo, and F. J. Carrilho. "Lactose Intolerance: Diagnosis, Genetic, and Clinical Factors." *Clinical and Experimental Gastroenterology* 5 (2012): 113–121. https://doi.org/10.2147/CEG.S32368.

Michaëlsson, K., et al. "Milk Intake and Risk of Mortality and Fractures in Women and Men: Cohort Studies." BMJ 349 (2014): g2015. https://doi.org/10.1136/bmj.g6015.

Moorman, P. G., and P. D. Terry. "Consumption of Dairy Products and the Risk of Breast Cancer: A Review of the Literature." *American Journal of Clinical Nutrition* 80, no. 1 (2004): 5–14. https://doi.org/10.1093/ajcn/80.1.5.

Wüthrich, B., A. Schmid, B. Walther, and R. Sieber. "Milk Consumption Does Not Lead to Mucus Production or Occurrence of Asthma." *Journal of the American College of Nutrition* 24, no. 6 Suppl (2005): 547S–555S.

Detox

Araujo, J. A. "Particulate Air Pollution, Systemic Oxidative Stress, Inflammation, and Atherosclerosis." *Air Quality, Atmosphere & Health* 4, no. 1 (2011): 79–93. https://link.springer.com/article/10.1007/s11869-010-0101-8.

Aschbacher, K., et al. "Good Stress, Bad Stress and Oxidative Stress: Insights from Anticipatory Cortisol Reactivity." *Psychoneuroendocrinology* 38, no. 9 (2013): 1698–1708. https://doi.org/10.1016/j.psyneuen.2013.02.004.

Choi, I., S. Lee, and Y. K. Hong. "The New Era of the Lymphatic System: No Longer Secondary to the Blood Vascular System." *Cold Spring Harbor Perspectives in Medicine* 2, no. 4 (2012): a006445. http://doi.org/10.1101/cshperspect.a006445.

Doi, K., and Uetsuka, K. "Mechanisms of Mycotoxin-Induced Neurotoxicity Through Oxidative Stress-Associated Pathways." *International Journal of Molecular Sciences* 12, no. 8 (2011): 5213-37. https://doi.org/10.3390/ijms12085213.

Hussain-Lukaszewicz, A. "Role of Oxidative Stress in Organophosphate Insecticide Toxicity— Short Review." *Pesticide Biochemistry and Physiology* 98, no. 2 (2010): 145–150. https://doi.org/10.1016/j.pestbp.2010.07.006.

Endocrine System

Baranowska, B., et al. "Evaluation of Neuroendocrine Status in Longevity." *Neurobiology of Aging* 28, no. 5 (2007): 774–783. https://doi.org/10.1016/j.neurobiolaging.2006.03.014.

Forslund, K. B., Ö. A. Lyungvall, and B. V. Jones. "Low Cortisol Levels in Blood from Dairy Cows with Ketosis: A Field Study." *Acta Veterinaria Scandinavica* 52, no. 31 (2010). https://doi.org/10.1186/1751-0147-52-31.

Fourman, L. T., and P. K. Fazeli. "Neuroendocrine Causes of Amenorrhea—An Update." *Journal of Clinical Endocrinology and Metabolism* 100, no. 3 (2015): 812–824. https://doi.org/10.1210/jc.2014-3344.

Holtorf, Kent. "Hormone Study Confusion." Holtorf Medical Group. www.holtorfmed.com/download/natural-hormone-replacement/Hormone_Study_Confusion.pdf.

Holtorf, Kent. "Natural (Bio-identical) vs. Synthetic HRT." Holtorf Medical Group. www.holtorfmed.com/download/natural-hormone-replacement/Natural_vs_Synthetic_HRT_Literature_Review.pdf.

Holtorf, Kent. "The Bioidentical Hormone Debate: Are Bioidentical Hormones (Estradiol, Estriol, and Progesterone) Safer or More Efficacious Than Commonly Used Synthetic Versions in Hormone Replacement Therapy?" *Postgraduate Medicine* 121, no. 1 (2009): 73–85. https://doi.org/10.3810/pgm.2009.01.1949.

Kinzig, K. P., and R. J. Taylor. "Maintenance on a Ketogenic Diet: Voluntary Exercise, Adiposity, and Neuroendocrine Effects." *International Journal of Obesity* 33, no. 8 (2005): 824–830. https://doi.org/10.1038/ijo.2009.109.

Kwa, M., C. S. Plottel, M. J. Blaser, and S. Adams. "The Intestinal Microbiome and Estrogen Receptor-Positive Female Breast Cancer." *Journal of the National Cancer Institute* 108, no. 8 (2016). https://doi.org/10.1093/jnci/djw029.

Mavropoulos, J. C., W. S. Yancy, Jr., J. Hepburn, and E. C. Westman. "The Effects of a Low-Carbohydrate, Ketogenic Diet on the Polycystic Ovary Syndrome: A Pilot Study." *Nutrition & Metabolism* 2 (2005): 35. https://doi.org/10.1186/1743-7075-2-35.

Pardridge, W. M. "Transport of Nutrients and Hormones Through the Blood-Brain Barrier." *Diabetologia* 20, no. 1 (1981): 246–254. https://doi.org/10.1007/BF00254490.

Spencer, Charles. "Estrogen's Role Focus of Work on Brain." American University. December 13, 2011. www.american.edu/americantoday/campus-news/20121213.cfm.

Wiley, T. S. "Bio-identical Hormones Replacement Therapy and the Quality of Life for Breast Cancer Patients." *Journal of Clinical Oncology* 33, no. 28_suppl (2015): 87. https://doi.org/10.1200/jco.2015.33.28_suppl.87.

Epilepsy

Barañano, K. W., and A. L. Hartman. "The Ketogenic Diet: Uses in Epilepsy and Other Neurologic Illnesses." *Current Treatment Options in Neurology* 10, no. 6 (2008): 410–419. www.ncbi. nlm.nih.gov/pmc/articles/PMC2898565/.

Lennox, W. G., and S. Cobb. "Epilepsy: From the Standpoint of Physiology and Treatment." *Medicine* 7, no. 2 (1928): 105–290. https://journals.lww.com/md-journal/Citation/1928/05000/EPILEPSY__FROM_THE_STANDPOINT_OF_PHYSIOLOGY_AND.1.aspx.

Lennox, W. G., and S. Cobb. "Studies in Epilepsy: VIII. The Clinical Effects of Fasting." *Archives of Neurology & Psychiatry* 20, no. 4 (1928): 771–779. https://doi.org/10.1001/archneurpsyc.1928.02210160112009.

Lutas, A., and G. Yellen. "The Ketogenic Diet: Metabolic Influences on Brain Excitability and Epilepsy." *Trends in Neuroscience* 36 (2013): 32–40.

Neal, E. G., et al. "A Randomized Trial of Classical and Medium-Chain Triglyceride Ketogenic Diets in the Treatment of Childhood Epilepsy." *Epilepsia* 50, no. 5 (2009): 1109–1117. https://doi.org/10.1111/j.1528-1167.2008.01870.x.

Palop, J. J., and L. Mucke. "Epilepsy and Cognitive Impairments in Alzheimer Disease." *Archives of Neurology* 66, no. 4 (2009): 435–440. https://doi.org/ 10.1001/archneurol.2009.

Roopra, A., R. Dingledine, and J. Hsieh. "Epigenetics and Epilepsy." *Epilepsia* 53, Suppl 9 (2012): 2–10. https://doi.org/10.1111/epi.12030.

Gut Microbiome

Bailey, M. T., et al. "Exposure to a Social Stressor Alters the Structure of the Intestinal Microbiota: Implications for Stressor-Induced Immunomodulation." *Brain, Behavior, and Immunity* 25, no. 3 (2011): 397–407. https://doi.org/10.1016/j.bbi.2010.10.023.

Bendtsen, K. M. B., et al. "Gut Microbiota Composition Is Correlated to Grid Floor Induced Stress and Behavior in the BALB/c Mouse." *PloS one* (2012). https://doi.org/10.1371/journal.pone.0046231.

Jiang, H., et al. "Altered Fecal Microbiota Composition in Patients with Major Depressive Disorder." *Brain, Behavior, and Immunity* 48 (2015): 186–194. https://doi.org/10.1016/j.bbi.2015.03.016.

Inflammation

Bruun, J. M., et al. "Consumption of Sucrose-Sweetened Soft Drinks Increases Plasma Levels of Uric Acid in Overweight and Obese Subjects: A 6-Month Randomised Controlled Trial." *European Journal of Clinical Nutrition* 69, no. 8 (2015): 949–953. https://doi.org/10.1038/ejcn.2015.95.

Cefalu, W. T. "Inflammation, Insulin Resistance, and Type 2 Diabetes: Back to the Future?" *Diabetes* 58, no. 2 (2009): 307–308. https://doi.org/10.2337/db08-1656.

Faraut, B., K. Z. Boudjeltia, L. Vanhamme, and M. Kerkhofs. "Immune, Inflammatory and Cardiovascular Consequences of Sleep Restriction and Recovery." *Sleep Medicine Reviews* 16, no. 2 (2012): 137–149. https://doi.org/10.1016/j.smrv.2011.05.001.

Herbort, C. P., L. Zografos, M. Zwingli, and M. Schoeneich. "Topical Retinoic Acid in Dysplastic and Metaplastic Keratinization of Corneoconjunctival Epithelium." *Graefe's Archive for Clinical and Experimental Ophthalmology* 226, no. 1 (1988): 22–26.

Jameel, F., M. Phang, L. G. Wood, and M. L. Garg. "Acute Effects of Feeding Fructose, Glucose and Sucrose on Blood Lipid Levels and Systemic Inflammation." *Lipids in Health and Disease* 13 (2014): 195. https://doi.org/10.1186/1476-511X-13-195.

Libby, P., P. M. Ridker, and A. Maseri. "Inflammation and Atherosclerosis." *Circulation* 105, no. 9 (2002): 1135–1143. https://doi.org/10.1161/hc0902.104353.

Miller, A. H., and C. L Raison. "The Role of Inflammation in Depression: From Evolutionary Imperative to Modern Treatment Target." *Nature Reviews Immunology* 16, no. 1 (2016): 22–34. https://doi.org/10.1038/nri.2015.5.

Quicksilver Scientific. "Bitters: Balancing Agents for the Gut, and Support for Liver/Kidney Detoxification." Quicksilver Scientific blog. March 17, 2017. www.quicksilverscientific.com/blog/bitters-balancing-agents-for-the-gut-and-support-for-liver-kidney-detoxification.

Wyss-Coray, T., and J. Rogers. "Inflammation in Alzheimer Disease—A Brief Review of the Basic Science and Clinical Literature." *Cold Spring Harbor Perspectives in Medicine* 2, no. 1 (2012): a006346. https://doi.org/10.1101/cshperspect.a006346.

Metabolism

Fontana, L., S. Klein, J. O. Holloszy, and B. N. Premachandra. "Effect of Long-Term Calorie Restriction with Adequate Protein and Micronutrients on Thyroid Hormones." *Journal of Clinical Endocrinology & Metabolism* 91, no. 8 (2006): 3232–3235. https://doi.org/10.1210/jc.2006-0328.

Kealy, R. D., et al. "Effects of Diet Restriction on Life Span and Age-Related Changes in Dogs." *Journal of the American Veterinary Medical Association* 220, no. 9 (2002): 1315–1320. https://doi.org/10.2460/javma.2002.220.1315.

Kennedy, A. R., et al. "A High-Fat, Ketogenic Diet Induces a Unique Metabolic State in Mice." *American Journal of Physiology-Endocrinology and Metabolism* 292, no 6 (2007): E1724–E1739.

Manninen, A. H. "Very-Low-Carbohydrate Diets and Preservation of Muscle Mass." *Nutrition & Metabolism* 3, no. 9 (2006). https://doi.org/10.1186/1743-7075-3-9.

Mathieson, R. A., et al. "The Effect of Varying Carbohydrate Content of a Very-Low-Caloric Diet on Resting Metabolic Rate and Thyroid Hormones." *Metabolism* 35, no 5 (1986): 394–398. https://doi.org/10.1016/0026-0495(86)90126-5.

Redman, L. M., and E. Ravussin. "Caloric Restriction in Humans: Impact on Physiological, Psychological, and Behavioral Outcomes." *Antioxidants & Redox Signaling* 14, no. 2 (2011): 275–287. https://doi.org/10.1089/ars.2010.3253.

Willcox, B. J., et al. "Caloric Restriction, the Traditional Okinawan Diet, and Healthy Aging." *Healthy Aging and Longevity: Third International Conference* 1114, no. 1 (2007): 434–455. https://doi.org/10.1196/annals.1396.037.

Minerals & Vitamins

Ahad, F., and S. A. Garnie. "Iodine, Iodine Metabolism and Iodine Deficiency Disorders Revisited." *Indian Journal of Endocrinology and Metabolism* 14, no. 1 (2010): 13–17. www.ncbi.nlm.nih.gov/pmc/articles/PMC3063534/.

Bolland, M. J., et al. "Effect of Calcium Supplements on Risk of Myocardial Infarction and Cardiovascular Events: Meta-Analysis." BMJ 341 (2010): c3691. https://doi.org/10.1136/bmj.c3691.

"Calcium-D-Glucarate." *Alternative Medicine Review* 7, no. 4 (2002): 336–339. www.ncbi.nlm.nih.gov/pubmed/12197785.

Delange, F., and P. Lecomte. "Iodine Supplementation: Benefits Outweigh Risks." *Drug Safety* 22, no. 2 (2000): 89–95. https://doi.org/10.2165/00002018-200022020-00001.

Lewis, J. R., et al."The Effects of Calcium Supplementation on Verified Coronary Heart Disease Hospitalization and Death in Postmenopausal Women: A Collaborative Meta-Analysis of Randomized Controlled Trials." *Journal of Bone and Mineral Research* 30, no. 1 (2015): 165–175. http://doi.org/10.1002/jbmr.2311.

National Institutes of Health. "Iodine: Fact Sheet for Health Professionals." September 26, 2018. https://ods.od.nih.gov/factsheets/Iodine-HealthProfessional/.

Patel, C., L. Edgerton, and D. Flake. "What Precautions Should We Use with Statins for Women of Childbearing Age?" *Journal of Family Practice* 55, no. 1 (2006): 75–77. www.mdedge.com/jfponline/article/62005/cardiology/what-precautions-should-we-use-statins-women-childbearing-age.

Shiraki, M., Y. Shiraki, C. Aoki, and M. Mirura. "Vitamin K2 (Menatetrenone) Effectively Prevents Fractures and Sustains Lumbar Bone Mineral Density In Osteoporosis." *Journal of Bone and Mineral Research* 15, no. 3 (2010): 515–521. https://doi.org/10.1359/jbmr.2000.15.3.515.

Smyth, P. P. A. "The Thyroid, Iodine and Breast Cancer." *Breast Cancer Research* 5, no.5 (2003): 235–238. https://doi.org/10.1186/bcr638.

Mitochondria/Energy

Calì, T., D. Ottolini, and M. Brini. "Mitochondrial Ca(2+) and Neurodegeneration." *Cell Calcium* 52, no. 1 (2012): 73–85. https://doi.org/10.1016/j.ceca.2012.04.015.

de Castro, I. P., L. M. Martins, and R. Tufi. "Mitochondrial Quality Control and Neurological Disease: An Emerging Connection." *Expert Reviews in Molecular Medicine* 12 (2010): e12. https://doi.org/0.1017/S1462399410001456.

Gano, L. B., M. Patel, and J. M. Rho. "Ketogenic Diets, Mitochondria, and Neurological Diseases." *Journal of Lipid Research* 55, no. 11 (2014): 2211–2228. https://doi.org/10.1194/jlr.R048975.

Johri, A., and M. F. Beal. "Mitochondrial Dysfunction in Neurodegenerative Diseases." *Journal of Pharmacology and Experimental. Therapeutics* 342, no. 3 (2012): 619–630. https://doi.org/10.1124/jpet.112.192138.

Lin, M. T., and M. F. Beal. "Mitochondrial Dysfunction And Oxidative Stress in Neurodegenerative Diseases." Nature 443, no. 443, no. 7113 (2006): 787–795. https://doi.org/10.1038/nature05292.

Mattson, M. P. "Energy Intake and Exercise as Determinants of Brain Health and Vulnerability to Injury and Disease." *Cell Metabolism* 16, no. 6 (2012): 706–722. https://doi.org/10.1016/j.cmet.2012.08.012.

Milder, J., and M. Patel. "Modulation of Oxidative Stress and Mitochondrial Function by the Ketogenic Diet." *Epilepsy Research* 100, no. 3 (2012): 295–303. https://doi.org/10.1016/j.eplepsyres.2011.09.021.

Pathak D., A. Berthet, and K. Nakamura. "Energy Failure: Does It Contribute to Neurodegeneration?" *Annals of Neurology* 74, no. 4 (2013): 506–516. http://doi.org/10.1002/ana.24014.

Schiff, M., et al. "Mitochondrial Response to Controlled Nutrition in Health and Disease." *Nutrition Reviews* 69, no. 2 (2011): 65–75. https://doi.org/10.1111/j.1753-4887.2010.00363.x.

Waldbaum, S., and M. Patel. "Mitochondrial Dysfunction and Oxidative Stress: A Contributing Link to Acquired Epilepsy?" *Journal of Bioenergetics and Biomembranes* 42, no. 6 (2010): 449–455. https://doi.org/10.1007/s10863-010-9320-9.

Mood, Anxiety & Depression

Ari, C., et al. "Exogenous Ketone Supplements Reduce Anxiety-Related Behavior in Sprague-Dawley and Wistar Albino Glaxo/Rijswijk Rats." *Frontiers in Molecular Neuroscience* 9 (2016): 137. https://doi.org/10.3389/fnmol.2016.00137.

Brinkworth, G. D., et al. "Long-Term Effects of a Very Low-Carbohydrate Diet and a Low-Fat Diet on Mood and Cognitive Function." *Archives of Internal Medicine* 169, no. 20 (2009): 1873–1880. https://doi.org/10.1001/archinternmed.2009.329.

El-Mallakh, R. S., and M. E. Paskitti. "The Ketogenic Diet May Have Mood-Stabilizing Properties." *Medical Hypotheses* 57, no. 6 (2001): 724–726. https://doi.org/10.1054/mehy.2001.1446.

McClernon, F. J., et al. "The Effects of a Low-Carbohydrate Ketogenic Diet and a Low-Fat Diet on Mood, Hunger, and Other Self-Reported Symptoms." *Obesity* 15, no. 1 (2007): 182–187. https://doi.org/10.1038/oby.2007.516.

National Institute of Mental Health. "Anxiety Disorders." Last revised July 2018. www.nimh.nih.gov/health/topics/anxiety-disorders/index.shtml.

Rao, A. V., et al. "A Randomized, Double-Blind, Placebo-Controlled Pilot Study of a Probiotic in Emotional Symptoms of Chronic Fatigue Syndrome." *Gut Pathogens* 1, no. 1 (2009): 6. https://doi.org/10.1186/1757-4749-1-6.

Sussman, D., J. Germann, and M. Henkelman. "Gestational Ketogenic Diet Programs Brain Structure and Susceptibility to Depression & Anxiety in the Adult Mouse Offspring." *Brain and Behavior* 5, no. 2 (2015): e00300. https://doi.org/10.1002/brb3.300.

Physical Activity

Gleeson, M. "Biochemical and Immunological Markers of Over-Training." *Journal of Sports Science & Medicine* 1, no. 2 (2002): 31–41. www.ncbi.nlm.nih.gov/pmc/articles/PMC3963240/.

O'Connor, P. J., et al. "Mood State and Salivary Cortisol Levels Following Overtraining in Female Swimmers." *Psychoneuroendocrinology* 14, no. 4 (1989): 303–310. https://doi.org/10.1016/0306-4530(89)90032-2.

Paoli, A., et al. "Ketogenic Diet Does Not Affect Strength Performance in Elite Artistic Gymnasts." *Journal of the International Society of Sports Nutrition* 9, no. 34 (2012). https://doi.org/10.1186/1550-2783-9-34.

Pauli, S. A., and S. L. Berga. "Athletic Amenorrhea: Energy Deficit or Psychogenic Challenge?" *Annals of the New York Academy of Sciences* 1205, no. 1 (2010): 33–38. https://doi.org/10.1111/j.1749-6632.2010.05663.x.

Samadi, Z., F. Taghian, and M. Valiani. "The Effects of 8 Weeks of Regular Aerobic Exercise on the Symptoms of Premenstrual Syndrome in Non-athlete Girls." *Iranian Journal of Nursing and Midwifery Research* 18, no. 1 (2013): 14–19. www.ncbi.nlm.nih.gov/pmc/articles/PMC3748549/.

Urhausen, A., H. Gabriel, and W. Kindermann. "Blood Hormones as Markers of Training Stress and Overtraining." *Sports Medicine* 20, no. 4 (1995): 251–276. https://doi.org/10.2165/00007256-199520040-00004.

Protein

Bray, G. A., et al. "Effect of Dietary Protein Content on Weight Gain, Energy Expenditure, and Body Composition During Overeating: A Randomized Controlled Trial." *JAMA* 307, no. 1 (2012): 47–55. https://doi.org/10.1001/jama.2011.1918.

Daley, C. A., et al. "A Review of Fatty Acid Profiles and Antioxidant Content in Grass-Fed and Grain-Fed Beef." *Nutrition Journal* 9, no. 10 (2009). https://doi.org/10.1186/1475-2891-9-10.

Ponnampalam, E. N., N. J. Mann, and A. J. Sinclair. "Effect of Feeding Systems on Omega-3 Fatty Acids, Conjugated Linoleic Acid and Trans Fatty Acids in Australian Beef Cuts: Potential Impact on Human Health." *Asia Pacific Journal of Clinical Nutrition* 15, no. 1 (2006): 21–29.

University of Sydney. "Lack of Protein Causes Overeating." Science Alert. November 7, 2013. www.sciencealert.com/overeating-driven-by-lack-of-protein.

WebMD Health News. "High-Protein Diets Cause Dehydration." April 22, 2002. www.webmd.com/diet/news/20020422/high-protein-diets-cause-dehydration.

Sweeteners

Choi, T. B., and W. M. Pardridge. "Phenylalanine Transport at the Human Blood-Brain Barrier. Studies with Isolated Human Brain Capillaries." *Journal of Biological Chemistry* 261 (1985): 6536–6541. www.jbc.org/content/261/14/6536.short.

Humphries, P., E. Pretorius, and H. Naudé. "Direct and Indirect Cellular Effects of Aspartame on the Brain." *European Journal of Clinical Nutrition* 62 (2008): 451–462. www.nature.com/articles/1602866.

Simopoulos, A. P. "The Importance of the Ratio of Omega-6/Omega-3 Essential Fatty Acids." *Biomedicine & Pharmacotherapy* 56, no. 8 (2002): 365–379. https://doi.org/10.1016/S0753-3322(02)00253-6.

Thyroid

Danforth, Jr., E., et al. "Dietary-Induced Alterations in Thyroid Hormone Metabolism During Overnutrition." *Journal of Clinical Investigation* 64, no. 5 (1979): 1336–1347. https://doi.org/10.1172/JCI109590.

Flier, J. S., M. Harris, and A. N. Hollenberg. "Leptin, Nutrition, and the Thyroid: The Why, the Wherefore, and the Wiring." *Journal of Clinical Investigation* 105, no. 7 (2000): 859–861. https://doi.org/10.1172/JCI9725.

Gannon, J. M., P. E. Forrest, and K. N. R. Chengappa. "Subtle Changes in Thyroid Indices During a Placebo-Controlled Study of an Extract of *Withania Somnifera* in Person with Bipolar Disorder." *Journal Ayurveda and Integrative Medicine* 5, no. 4 (2014): 241–245. https://doi.org/10.4103/0975-9476.146566..

Khaleeli, A. A., D. G. Griffith, and R. H. T. Edwards. "The Clinical Presentation of Hypothyroid Myopathy and Its Relationship to Abnormalities in Structure and Function of Skeletal Muscle." *Clinical Endocrinology* 19, no. 3 (1983): 365–376. https://doi.org/10.1111/j.1365-2265.1983.tb00010.x.

Kose, E., O. Guzel, K. Demir, and N. Arslan. "Changes of Thyroid Hormonal Status in Patients Receiving Ketogenic Diet Due to Intractable Epilepsy." *Journal of Pediatric Endocrinology and Metabolism* 30, no. 4 (2017): 411–416. https://doi.org/10.1515/jpem-2016-0281.

Messina, M., and G. Redmond. "Effects of Soy Protein and Soybean Isoflavones on Thyroid Function in Healthy Adults and Hypothyroid Patients: A Review of the Relevant Literature." *Thyroid* 16, no. 3 (2006): 249–258. https://doi.org/10.1089/thy.2006.16.249.

O'Hearn, L. Amber. "The Effect of Ketogenic Diets on Thyroid Hormones." The Ketogenic Diet for Health. December 24, 2014. www.ketotic.org/2014/12/the-effect-of-ketogenic-diets-on.html.

Rozing, M. P., et al. "Low Serum Free Triiodothyronine Levels Mark Familial Longevity: The Leiden Longevity Study." *Journals of Gerontology* 65A, no. 4 (2010): 365–368. https://doi.org/10.1093/gerona/glp200.

Shao, S., et al. "Dietary High-Fat Lard Intake Induces Thyroid Dysfunction and Abnormal Morphology in Rats." *Acta Pharmacologica Sinica* 35, no. 11 (2014): 1411–1420. https://doi.org/10.1038/aps.2014.82.

Spaulding, S. W., I. J. Chopra, R. S. Sherwin, and S. S. Lyall. "Effect of Caloric Restriction and Dietary Composition of Serum T3 and Reverse T3 in Man." *Journal of Clinical Endocrinology & Metabolism* 42, no. 1 (1976): 197–200: https://doi.org/10.1210/jcem-42-1-197.

Weight Loss

Ebbeling, C. B., et al. "Effects of Dietary Composition on Energy Expenditure During Weight-Loss Maintenance." *JAMA* 307, no. 24 (2012): 2627–2634. https://doi.org/10.1001/jama.2012.6607.

Hession, M., et al. "Systematic Review Of Randomized Controlled Trials of Low-Carbohydrate vs. Low-Fat/Low-Calorie Diets in the Management of Obesity and Its Comorbidities." *Obesity Reviews* 10, no. 1 (2009): 36–50. https://doi.org/10.1111/j.1467-789X.2008.00518.x.

Pasquali, R., et al. "Effect of Dietary Carbohydrates During Hypocaloric Treatment of Obesity on Peripheral Thyroid Hormone Metabolism." *Journal of Endocrinological Investigation* 5, no. 1 (1982): 47–52. https://doi.org/10.1007/BF03350482.

Sumithran, P., et al. "Ketosis and Appetite-Mediating Nutrients and Hormones After Weight Loss." *European Journal of Clinical Nutrition* 67, no. 7 (2013): 759–764. https://doi.org/10.1038/ejcn.2013.90.

Thio, L. L., E. Erbayat-Altay, N. Rensing, and K. A. Yamada. "Leptin Contributes to Slower Weight Gain in Juvenile Rodents on a Ketogenic Diet." *Pediatric Research* 60 (2006): 413–417. https://doi.org/10.1203/01.pdr.0000238244.54610.27.

Wright, C., and N. L. Simone. "Obesity and Tumor Growth: Inflammation, Immunity, and the Role of a Ketogenic Diet." *Current Opinion in Clinical Nutrition and Metabolic Care* 19, no. 4 (2016): 294–299. https://doi.org/10.1097/MCO.0000000000000286.

Yancy, Jr., W. S., et al. "A Low-Carbohydrate, Ketogenic Diet Versus a Low-Fat Diet to Treat Obesity and Hyperlipidemia: A Randomized, Controlled Trial." *Annals of Internal Medicine* 140, no. 10 (2004): 769–777. https://doi.org/10.7326/0003-4819-140-10-200405180-00006.

Index

movement *(continued)*
    nervous system support and, 319
    suggested timing for, 209–211
    suggested workouts, 211–213
    thyroid support and, 372
MRI, 295
MTHFR gene, 242
MUFAs (monounsaturated fats), 96, 97, 154, 180
multiple sclerosis, 241
muscle aches/pains, stress and, 167
MyFlo app, 341

N
naturthyroid, 370
nausea, 113
near-infrared sauna, 113
neck, glands in, 325–326
negative environments, adrenal health and, 383
negativity, hormonal support and, 339
nervous system support
    about, 313
    ADD/ADHD, 314–315
    adjustments for, 318–320
    anxiety, 316–317
    diet adjustments for, 317–318
    epilepsy, 317
    role of mitochondria in neurological imbalances, 314
    supplements for, 320
nervousness, stress and, 168
net carbs, total carbs vs., 133
night sweats, menopause and, 363
nightshades
    about, 290–291
    AIP and, 245
    elimination protocol and, 278
    gut support and, 266

nitrates, 93
nitrites, 93
NMR LipoProfile test, 59
NMR (nuclear magnetic resonance) test, 308
nonalcoholic fatty liver disease, 57
nonalcoholic steatohepatitis, 57
non-starchy vegetables
    about, 94, 104, 110
    adrenal health and, 380
    carb-ups and, 190, 191
    cardiovascular health and, 311
    elimination protocol and, 279
    in Fat Fueled Food Pyramid, 85
    gallbladder support and, 296
    gut support and, 263
    high-FODMAP, 286
    inflammation reduction and, 253
    low-FODMAP, 287
    lymphatic system support and, 304
    menopause and, 365
    nervous system support and, 318
    thyroid support and, 371
    as ultra-healing foods, 248
nonsteroidal anti-inflammatory drugs (NSAIDs)
    AIP and, 245
    overuse of, 267
norepinephrine, 49
NSAIDs (nonsteroidal anti-inflammatory drugs)
    AIP and, 245
    overuse of, 267
nuclear magnetic resonance (NMR) test, 308
nutrient density
    amenorrhea and, 352
    nervous system support and, 319

nutrient stat, 32
nutrient-dense foods
    cravings and, 38
    gut support and, 264
    importance of, 246
nutritional deficiencies
    hormonal imbalances and, 334
    nervous system support and, 318
nutritional ketosis, 20
nuts, 154
nuts and seeds
    AIP and, 245
    candida support and, 271
    elimination protocol and, 278

O
oils, 97
omega-3 fatty acids, 17, 56, 97–98, 358
omega-6 fatty acids, 64, 97–98, 255
onions, preparing, 95
organ meats, 92
organic acids test, 268, 298
organic produce
    autoimmune support, 249
    hormonal support and, 356
osteopenia, 130
osteoporosis, 130
ovaries, 328
overeating, 114–115
overtraining
    about, 74
    adrenal health and, 383
    autoimmune support and, 250
    inflammation reduction and, 255
    kidney support and, 302
ox bile, gallbladder support and, 296
oxalates, 299, 301
oxidative stress, reducing, 60